BIOMEDICAL ENGINEERING PRINCIPLES

An Introduction to Fluid, Heat, and Mass Transport Processes

DAVID O. COONEY

Clarkson College of Technology
Potsdam, New York

Current affiliation:
University of Wyoming
Laramie, Wyoming

MARCEL DEKKER, INC. New York and Basel

MARCEL DEKKER, INC.

270 Madison Avenue, New York, New York 10016

LIBRARY OF CONGRESS CATALOG CARD NUMBER: 75-17034

ISBN: 0-8247-6347-5

Current printing (last digit):
15 14

PRINTED IN THE UNITED STATES OF AMERICA

To my parents

Edward and Kathleen Cooney

CONTENTS

PREFACE

The field of biomedical engineering is still a relatively new one, and not yet sharply defined. Whether it is, in fact, really a "new" discipline, underlain with principles and fundamentals unique to itself, is also not clear. Certainly, it is to a very large extent a sheer amalgamation of the life sciences and engineering. Whether it is somehow more than just a combination of these is a question that shall have to be answered by time. Emergent fields of activity have a habit of gaining definition and direction via feedback from the job market for graduating students. In biomedical engineering, this market is extremely varied at present, with both the kinds and numbers of positions available to new graduates uncertain. In a society that is becoming increasingly conscious of health care and that continues to grow increasingly technological, there is little doubt that a strong and consistent demand for some type of biomedical engineer will ultimately develop.

An important question in this regard concerns what sort of formal academic training such graduates should have. It is clear that a background involving classical courses in the biological sciences (especially physiology and anatomy), in chemistry and physics (particularly biochemistry and biophysics), and in basic engineering (with emphasis on fluid dynamics, heat transfer, and mass transfer) is desirable. What is not so clear is what should be the nature of the more advanced courses that attempt to *synthesize* information from the life sciences and from engineering (those courses usually called "biomedical engineering" courses).

The present work represents the particular approach taken by the author in constructing such a course. It is based on the following reasoning: (1) biology and physiology traditionally have amounted to little more than large compilations of observed facts; (2) engineering encompasses a set of general unifying principles and correlative tools; and (3) there is a great need to apply engineering principles and modes of analysis to life science systems.

This book is really what one might call a "quantitative physiology" text, accenting the use of principles most familiar to engineers in describing transport processes in the human body. Applications of these principles to the description of transport processes in certain biomedical systems (artificial organs, in this case) are also considered in some depth. The material should provide a reasonable advanced level one-semester course for many biomedical engineers. Because of the diverse and still emerging nature of the field, it is clear that a significant number of biomedical engineers will find that the present text clashes with their own views and/or needs. This is reason enough why a great variety of textbooks should continue to be developed—no other way exists to satisfy every valid curricular approach to biomedical engineering training.

This text is meant to be *introductory* in nature, and is aimed primarily at junior and senior level undergraduate biomedical engineers, although many parts could be used in a first-year graduate course (if supplemented with material from other, more advanced texts such as E.N. Lightfoot's *Transport Phenomena and Living Systems* or S. Middleman's *Cardiovascular Transport Phenomena)*. Applied physiologists at various levels may also find that certain chapters provide an introductory overview or review of topics of interest.

All areas of biomedical engineering not *directly* related to fluid dynamics, heat transport, and mass transport are excluded from the text. Thus, biocontrol theory and biomechanics, for example, are omitted. Electrical phenomena (like nerve impulse conduction) are not discussed, even though these often do involve mass transport processes. Even in the areas the book primarily attempts to cover, many subjects (e.g., capillary dynamics) or details, for lack of space, do not appear. The reader is reminded, therefore, that the book is truly introductory, and more detailed treatises should be consulted if an in-depth knowledge is desired.

After a brief summary of historical developments in medicine, the coverage begins with a basic quantitative characterization of the human body and with a detailed consideration of the physical, chemical, and flow properties of blood. This information is useful in virtually all that follows. Next we consider the modeling of fluid flow, heat transfer, and mass transfer processes in the human body (the last on a gross, or "compartmental" scale). Engineering principles (e.g., Bernoulli's equation), correlation methods (e.g., use of dimensionless groups), and mathematical modeling are stressed heavily throughout. Following this, a much more detailed consideration of mass transfer across biological membranes in general, and then in particular in the kidneys and lungs, is presented. Fundamental diffusion phenomena are quantified and modeled in these chapters. Finally, the text considers two major biomedical engineering developments, artificial kidneys and blood oxygenators. Mathematical modeling of mass transport in these devices is extensively treated. One should be struck here by the relative crudeness of these systems and how different they are from their natural counterparts. One should additionally be astonished at how well they actually do work.

A reasonable number of homework problems are included at the ends of chapters. These problems encompass a variety of important and realistic applications of the concepts and methods given in the text. In general, they may be solved without great difficultv A manual containing detailed solutions to all problems is available. Instructors may obtain copies directly from the author or publisher.

As with any book, many persons other than the author played a role. First thanks should go to the Department of Chemical Engineering at Clarkson for providing the atmosphere, time, and resources necessary. Secondly, there are the many students whose enthusiasm for biomedical subjects served as a constant impetus for developing the material in the book. I would like to express my thanks also to Marlene Wright and to Linda Delosh for their excellent and conscientious typing.

Potsdam, New York David O. Cooney

BIOMEDICAL ENGINEERING PRINCIPLES

An Introduction to Fluid, Heat, and Mass Transport Processes

Chapter 1

THE HISTORY OF BIOMEDICINE—A BRIEF REVIEW

The modern student should appreciate that the application of "nonbiological" scientific and engineering principles to the areas of physiology and medicine is not a new phenomenon. Although biomedical engineering is currently enjoying great popularity, its roots nevertheless go back many centuries. We wish here to review briefly the history of medicine, with emphasis on the contributions of engineers, chemists, and physicists.

I. THE SIXTEENTH CENTURY

We begin in the sixteenth century, the dawn of modern medicine, with Leonardo da Vinci (1452-1518). Medicine, during earlier medieval times and even further back, developed very slowly and was dominated by the influence of the theories of Galen (A.D. 130-200), who taught that the activity of all living things was associated with three types of spirits: natural, vital, and animal (created in the liver, heart, and brain, respectively). Da Vinci, artist, engineer, and scientist, essentially founded the science of anatomy, and studied the principles of the motions of bones and muscle in extensive detail. Later, Vesalius (1514-1564) produced, in 1543, a great treatise on human anatomy which initiated exuberant new scientific activity in medicine and transformed surgical practice.

Rising activity in the physical sciences, fostered by the Renaissance spirit, began to have an effect on medicine. Sanctorius (1561-1636) applied new measurement techniques to the human body and, by careful weighing of body inputs and outputs, was able to show that "insensible perspiration" occurs. This laid the foundation for the study of metabolism. Sanctorius also developed a crude fever thermometer and a rudimentary device for determining pulse rates.

The science of physiology began to blossom in this same era. William Harvey (1578-1657), the great English physiologist, discovered that blood is pumped in a circuit by the muscular contraction of the heart, and pointed out the differences in directions of flow in the arteries and veins. The first real physiology book, *De homine*, was written by the French philosopher-scientist René Descartes (1596-1650). Although wrong in many respects (e.g., he rejected Harvey's experiments and claimed that the heart propelled blood by creating thermal expansion), the book correctly stressed the importance of the nervous system and its role in coordinating bodily activities.

II. THE SEVENTEENTH CENTURY

During the seventeenth century, new theories of how the body works appeared. Three important ones dealt with "iatrophysics," "iatrochemistry," and "vitalism." Borelli (1608-1679) of Italy propounded the first view, which explains animal activity on a mechanical basis. Others, like Sylvius (1614-1672) of Holland, sought to explain bodily activity on a strictly chemical basis (iatrochemistry). Much knowledge of the chemical properties of various body fluids (e.g., saliva, digestive juices) was obtained in Sylvius' laboratory. Stahl (1660-1734), a German, believed in contrast that the body is not a machine, nor governed by physical and chemical laws, but is driven by a "sensitive soul," of which the chemical processes were only instruments. This view was called vitalism.

III. THE EIGHTEENTH CENTURY

After the great seventeenth century burst of knowledge spurred by advances in chemistry and physics, and by development of the microscope, research work seemed to pause and consolidate. New emphasis was placed on teaching. Boerhaave (1668-1738) revolutionized medical teaching by bringing it into the clinics, where direct observation of patients was possible. Albrecht von Haller (1708-1777), one of Boerhaave's students, also became a great eighteenth century figure, as a physiologist. Working in the areas of respiration, bone formation, embryology, and digestion, he exhibited consistent logic and rationality. Hales (1677-1761), an English physiologist, investigated the dynamics of the circulatory system by tying tubes into the arteries and veins of animals and manometrically measuring the pressures at various points. Circulation rates and velocities were also measured by Hales.

Other prominent men of the eighteenth century who advanced the physiological knowledge of digestive processes were Réaumer (1683-1757), Spallanzani (1729-1799), and Prout (1785-1850). Studies of electrical phenomena in the body were made by men such as Galvani (1737-1798) and Volta (1745-1827), who both showed, for example, that muscles can be made to contract by application of external currents. During the second half of the eighteenth century, important advances in respiratory physiology were made by Black (1728-1799), Priestley (1733-1804), and Lavoisier (1743-1794). These scientists demonstrated how plants and animals consume and produce carbon dioxide and oxygen.

Clinical medicine was aided in this general era with the development of the first good "pulse watch," the first safe and reliable thermometer, and with the invention of the stethoscope by Laënnec in 1819 (originally just a roll of paper). Public health conditions of cities were remarkably improved in the eighteenth century by the advent of civil engineering practices such as the covering of sewerage systems and the draining of open wetlands. It was about this same time that there occurred a strong movement to build many improved hospitals. Vaccination was introduced by Jenner (1749-1823) in 1796.

IV. THE NINETEENTH CENTURY

This period was marked by tremendous advances in physiology, led by the Frenchman Claude Bernard and several Germans (Müller, von Liebig, and Ludwig). New understandings of the brain and of the whole nervous system were brought about. The idea of the essential cellular nature of living things was established around 1840. Histology, the study of tissues, was elevated to the level of a separate science by Albrecht von Kölliker (1817-1905).

Poiseuille (1799-1869), a French physiologist, studied blood flow dynamics extensively and was the first to derive the laminar flow law which bears his name. He was also the first to investigate the viscometric properties of blood. Another eminent physiologist who lived in this general period and who likewise deduced a fundamental physical law was the German Adolf Fick (1829-1901), discoverer of the law of diffusion in liquids.

The concept that diseases can be caused by specific germs was a tremendous leap made in the nineteenth century. It was shown by Pasteur (1822-1895) and others that certain diseases are caused by microorganisms which cannot generate spontaneously but only from microorganisms of a like kind. Koch (1843-1910) was the first person to develop solid media for culturing bacteria. Soon after, specific disease-producing organisms (e.g., of leprosy and tuberculosis) were isolated. Bacteriology was now a new science by itself. Methods for obtaining weakened viruses for inoculation, to produce immunity to various diseases, were developed and applied (against typhoid in 1888, against diphtheria in 1894).

Another significant step in medical progress in this period was the discovery of general anesthetics (ether and chloroform) in 1846. The new knowledge of antiseptics (germ-killing agents) and anesthetics placed surgery on an entirely new footing. In addition, great advances in diagnosis and treatment followed the discovery of x-rays by Röntgen in 1895 and of radium by the Curies in 1898. The field of psychiatry was redirected by Freud (1856-1939).

V. THE TWENTIETH CENTURY

Our current era has seen such tremendous waves of discoveries and advances that all prior medical practice seems barely recognizable. We can do little more here than indicate some of the large new areas developed since 1900, such as chemotherapy, immunology, endocrinology, and the science of nutrition. Work in these fields has led to the discovery of antibiotics (e.g., penicillin), vaccines against influenza and polio, isolation of insulin (for treating diabetes) and of cortisone (valuable in alleviating arthritis and certain allergies), and identification of essential vitamins. Advances in surgical procedures in the last half-century are too numerous to mention here (many of these, ironically, resulted from the fact that World Wars I and II provided surgeons with a vast number of battlefield patients, on whom daring new techniques were justified).

Special mention should be made, however, of the development of implantable devices of various kinds (e.g., metals and plastics) and of artificial organs. Stainless steel has been used extensively to repair joints and bones, and tantalum metal has been used in wire or mesh form for many purposes (e.g., strengthening vertebrae). Ceramic materials are commonly used to replace jawbones and hip joints. Plastics such as Orlon and Dacron, fashioned into tube form, have been implanted in place of arteries. Nylon thread is a widely used surgical material. Other plastics (clear ones) have found use as artificial corneas for eyes. Silastic, a silicone rubber that has an enormous range of flexibility and consistency, has been employed as imitation body fat in breasts, cartilage in ear and nose repair, and as the main material for artificial heart devices.

Artificial organs are a comparatively recent development. The first artificial kidney treatment was carried out on a dog by Able, Rountree, and Turner in 1913. In 1943 the first applications to humans were made. Heart-lung devices, which oxygenate blood outside of the body and pump it back to the patient, were developed and used in the early 1950s. The use of artificial heart valves and implantable partial hearts has also been relatively recent, occurring since about 1960. A more detailed discussion of artificial organs is deferred to later chapters.

This brief review demonstrates, we hope, that the history of biomedicine is a long one, and that present-day efforts are but an extension or refinement of previous breakthroughs. Many excellent accounts of the fascinating history of medicine are available (see references below) and the student is urged to read through some of these in order to gain additional perspectives, especially on twentieth century developments.

REFERENCES

Garrison, F. H., *History of Medicine*, 4th ed., Saunders, Philadelphia, Pennsylvania, 1960.

Major, R. H., *History of Medicine*, 2 vols., Thomas, Springfield, Illinois, 1955.

Singer, C., and Underwood, A. E., *Short History of Medicine*, 2nd ed., Oxford Univ. Press, London and New York, 1962.

Walker, K., *Story of Medicine*, Oxford Univ. Press, London and New York, 1955.

Chapter 2

OVERALL DESCRIPTION OF THE HUMAN BODY

In this chapter we present basic information and data on the human body. Both a qualitative and a quantitative knowledge of the body are required as a basis for subsequent reading and discussion.

I. ANATOMY (GROSS)

We will not consider here the field of microscopic anatomy, but only that of macroscopic, or gross, anatomy. Figures 2.1 through 2.6 (taken from L. L. Langley and E. Cheraskin, *The Physiology of Man*, 2nd ed., McGraw-Hill, New York, 1958) summarize the gross anatomical features of the human body quite well.

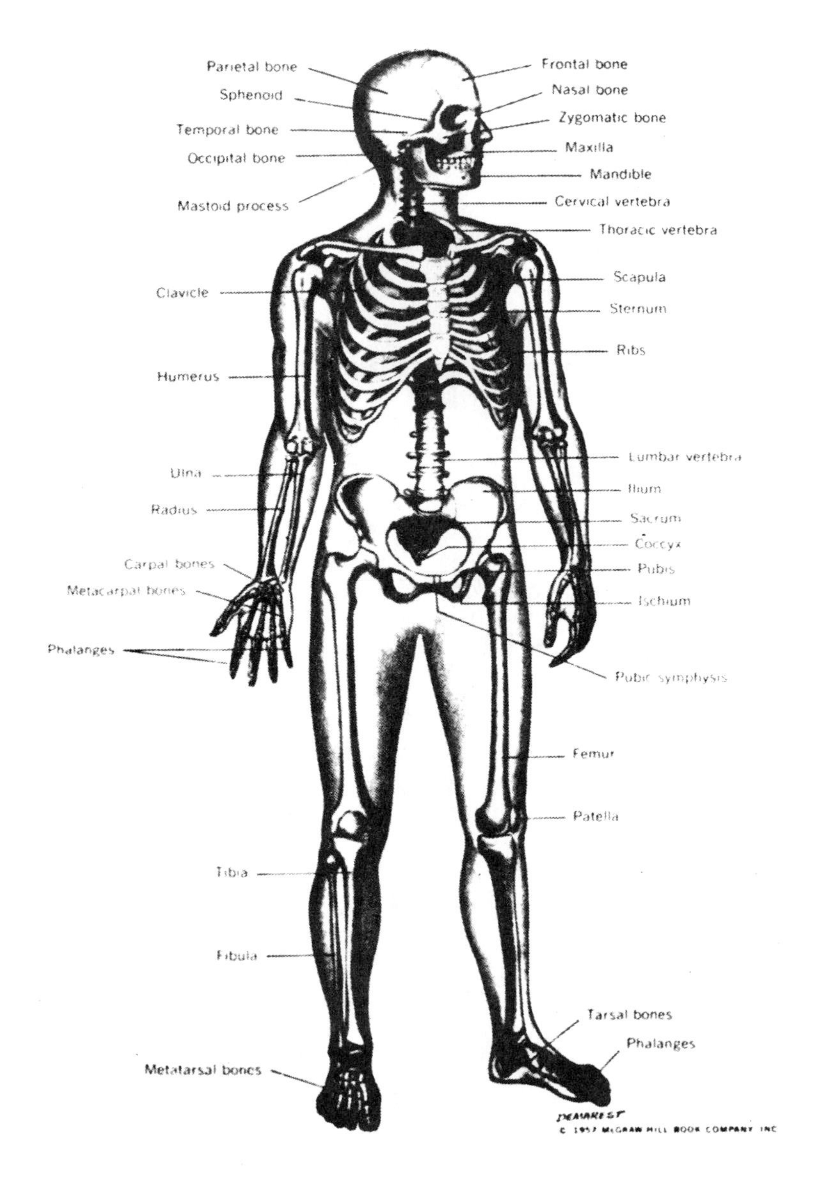

FIG. 2.1. Skeletal system (anterior view). [Copyright 1957, McGraw-Hill Book Company. Reprinted with permission.]

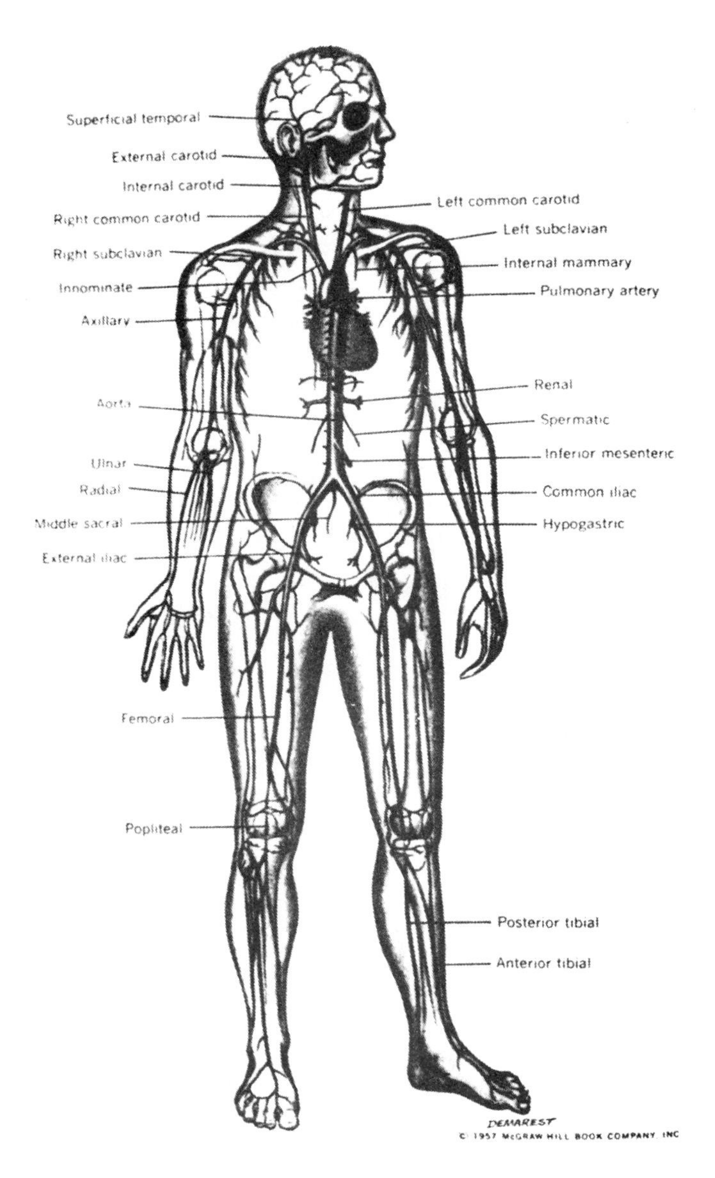

FIG. 2.2. Arterial system. [Copyright 1957, McGraw-Hill Book Company. Reprinted with permission.]

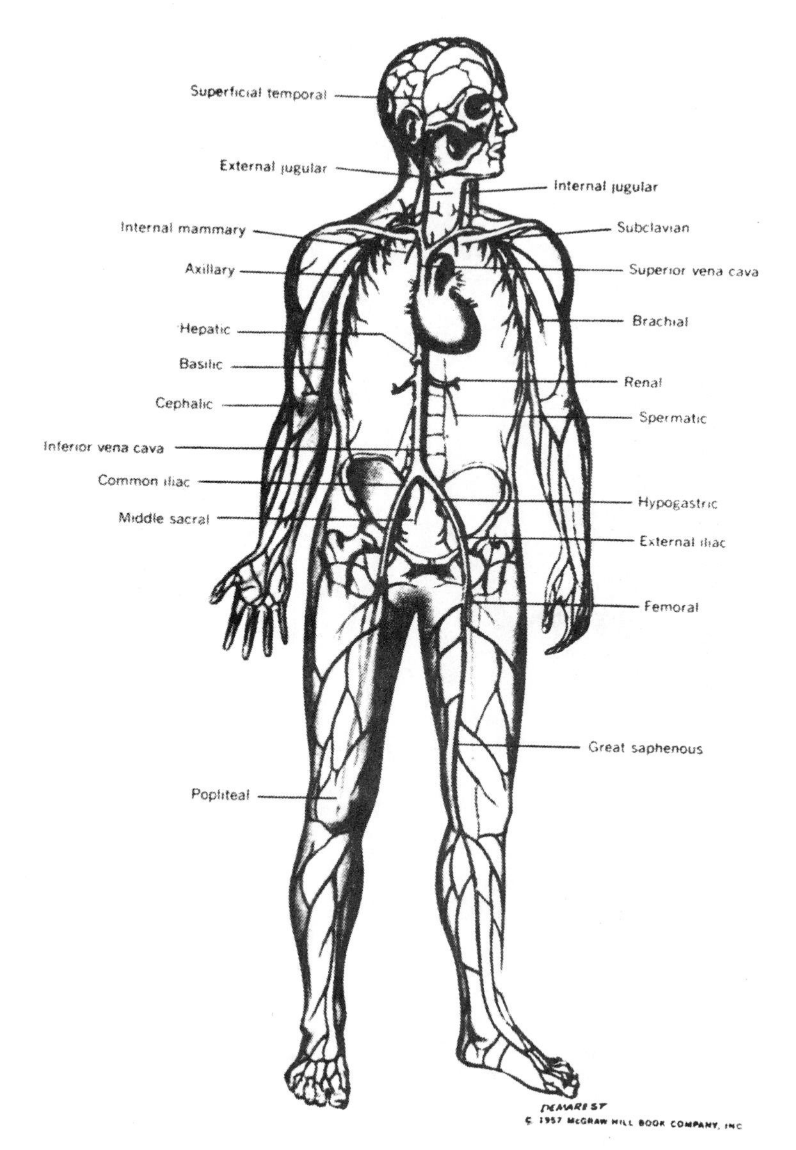

FIG. 2.3. Venous system. [Copyright 1957, McGraw-Hill Book Company. Reprinted with permission.]

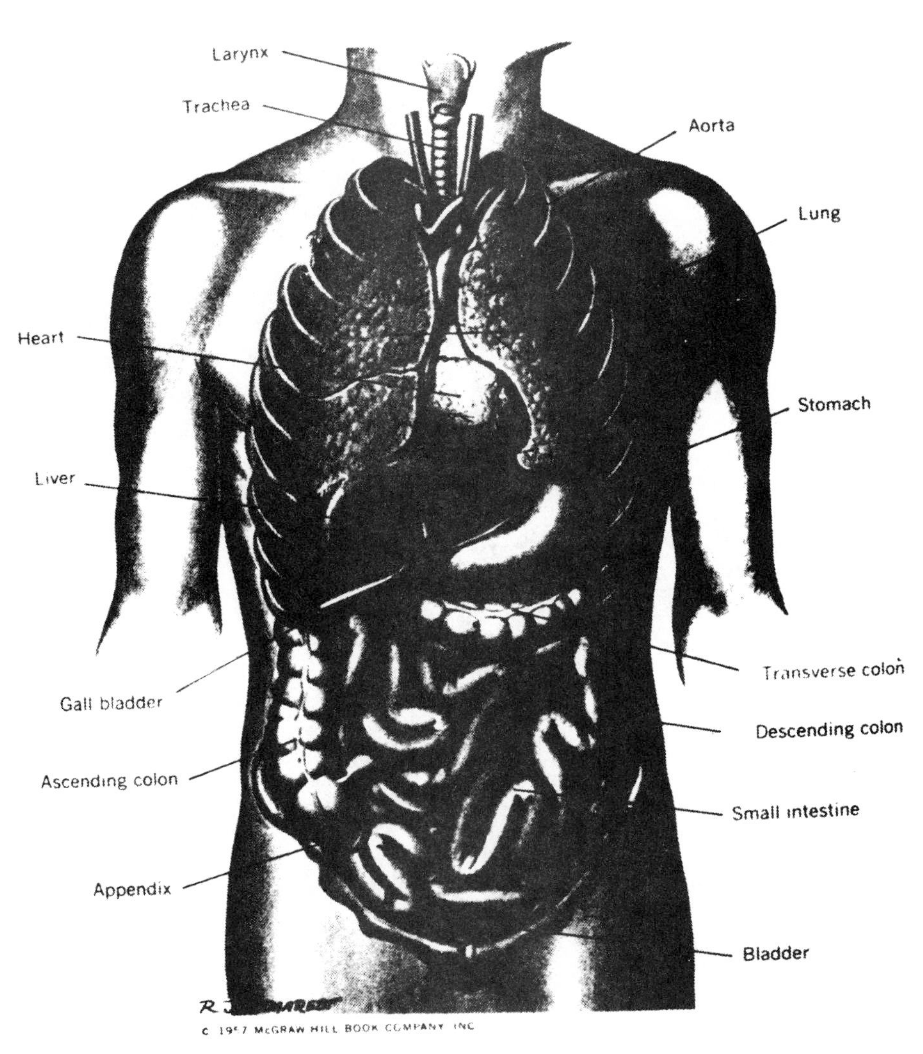

FIG. 2.4. Viscera. [Copyright 1957, McGraw-Hill Book Company. Reprinted with permission.]

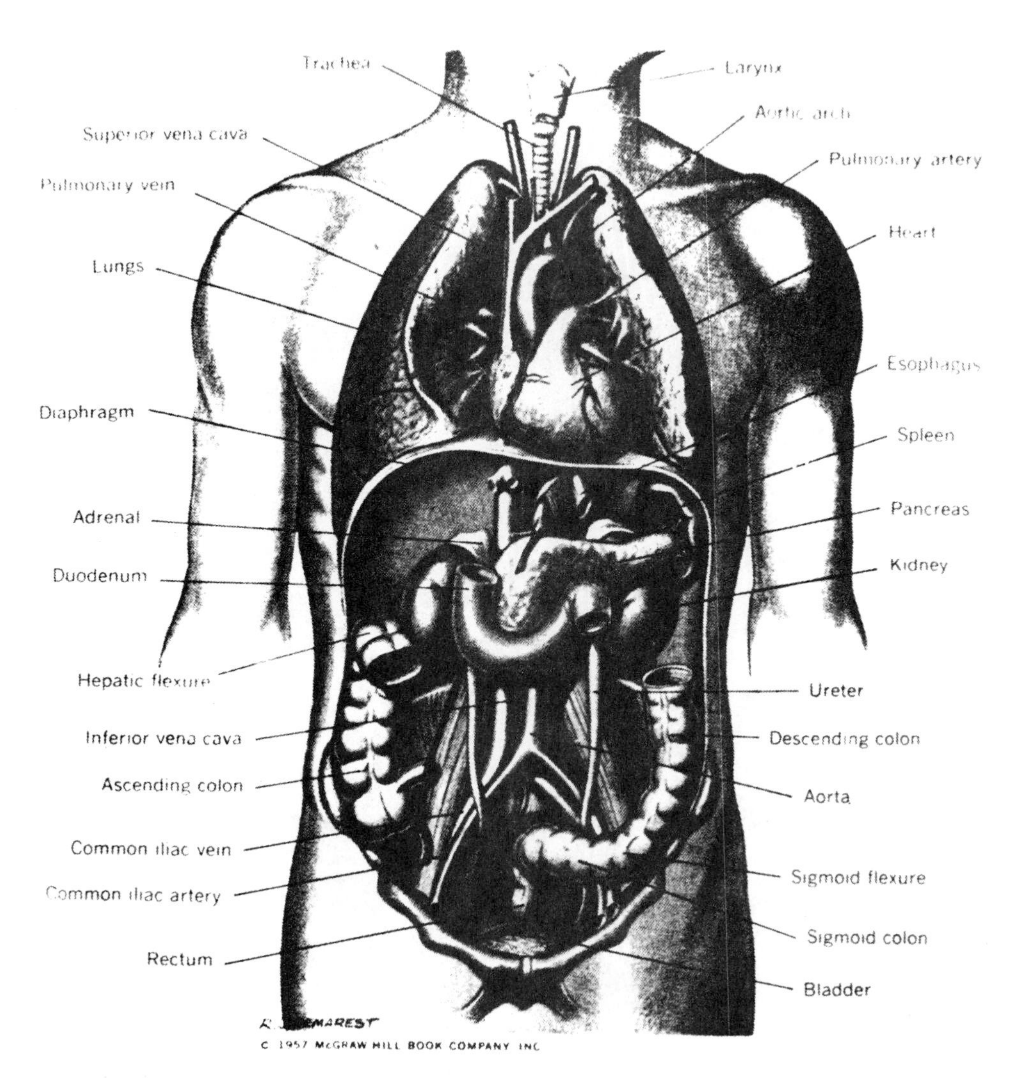

FIG. 2.5. Viscera (deep structures). [Copyright 1957, McGraw-Hill Book Company. Reprinted with permission.]

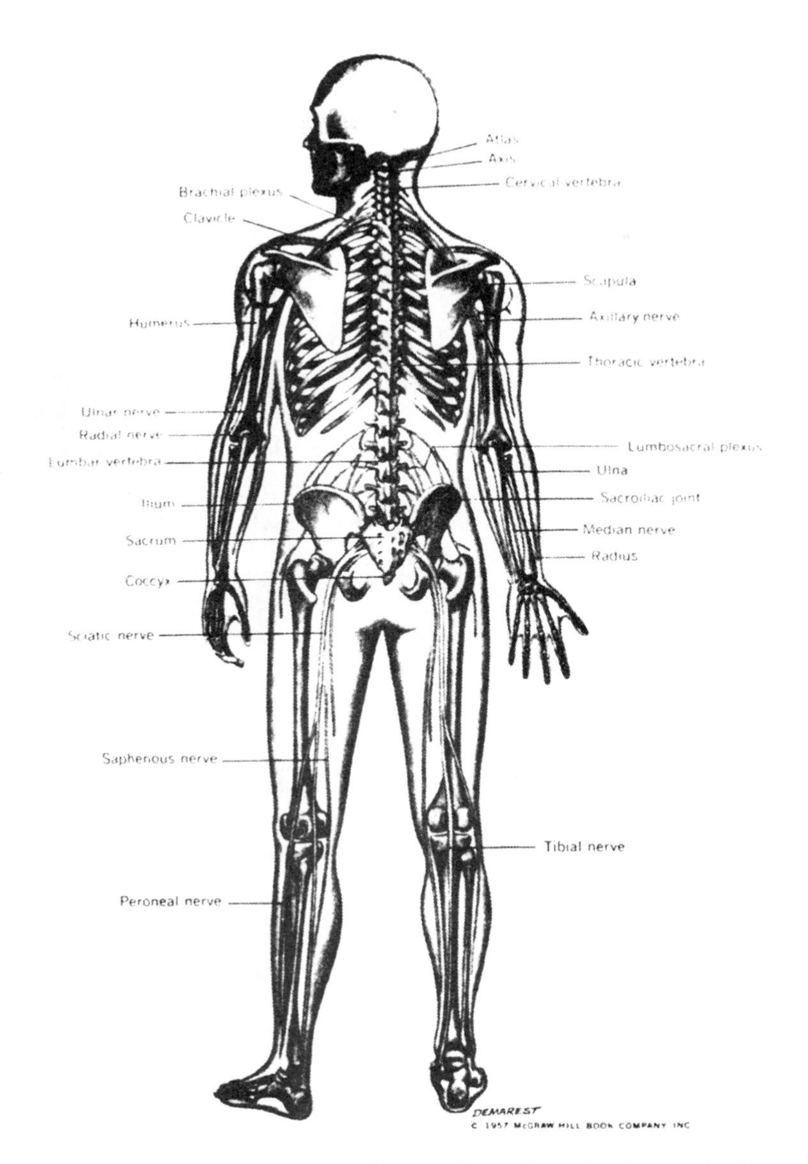

FIG. 2.6. Skeletal system (posterior view showing spinal nerves). [Copyright 1957, McGraw-Hill Book Company. Reprinted with permission.]

A. *Skeletal System*

The functions of the skeletal system (Figures 2.1 and 2.6) are primarily to provide a somewhat rigid protective and supportive structure (e.g., the rib cage protects the lungs) and a framework for muscle attachment. This framework permits turning, extension, and flexing motions through incorporation of hinge joints (elbow), ball-and-socket joints (hips), and other connections. Note how the large bones of the extremities (humerus, femur) branch to give greater flexibility of motion (ulna and radius; tibia and fibula). These extremities end in exceptionally flexible members, hands and feet, which are constituted of very many bones. For example, each hand contains 27 bones and each foot 26 bones; in fact, of the 206 bones in the body, over 50 percent are contained simply in hands and feet.

The skull consists of many separate bones joined along jagged interfaces (sutures). This arrangement allows for convenient expansion of the cranial cavity during growth and yet firm overall rigidity and cohesion. Other major bones are the clavicles (collarbones), which provide considerable protection to the arteries, veins, lungs, etc., that underlie them, and the scapulae (shoulder blades), which provide broad surfaces for the attachment of large muscles. The spinal column is another mechanical marvel, flexible yet strong, comprised of alternating collagenous discs and bones (vertebrae). Support for the body and protection of the great nerve bundles running inside the column are two prime functions. The coccyx, a vestigial tail, reminds us of our distant ancestors.

B. *Arterial and Venous Systems*

The arterial and venous systems (Figures 2.2 and 2.3) are similar in many respects. Figure 2.7 shows schematically the nature of the circulatory system. Starting with the left ventricle, blood is squeezed into the large arteries which feed all parts of the

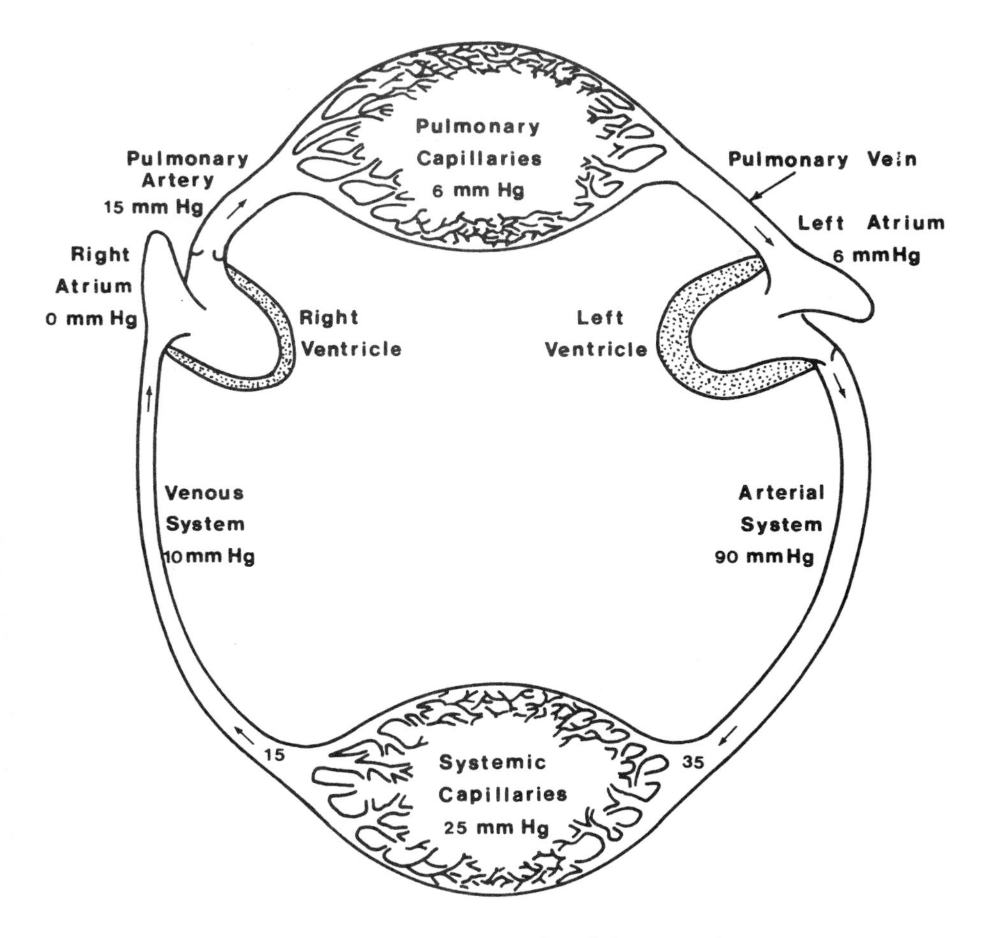

FIG. 2.7. The human circulatory system.

body except the lungs. Blood flows through a branching network of smaller and smaller diameter vessels until it finally reaches the very numerous capillaries, where exchange of nutrients, O_2, and CO_2 takes place. Leaving these capillaries the blood flows from a converging branched network into successively larger veins and finally empties into the right atrium of the heart. This loop, from left ventricle to right atrium, is termed the "systemic circulation."

Blood from the right atrium flows, during each heartbeat cycle, into the right ventricle. From here it is squeezed through the "pulmonary circulation," another sequence of arteries-capillaries-veins, and returns to the left atrium of the heart. As shown in Figure 2.7, the pulmonary system pressure levels are much lower than the systemic circulation pressures. The heart is thus a four-chambered duplex pump, with two inflow receivers (the atria) and two chambers which provide the pumping action (the ventricles).

The main arteries coming from the heart are shown in Figure 2.2: the aorta and the pairs of pulmonary, subclavian, carotid, and iliac arteries. Other branches, such as the renal arteries (which lead to the kidneys), are also shown. The venous system (Figure 2.3) is analogous in all major respects of configuration. Combining near the right atrium are the two major veins which carry blood back to the heart from the upper and lower parts of the body: the superior vena cava and the inferior vena cava, respectively. In other respects, however, the venous system is very different (e.g., total volume) from the arterial system, as we shall see later. The veins normally run near the surface of the body, whereas the arteries lie deeper. The evolutionary reason for this is obvious: The blood loss rate from a low pressure system (venous) would be much less, if the system is accidentally cut, than from a high pressure system (arterial).

A unique feature of the systemic circulation is the portion known as the portal circulation, illustrated in Figure 2.8. This consists of the hepatic artery which goes directly to the liver and portal vein which feeds blood from the digestive organs, the spleen, the pancreas, and the gallbladder to the liver. This system offers some protection to the body, as it permits the liver to detoxify any harmful substances that might have been picked up in the gastrointestinal tract before entry into the rest of the circulation is gained.

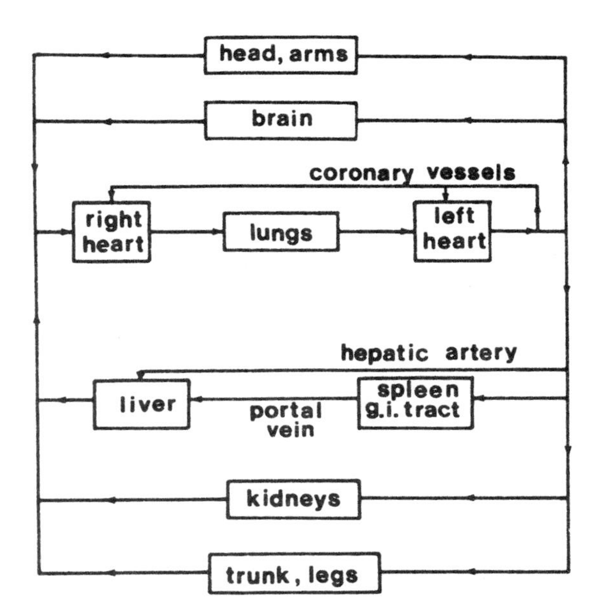

FIG. 2.8. The adult circulatory system. [From Ganong, W. F., *Review of Medical Physiology*, 5th ed., Lange Med. Publ., Los Altos, California, 1971, p. 415.]

C. *The Viscera*

The viscera are the large organs in the interior cavities of the body (the thoracic, abdominal, and pelvic cavities). Configurations and locations are shown in Figures 2.4 and 2.5. The most important of these organs are the heart, lungs, liver and gallbladder, kidneys, pancreas, spleen, stomach, small intestines, large intestines, bladder, and ureters. Specific functions can be identified with each organ and related strongly to their corresponding structures. We mention here briefly the functions of several of these organs, with special attention to those that are least familiar to the typical student.

The spleen is a flattened, oblong, purplish, glandlike organ about 5 in. long, located in the upper part of the abdominal cavity. Its prime function is to remove old red blood cells from the circulation and set free the contained hemoglobin (which the liver converts to bilirubin). The spleen also forms certain blood cells (lymphocytes, monocytes, and, in infants, red blood cells) and manufactures antibodies. As other organs in the body also perform these same functions, the spleen can be removed without any dire effects. Many of the more subtle functions of this organ have not been identified.

The pancreas, a large elongated gland located behind the stomach, secretes fluid containing a variety of digestive enzymes into the small intestine (duodenum), via the pancreatic duct. Internally, the pancreas also secretes into the blood the hormone insulin, which is important in the regulation of carbohydrate (sugar) metabolism.

Functions of the stomach include primarily the storage of food, the mixing of food with gastric secretions to form a mushy mixture called chyme, and the slow release of this semifluid into the small intestine. In the small intestine, food is mixed with the pancreatic juice, bile, and other secretions. Digestion, begun in the mouth and stomach, is essentially completed in the small intestine, and the end products are absorbed into the blood and lymph. The upper part of the small intestine is the duodenum ($\sim$22 cm long) and the lower part (258 cm long) is divided somewhat arbitrarily into the jejunum (first 2/5) and the ileum (last 3/5). The ileum joins the large intestine, which is comprised of the ascending, transverse, descending, and sigmoid colons and ends with the rectum. Functionally, the colons' main purpose is to permit reabsorption of water and other items from the entering 500 ml or so of chyme and produce about 250 g of semisolid feces (daily basis).

The liver, the largest gland in the body, has many complex functions. These include the formation of bile (which is stored in the gallbladder connected to the liver and secreted into the duodenum when needed for digestion), the storage of carbohydrates, the manufacture of plasma proteins, urea formation, and a vast number of other chemical syntheses and degradations. This organ is of prime importance in nearly all facets related to the body's chemistry: metabolism, hormonal aspects, etc.

The kidneys, about which much more will be said in Chapter 8, are two organs, each about 4 in. by 2 in. by 1-in. thick, located in the back center of the abdominal cavity. By secreting a urine containing metabolic waste products (urea, creatinine, etc.), electrolytes, and other species, the kidneys accurately control the compositions and volumes of the body's fluids at desired values. Although the kidneys are really fairly small organs, they process as much as 1500 cc of blood each minute.

The lungs, which shall also be further treated in detail (Chapter 10), consist of two spongy organs in the chest cavity. Exchange of oxygen and carbon dioxide is the prime function of the lungs. The upper portions of the airways leading to the lungs contain the trachea, a large single tube, and, above it, the larynx, another section of cartilaginous tube which functions also as the organ of voice.

II. THE "STANDARD" MAN

Table 2.1 shows some basic data for a standard male person. Given here are weight, dimensions, physical properties, and steady-state operating parameter values.

Note the great proportion of the body weight comprised by fluids (∿60%). The volume of blood of 5 liters consists of about 3 liters of plasma and about 2 liters of cells (mostly red blood cells), which are full of intracellular fluid. Hence, the cells in blood are included in with the other intracellular fluids of the body (as in muscle cells, nerve cells, etc). The interstitial fluid is the fluid occupying the spaces between cells. It flows slowly through the tissue interstices and bathes the cells, but is in near equilibrium

TABLE 2.1

Standard Man Data[a]

Age			30 yr
Height			5 ft 8 in. or 1.73 m
Weight			150 lb or 68 kg
Surface area			1.80 m^2 or 19.5 ft^2
Normal body core temperature			37.0°C
Normal mean skin temperature			34.2°C
Heat capacity			0.86 kcal/kg °C
Percent body fat			12% (8.2 kg)
Subcutaneous fat layer			5 mm
Body fluids			41 liters (60 wt% of body)
Intracellular	28.0 liters	40%	
Interstitial	10.0 liters	15%	
Transcellular	———	—	
Plasma	3.0 liters	5%	
	41.0 liters	60%	
Basal metabolism			40 kcal/m^2 hr, 72 kcal/hr, 1730 kcal/day
Oxygen consumption			250 ml/min } at STP (standard temperature and pressure, 0°C and 1 atm)
CO_2 production			200 ml/min } at STP (standard temperature and pressure, 0°C and 1 atm)
Respiratory quotient			0.80
Blood volume			5 liters
Resting cardiac output			5 liters/min
Systemic blood pressure			120/80 mm Hg
Heart rate at rest			65/min
General cardiac output			3.0 + 8M liters/min (M = liters O_2 consumed/min at STP)
Total lung capacity			6000 ml } at BTP (body temperature and pressure, 37°C and 1 atm)
Vital capacity			4200 ml } at BTP
Ventilation rate			6000 ml/min } at BTP
Alveolar ventilation rate			4200 ml/min } at BTP
Tidal volume			500 ml } at BTP
Dead space			150 ml } at BTP
Breathing frequency			12/min
Pulmonary capillary blood volume			75 ml
Arterial O_2 content			0.195 ml O_2/ml blood } at STP
Arterial CO_2 content			0.492 ml CO_2/ml blood } at STP
Venous O_2 content			0.145 ml O_2/ml blood } at STP
Venous CO_2 content			0.532 ml CO_2/ml blood } at STP

[a]Adapted from R. C. Seagrave, *Biomedical Applications of Heat and Mass Transfer*, Iowa State Univ. Press, Ames, 1971, p. 66.

with the blood plasma. Lymph is one type of interstitial fluid. Transcellular fluids are special fluids identified with specific compartments apart from the ordinary tissues, and include the cerebrospinal, intraocular, pleural, pericardial, synovial, sweat, and digestive fluids.

The "basal" (at rest) metabolic rate of 72 kcal/hr represents a substantial amount of energy production, and the body's surface area of 19.5 ft^2 is an important factor in dissipating this heat, as we shall see in Chapter 5. Terms associated with the lungs, such as "tidal volume," are defined in the chapter on lung physiology.

Other data in Table 2.1 indicate that the body uses more O_2 than appears ultimately in the form of CO_2 given off (the rest of the O_2 appears as part of H_2O created) and that the mean circulation time of blood in the body is only about 1 min.

III. COMPOSITION OF THE BODY

Table 2.2 gives a gross breakdown of the human body composition in terms of major organic and inorganic components. Note that water

TABLE 2.2

Content in Grams of a 70-kg Adult Man[a]

Water	41,400	Mg	21
Fat	12,600	Cl	85
Protein	12,600	P	670
Carbohydrate	300	S	112
Na	63	Fe	3
K	150	I	0.014
Ca	1,160		

[a]From A. C. Guyton, *Function of the Human Body*, 3rd ed., Saunders, Philadelphia, Pennsylvania, 1969, p. 393.

accounts for about 60% of the total, and that the amounts of fat and protein are similar (each individual would show varied proportions, but the rough equivalence is correct). Carbohydrates, existing as stored derivatives such as glycogen, account for little "permanent" weight since they are a prime energy source, more like energy in transit. The substantial amount of calcium derives primarily from the skeletal system. Many items not listed occur in small amounts but are nevertheless vital for life. The total "ash" content of a 70-kg person would be about 3000 g.

The compositions of the body fluids are shown in Table 2.3. Plasma and interstitial fluid are quite similar except for protein content. The reason for this is that interstitial fluids are formed by filtration of blood plasma outward from the capillaries into the tissues. The walls of the capillaries are porous enough to let all low molecular weight solutes through, but only a portion of higher molecular weight solutes are able to pass. Intracellular fluid is very different, especially in terms of Na^+ and K^+ contents, which are almost the reverse of the Na^+ and K^+ levels in the other two types of fluids. Cl^- contents also differ widely. Such concentration gradients are maintained only by the expenditure of large amounts of biochemical energy, as we shall see later. Certain items involved with cell metabolism (phosphocreatine, hexose monophosphate, Mg^{2+}, adenosine triphosphate, etc.) are found only or primarily in the intracellular fluid environment.

The various fluids are essentially equal in terms of osmolarity, which means that no shift of water will occur if they are separated by semipermeable membranes (which they are). "Osmolarity" actually refers to water activity, and a one osmolar solution has the water activity of a 1M solution of a nondissociating solute. Hence, body fluids correspond roughly to the osmolarity one would obtain with a 0.15N solution of NaCl, which dissociates into two species. The concentration of seawater is about 0.52N by contrast (which has evolutionary significance).

TABLE 2.3

Osmolar Substances in Extracellular and Intracellular Fluids[a]

	Plasma (mOsm./ liter of H_2O)	Interstitial (mOsm./ liter of H_2O)	Intracellular (mOsm./ liter of H_2O)
Na^+	144	137	10
K^+	5	4.7	141
Ca^{2+}	2.5	2.4	0
Mg^{2+}	1.5	1.4	31
Cl^-	107	112.7	4
HCO_3^-	27	28.3	10
$HPO_4^{2-}, H_2PO_4^-$	2	2	11
SO_2^{2-}	0.5	0.5	1
Phosphocreatine			45
Carnosine			14
Amino acids	2	2	8
Creatine	0.2	0.2	9
Lactate	1.2	1.2	1.5
Adenosine triphosphate			5
Hexose monophosphate			3.7
Glucose	5.6	5.6	
Protein	1.2	0.2	4
Urea	4	4	4
Total (mOsm)	303.7	302.2	302.2
Corrected osmolar activity (mOsm)	282.6	281.3	281.3
Total osmotic pressure at 37° C (mm Hg)	5454	5430	5430

[a]From A. C. Guyton, *Textbook of Medical Physiology*, 4th ed., Saunders, Philadelphia, Pennsylvania, 1971, p. 387.

The body fluids are also essentially electrically neutral. It should be pointed out that proteins, at the body's pH of ∿7.4, are predominantly anions, i.e., have the form shown on the far right below:

$$\text{R-CH}(\text{NH}_3^+)\text{-C}(=\text{O})\text{OH} \rightleftarrows \text{R-CH}(\text{NH}_3^+)\text{-C}(=\text{O})\text{O}^- \rightleftarrows \text{R-CH}(\text{NH}_2)\text{-C}(=\text{O})\text{O}^-$$

This is called amphoteric behavior, and the species in the middle is a zwitterion. The so-called isoelectric point (pI) is the pH of the fluid at which electrical balance between the anionic and cationic forms is achieved. For each ionic group ($-NH_3^+$, $-COO^-$, etc.) the value of pH at which half of the group is dissociated and half undissociated is termed the pK_a of that group. Values of pK and pI for selected amino acids are given in Table 2.4.

TABLE 2.4

pK and pI Values of Representative Amino Acids[a]

Amino acid	pK_{a_1}	pK_{a_2}	pK_{a_3}	pI
Glycine	2.34 (COOH)	9.60 (NH_3^+)	—	5.97
Aspartic acid	1.88 (COOH)	3.65 (COOH)	9.60 (NH_3^+)	2.77
Glutamic acid	2.19 (COOH)	4.28 (COOH)	9.66 (NH_3^+)	3.20
Tyrosine	2.20 (COOH)	9.11 (NH_3^+)	10.07 (OH)	5.66
Cysteine	1.96 (COOH)	8.18 (NH_3^+)	10.28 (SH)	5.07
Lysine	2.18 (COOH)	8.95 (α-NH_3^+)	10.53 (ε-NH_3^+)	9.74

[a]From A. Mazur and B. Harrow, *Textbook of Biochemistry*, 10th ed., Saunders, Philadelphia, Pennsylvania, 1971, p. 45.

The weights and water contents of the various organs of the human body are shown in Table 2.5. The low water content of the skeletal system is notable, as are the relatively large weights of the brain and liver (e.g., more than 3 lb each for a 150-lb man).

IV. OVERALL MASS BALANCES ON THE BODY

A. *Water*

Table 2.6 shows approximate steady-state values (actually time-averaged values) for water intake, production, and excretion for an adult under average conditions. "Water of oxidation" refers to the

TABLE 2.5

Weights and Water Contents of Organs in the Human Body[a]

Organs	Amount of Water in Organ (Wt%)	Organ Weight Relative to Body Weight (%)	Organ Weight For a 70-kg Man (lb)
Skin	72.03	18	27.8
Muscles	75.67	41.7	64.3
Skeleton	22.04	15.9	24.5
Brain	74.84	2.01	3.10
Spinal cord	—	—	—
Liver	68.25	2.26	3.48
Heart	79.21	0.47	0.72
Lungs	78.96	1.34	2.07
Kidneys	82.68	0.37	0.57
Spleen	75.77	0.43	0.66
Blood	83	4.9	7.56
Intestines	74.54	2.25	3.47
Rest of body	—	10.37	15.96
Entire body	63	100.00	154.2

[a]Adapted from M. Skelton, *Arch. Intern. Med.*, 40, 140 (1927).

TABLE 2.6

Average Daily Water Balance[a]

Water intake (approximate) (ml)		Water excretion (approximate) (ml)	
Drinking water	1200	Urine	1400
Water content of food	1000	Insensible water loss	700
Water of oxidation	300	Sweat	200
	2500	Stool	200
			2500

[a]Adapted from T. C. Ruch and H. D. Patton, *Physiology and Biophysics*, 19th ed., Saunders, Philadelphia, Pennsylvania, 1965, p. 894.

water produced by metabolism of food (e.g., glucose → CO_2 + H_2O). The insensible water loss refers to losses by diffusion through the skin (as opposed to water exuded by the sweat glands) and by evaporation from the lungs (expired air is normally saturated with water at body temperature). Shown in Table 2.7 are figures that indicate the effects of hot weather and heavy exercise on water loss (which must ultimately be matched by water input, mainly by drinking). Note the shift of water from urine to sweat under the hot exercise conditions. The tremendous increase in the sweating response is clear. On the other hand, the water loss via the lungs does not change much, dropping some in hot weather (inspired air is usually more humid, and the expired air may be less than saturated), and rising with exercise (increased breathing rate).

The figure in Table 2.7 for water loss from the lungs is easily checked by assuming the average person inspires 12 breaths of 500 ml each per minute (referred to body temperature, 37°C) of bone-dry inlet air, and assuming saturated expired air at a body temperature of 37°C (partial pressure of H_2O is 47 mm Hg). Simple calculations indicate a water loss rate of 403 g/day. Of course, since inspired air is

TABLE 2.7

Daily Loss of Water[a]

(in milliliters)

	Normal temperature	Hot weather	Prolonged heavy exercise
Insensible loss:			
Skin	350	350	350
Lungs	350	250	650
Urine	1400	1200	500
Sweat	200	1400	5000
Feces	200	200	200
Total	2500	3400	6700

[a]Adapted from A. C. Guyton, *Textbook of Medical Physiology*, op. cit., p. 420.

seldom bone dry, the loss rate will normally be lower (e.g., for an air temperature of 70°F and relative humidity of 30%, $P_{H_2O} \cong 19$ mm Hg and thus the loss rate becomes roughly 240 g/day).

B. Gases

As given in Table 2.1, an average male at rest breathes about 12 times per minute, each breath moving about 500 ml of gas (tidal volume) in and out. Oxygen consumption is about 250 ml O_2 (STP) per minute and CO_2 rejection about 200 ml CO_2 (STP) per minute. These figures correspond to time averaged flow rates of 515 g O_2 and 565 g CO_2 per day, or a net mass loss of 50 g. Water is normally lost from the skin and lungs in gaseous form, although at high sweating rates sweat loss by direct liquid runoff can occur, especially under humid conditions. The figures for water have been discussed above.

C. Solids

The feces are normally about 3/4 water by weight and 1/4 solid matter. Since the water loss per day in the feces is ∿200 g, the corresponding solids loss is about 70 g/day. We should perhaps also include here the solute content of the urine. Assuming the urine to be a 0.14N NaCl solution and its excretion rate to be 1400 ml/day, the solute content becomes roughly 12 g/day.

Food is, of course, a variable item but for the average person it amounts to about 430 g/day (solid part only—food, like the human body, has much water). Another regular but fairly small loss of mass from the body occurs as the result of the sloughing off of dead epithelial cells from the outer surfaces of the body. However, no numbers seem to be available regarding the total grams per day lost by this means.

A schematic diagram of steady-state mass balances on the body is shown in Figure 2.9.

V. CORRELATIONS OF PHYSIOLOGICAL VARIABLES IN MAN

While data pertinent to a "standard" man (Table 2.1) are interesting, it is of value to determine how important physiological parameters vary among all men. Table 2.8 presents a few basic correlations from the literature (additional correlations are discussed in later chapters on heat transfer, pulmonary physiology, etc.).

Surface area has traditionally been used as a primary variable for correlating metabolic rates versus body "size." Experimentally it is found that persons may vary considerably in body proportions and yet usually possess about the same metabolic rate per unit area of surface. However, other correlations of metabolic rate, with "lean body mass," weight alone, and with height and weight (like that given in Table 2.8) are also very common. Surface area is easily measured by wrapping a person completely with inelastic tape of uniform width and measuring the length of tape required.

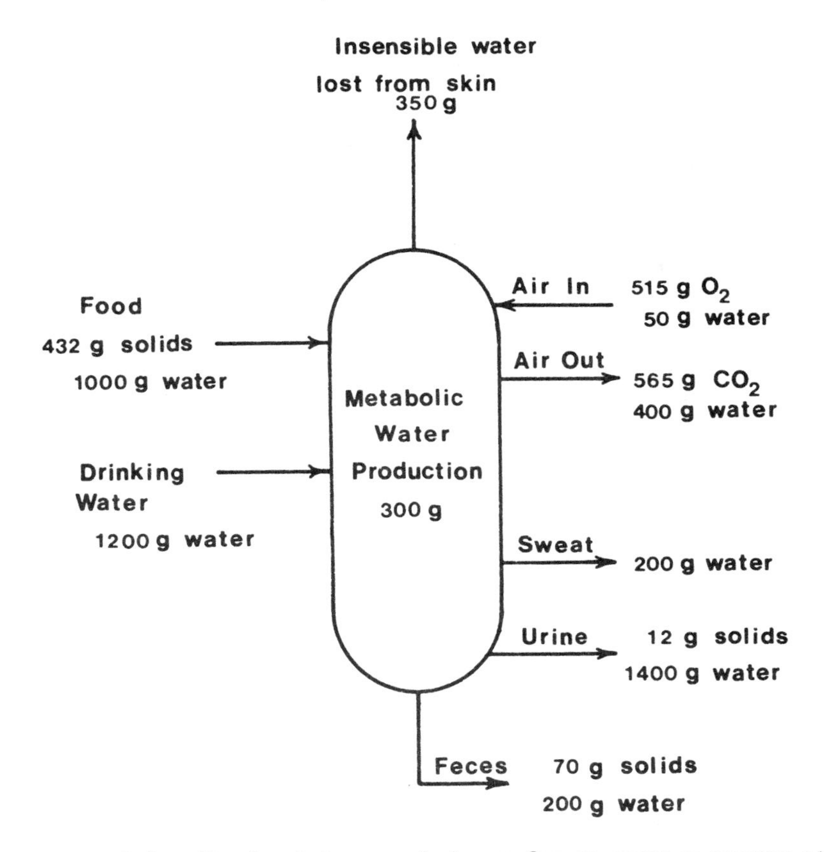

FIG. 2.9. Steady-state mass balance for an average person at rest (per day), where the solids content of sweat (probably less than 2 g) has been neglected. A general mass balance can be written as $\Sigma\dot{m}_{in} - \Sigma\dot{m}_{out} = dm_{tot}/dt$ (zero at steady state), where $\dot{m}$ is the mass flow rate, and m_{tot} is the total body mass at any time t. The terms in the mass balance must in general be time averaged over a reasonable period to have significance.

Body densities, which can be correlated with height and weight as shown, are normally expressed as weight per body volume exclusive of the volume of gas contained in the lungs. When densities are measured by the "underwater weighing" technique, a correction for the lung gas volume remaining after a forceful expiration is involved. For an average person, the correction for a 1.2-liter residual volume

TABLE 2.8

Some Correlations for Physiological Variables in Man[a]

Surface area (m^2) (DuBois and DuBois, 1916)

Area = $71.84W^{0.425}H^{0.725}$

Basal metabolic rate (kcal/hr) (Carpenter, 1939)

BMR (newborn) = $0.054W^{1.5}H$

BMR (males) = $2.77 + 0.57W + 0.21H - 0.28\text{Age}$

BMR (females) = $2.71 + 0.40W + 0.08H - 0.19\text{Age}$

Body density (g/cc) (Cowgill, 1957)

ρ (males) = $0.0277W^{-0.3}H^{0.725} + 0.75$

maximum ρ (zero fat) $\cong$ 1.100

average ρ (12% fat) $\cong$ 1.073[b]

(density of fat $\cong$ 0.92)

Blood volume (liters) (Allen et al., 1956)

Blood (males) = $4.17 \times 10^{-7}H^3 + 0.045W - 0.03$

Blood (females) = $4.14 \times 10^{-7}H^3 + 0.033W - 0.03$

Energy expenditure (kcal/hr) (Durnin and Edwards, 1955)

Energy = $10.38VR - 0.52$, where

VR is ventilation rate at body temperature (liters/min)

---

[a]In all formulas, W is body weight in kilograms, H is height in centimeters.

[b]Keys et al. (1951) found that the average percentage of fat in men was 10% at age 20 but that it increased steadily to 25% at age 55.

has the effect of raising the body density value from an "apparent" value of about 1.053 g/cc to a true value of 1.073 g/cc. Simple computations also reveal that for an average person, the body will have an apparent density of only 0.985 g/cc if maximum air inspiration (5.7 liters of gas in the lungs) is achieved. This explains why an average person can float on water if a deep breath is taken.

Other body density correlations have been developed in terms of "skinfold thicknesses," i.e., thicknesses of skin and subcutaneous fat measured when calipers are used to pinch a body surface at a prescribed tension (usually 10 g/mm^2 of caliper face area). One such correlation, for men aged 18 to 26, is (Brožek and Keys, 1951)

$$\rho\ (g/cc) = 1.0017 - 0.000282A - 0.000736B - 0.000883C$$

where A, B, and C are skinfold thickness in millimeters at certain locations in the abdomen, chest, and arm.

It should be noted that in some cases significant differences exist between males and females, depending on the variable being measured.

PROBLEMS

1. Verify the following figures given in the text:

   (a) water lost by breathing bone-dry air = 403 g/day
   (b) O_2 consumed and CO_2 produced = 515 and 565 g/day, respectively
   (c) solids lost in the urine = 12 g/day.

2. Table 2.1 indicates that an average man, 5 ft 8 in. tall, has a body surface area of 19.5 ft^2 and a weight of 150 lb.

   (a) If the body were modeled as an equivalent cylinder of the same height and surface area, what would its diameter be?
   (b) If the body were modeled as an equivalent cylinder having the same height and weight, what would its diameter be? Use an average overall body density value of 1.053 g/cc.

   Such cylinders can be used to estimate heat transfer (see p. 109).

3. What would be the daily loss of solids (in grams) by sweating under normal conditions, if one assumes sweat to be a 0.14N NaCl solution? Note that in dry weather, when sweat readily evaporates, one does not actually "lose" the solids until they are washed off in the shower, or such.

4. Show that if an average person inspires enough air to give 5.7 liters of gas in his lungs, then the apparent density of his body in water will be around 0.985 g/cc. Assume a "true" density (zero gas in lungs) of 1.073 g/cc.

5. If a person is exercising at a rate such that his metabolic rate is six times its basal value, what will his cardiac output be (see Table 2.1)? If his pulse under such conditions is 130 beats per minute, what does this imply about the amount of blood pumped by the heart per beat (i.e., the "stroke volume")?

DISCUSSION QUESTIONS

1. Table 2.2 indicates that iodine is present in the human body in only a trace amount. Is iodine nevertheless important? If so, why? Name a normal source for iodine in the diet.

2. Glutamic acid is in aqueous solution at a pH of 5. Which dissociable groups will be more than half dissociated under these conditions; which will be less than half dissociated? Will this amino acid carry a net positive charge or net negative charge? The formula for glutamic acid is

```
H2N-CH-CH2-CH2
    |      |
   COOH   COOH
```

3. Table 2.8 indicates that for two males having the same weight, the taller one will have the greater body density. Why would you expect this to be so?

REFERENCES

Allen, T. H., Peng, M. T., Chen, K. P., Huang, T. F., Chang, C., and Fang, H. S., *Metabolism*, 5, 328 (1956).

Brožek, J., and Keys, A., *Br. J. Nutr.*, 5, 194 (1951).

Carpenter, T. M., *Tables, Factors, and Formulas for Computing Respiratory Exchange and Biological Transformations of Energy*, 3rd ed., Carnegie Institution of Washington, 1939.

Cowgill, G. R., *Am. J. Clin. Nutr.*, 5, 601 (1957).

DuBois, D., and DuBois, E. F., *Arch. Intern. Med.*, 17, 863 (1916).

Durnin, J. V. G. A., and Edwards, R. G., *Q. J. Exp. Physiol.*, 40, 370 (1955).

Keys, A., Anderson, J., and Brožek, J., *Am. J. Physiol.*, 167, 802 (1951).

BIBLIOGRAPHY

Consolazio, C. F., Johnson, R. E., and Pecora, L. J., *Physiological Measurements of Metabolic Functions in Man*, McGraw-Hill, New York, 1963.

Biological handbooks published by the Federation of American Societies for Experimental Biology, Bethesda, Maryland, P. L. Altman and D. S. Dittmer, eds.:
Blood and Other Body Fluids 1961
Growth, Including Reproduction and Morphological Development 1962
Biology Data Book 1964
Metabolism 1968

Chapter 3

PHYSICAL, CHEMICAL, AND RHEOLOGICAL PROPERTIES OF BLOOD

A thorough knowledge of the physical, chemical, and flow properties of blood is essential for understanding and modeling capillary transport phenomena and circulatory system dynamics in the body. Similarly, in the design and development of extracorporeal devices (i.e., those external to the body) such as artificial kidneys, blood oxygenators, and blood pumps, the same knowledge is critical. Many of the major practical problems involved in artificial organ applications result, in fact, from the sensitivity of blood to the unfamiliar shear stresses imposed by such devices, stresses that cause blood cell rupture and clotting problems. In this chapter, we consider, in a general way, the various properties of blood and phenomena that occur during the extracorporeal handling of blood, without reference to particular devices.

I. PHYSICAL PROPERTIES

Table 3.1 summarizes the important physical properties of blood. Whole blood, which is slightly alkaline (pH $\cong$ 7.4), can be divided into about 55 vol% plasma, and about 45 vol% cells, or "formed elements." The hematocrit, a quantity of significant physiological importance, is defined as the volume percentage of cells, and is easily measured by centrifugation of a small blood sample.

The cells consist of about 95% (by number) red blood cells (RBCs), or erythrocytes. White cells comprise another 0.13% by number, and the remainder, about 4.9%, consists of platelets. The plasma portion of the blood is essentially a dilute (0.15N) electrolyte solution containing about 8 wt% proteins. Note that the RBCs are heavier than the plasma. In nonflowing blood the RBCs therefore tend to settle. In fact, an elevation of the so-called sedimentation rate is often correlated strongly with various diseased states.

Dimensions of a typical RBC are shown in Figure 3.1. The cell has the shape of a biconcave disc which can deform, however, into a bullet-shaped entity during passage through small capillaries. Prime functions of the RBCs are the transport of O_2 and CO_2 throughout the body and buffering the blood so as to regulate pH. As the physical solubility of O_2 and CO_2 in blood plasma is rather low, the requirements for O_2 and CO_2 transport by the blood are ingeniously met by the reversible binding of O_2 and CO_2 with the hemoglobin contained in the RBCs. Under normal conditions about 60 times as much O_2 and about 20 times more CO_2 can be bound by hemoglobin than can physically dissolve in the plasma. Hemoglobin, which is present to the extent of more than 33 wt% inside the RBCs, consists of four long protein chains to which are bound four "heme" groups (a ferroprotoporphyrin, a chelating structure composed, in turn, of four pyrrole rings) and has a molecular weight of 68,000. Figure 3.2 shows the structure of hemoglobin, with and without bonded O_2. The globin portion (protein chain) does not bind O_2 or CO_2 but is important as a buffering agent (recall our previous discussion of the amphoteric behavior of amino acids).

TABLE 3.1

Physical Properties of Human Blood

(Normal Adult Mean Values)

Whole blood	
pH	7.35-7.40
Viscosity (37°C)	3.0 cP (at high shear rates)
Specific gravity (25/4°C)	1.056
Venous hematocrit—Male	0.47
Female	0.42
Whole blood volume	∿78 ml/kg body wt
Plasma or serum	
Colloid osmotic pressure	∿330 mm H_2O
pH	7.3-7.5
Viscosity (37°C)	1.2 cP
Specific gravity (25/4°C)	1.0239
Formed elements	
Erythrocytes	
pH	7.396
Specific gravity (25/4°C)	1.098
Count—Male	5.4×10^9/ml whole blood
Female	4.8×10^9/ml whole blood
Mean corpuscular volume	87 μm^3
Diameter	8.4 μm
Maximum thickness	2.4 μm
Minimum thickness	1.0 μm
Surface area	163 μm^2
Life span	120 days
Production rate	4.5×10^7/ml whole blood per day
Hemoglobin concentration	0.335 g/ml erythrocyte
Leukocytes	
Count	$\sim 7.4 \times 10^6$/ml whole blood
Diameter	7-20 μm
Platelets	
Count	$\sim 2.8 \times 10^8$/ml whole blood
Diameter	∿2-5 μm

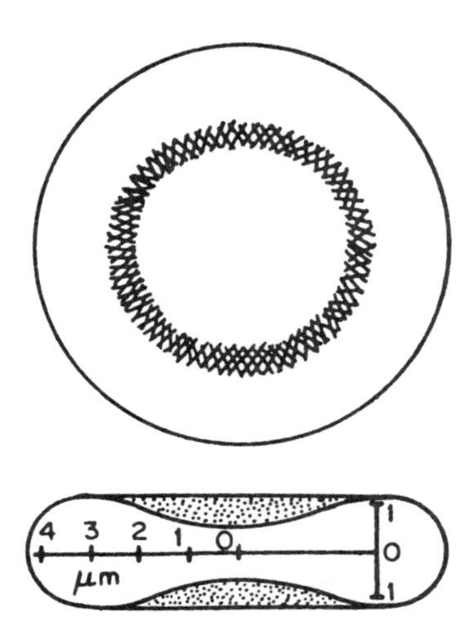

FIG. 3.1. An idealized human red cell.

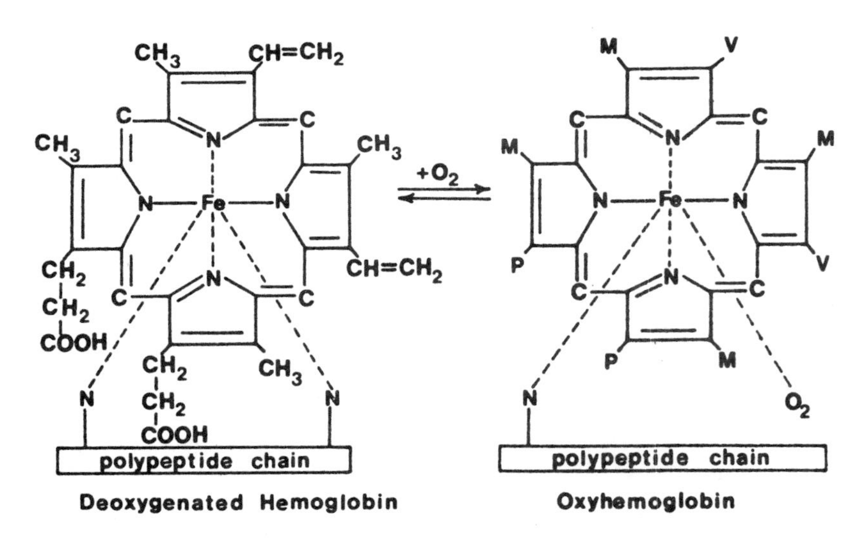

FIG. 3.2. Chemistry of hemoglobin. The hemoglobin molecule is made up of four of the units shown on the left. The abbreviations M, V, and P stand for the groups shown on the molecule on the left. [From Ganong, W. F., *Review of Medical Physiology*, 5th ed., Lange Med. Publ., Los Altos, California, 1971, p. 379.]

White blood cells are of several types, but are generally round and somewhat larger than RBCs. Lymphocytes, monocytes, eosinophils, neutrophils, and basophils are the major WBCs. Although present in much smaller numbers than the RBCs, the WBCs are important in combating infections by production of antibodies or by the direct engulfment and digestion of bacteria. The life spans of WBCs (somewhat uncertain) appear to be on the orders of a few hours or days.

Platelets, small flat cells of about 3 μm diameter, are present in fair numbers and play an important role in the processes of blood coagulation and clotting. Platelet lives average less than four days.

II. CHEMICAL PROPERTIES

The solute contents of plasma and intracellular fluids were given earlier in Table 2.3, in terms of milliosmoles per liter. The intracellular values apply to the formed elements of blood, as well as to the cells of muscle tissue, etc. Since large molecular weight molecules can be present in significant proportions by weight and yet in minor amounts when expressed as moles, a breakdown of plasma constituents by weight is presented in Table 3.2. Note that proteins account for over 8 wt% of the plasma, and that the total solutes equal 9.77 g/100 ml (102.4 g) of plasma, or 9.55 wt%. The carbohydrates include mainly glucose and other sugars, while the nonprotein nitrogenous compound category includes primarily urea, uric acid, and creatinine.

A further breakdown of the proteins typically shows the following results (per 100 ml of plasma):

Albumins	4.8 g	mol wt = 69,000
Globulins	2.5 g	mol wt = 35,000-1,000,000
Fibrinogen	0.3 g	mol wt = 330,000

The globulin class is actually rather broad. For example, it includes lipoproteins (proteins conjugated with lipids). In general, albumin functions primarily to regulate plasma volume and pH. The globulins

TABLE 3.2

Overall Breakdown of Plasma Constituents

Type of compound	Concentration (mg/100 ml plasma)
Proteins	8218
Electrolytes	745
Carbohydrates	577
Organic acids	96
Nonprotein nitrogenous compounds	79.5
Free lipids	∿30
Vitamins	∿28
Hormones	0.11
Enzymes	(trace)
Total dissolved compounds	9770

exhibit various immunological (antigen-antibody) reactions. Fibrinogen plays a key part in the blood clotting process, during which it is converted into long fibrin strands which intertwine, trap cells and other debris, and thereby form clots. Figure 3.3 illustrates the relative sizes and shapes of these proteins (not to be taken too literally) compared to hemoglobin and some smaller molecules.

III. THE RHEOLOGICAL PROPERTIES OF BLOOD

Blood, as we have seen, is a rather complex fluid, containing a fair number of relatively small molecules and a large variety of macromolecules. As one might suppose, the rheological behavior of blood—that is, its deformation and flow behavior, or more specifically the dependence of its apparent viscosity on flow rate, temperature, etc.—is not simple. In this section we shall discuss how the

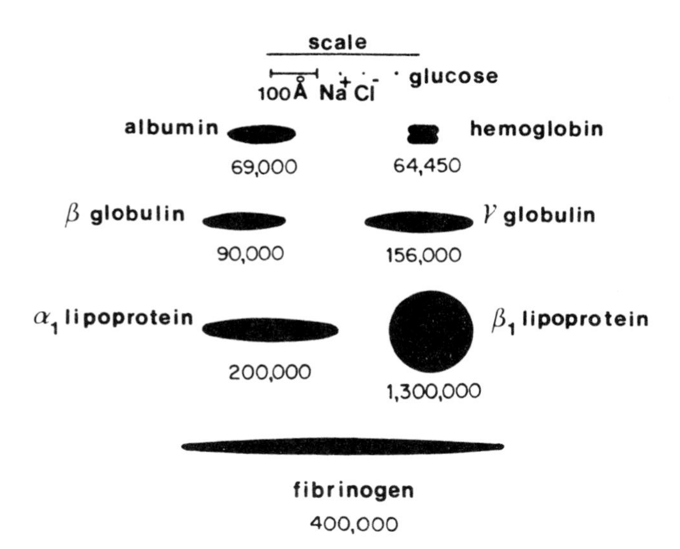

FIG. 3.3. Relative dimensions and molecular weights of some of the protein molecules in the blood. [From Harper, J. L., *Review of Physiological Chemistry*, 13th ed., Lange Med. Publ., Los Altos, California, 1971.]

apparent viscosity of blood is affected by shear rate (meaning, in essence, the magnitude of the velocity gradient, $\dot{\gamma} = dv/dx$), temperature, the apparatus used for the viscosity determinations, and the chemical composition of the blood (especially protein content).

Table 3.1 indicates that the relative viscosity of plasma or serum (plasma with fibrinogen removed) is 1.2 at 37°C. By relative viscosity we mean the viscosity relative to that of water, at the same temperature. For plasma, this value (1.2) is nearly constant with shear rate; that is, plasma seems to behave in a Newtonian fashion (it is also insensitive to temperature). Such is not true for whole blood (the value of 3.0 in Table 3.1 is the value asymptotically approached as the shear rate becomes large). Let us now see how the viscosity of whole blood has been found to depend on a variety of parameters.

A. Definition and Measurement of Viscosity

Viscosity is defined, for a fluid, as the ratio of shear stress to shear rate (or velocity gradient). In the present exposition, we assume the reader to have had previous acquaintance with the concept of viscosity and therefore offer no review here. Figure 3.4 shows typical shear stress versus shear rate curves for various materials. As the viscosity equals the slope of these curves, the constant-slope line corresponds to Newtonian behavior, i.e., a fluid having a viscosity that is independent of shear rate. Many kinds of non-Newtonian fluids exist. One, the "power law" type, is characterized by a viscosity that depends on shear rate raised to a power not equal to unity. A Bingham plastic fluid demonstrates a "yield stress"; i.e., it will not begin to flow at all until a shear stress τ_y or greater has been imposed on it. Whole blood seems to follow the "Casson" type of curve, as will be discussed later in detail.

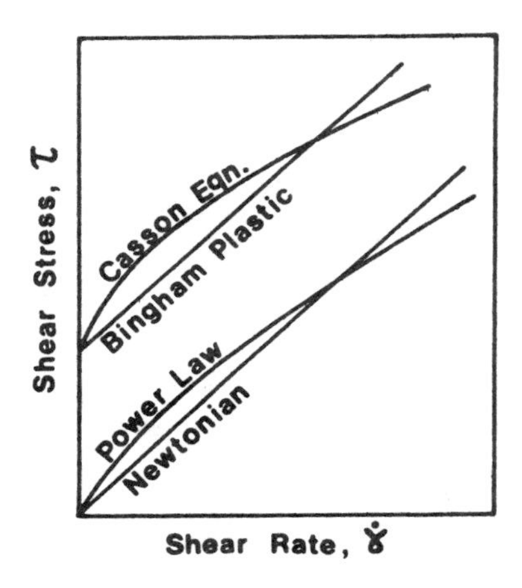

FIG. 3.4. Flow curves of various model materials. [From Whitmore (1968), p. 6.]

Viscosity measurements of blood are commonly made in either Couette viscometers (two concentric cylinders, outer cylinder rotating, blood in the annulus) or capillary tube viscometers. The former is convenient because a nearly uniform shear rate prevails in the fluid; the latter is cheaper, easier to use, and requires much smaller fluid volumes. In working with blood, Couette instruments have the disadvantage of a large gas-liquid interface, where stiff monolayers of denatured protein and other materials can accumulate, causing errors. Tube instruments suffer from the fact that blood viscosity is, for small diameters, a function of the tube diameter itself (the Fahraeus-Lindqvist effect, discussed later).

Blood viscosity measurement is also complicated by the requirement that an anticoagulant (heparin, citrates) be added to the blood to prevent clot formation. Although adding such materials may not create a chemical effect which alters blood viscosity, a dilution effect, caused simply by mixing two fluids of different viscosities, does occur and must be accounted for (even though the blood volume/anticoagulant solution volume ratio may be fairly high). The great variability of blood composition between individuals also makes it difficult to reach general conclusions from experiments.

B. Effect of Shear Rate

Figure 3.5 shows the observed dependence of the apparent absolute viscosity of blood on shear rate. The very large rise in viscosity as shear rate decreases is believed to result from the formation of "rouleaux," or aggregates of RBCs, under conditions of low shear; these aggregates are gradually broken up under the influence of larger velocity gradients, so that above a shear rate of about 50 sec^{-1} practically no aggregates remain, and an asymptotic value of blood

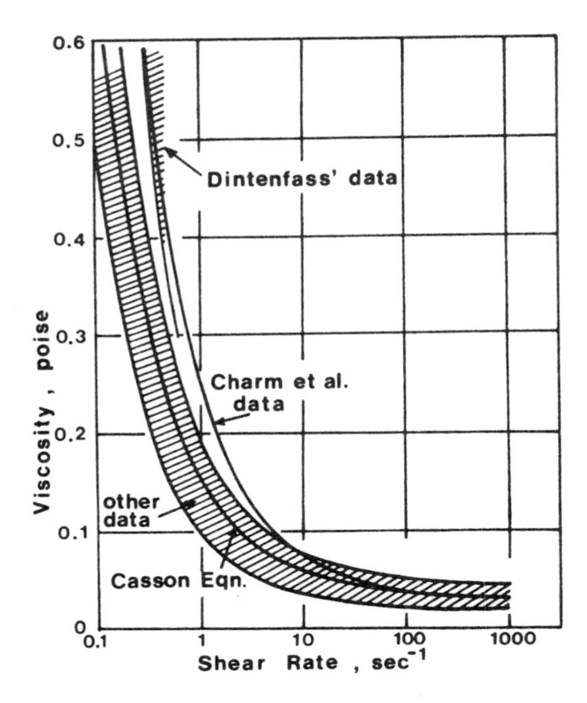

FIG. 3.5. Variation of apparent viscosity of human blood with rate of shear. The Casson equation is plotted on the assumption that the viscosity of plasma is 1.2 cP. [From Whitmore (1968), p. 67.]

viscosity is closely approached. Figure 3.6 shows sketches derived from actual photomicrographs of rouleaux.

C. *Effect of Hematocrit*

Figure 3.7 shows the effect of hematocrit on relative blood viscosity (here relative to plasma, not water), for shear rates which are high enough so that low shear rouleaux effects are negligible; i.e., the values are essentially asymptotic with respect to shear rate. This plot suggests a linear relation between viscosity and

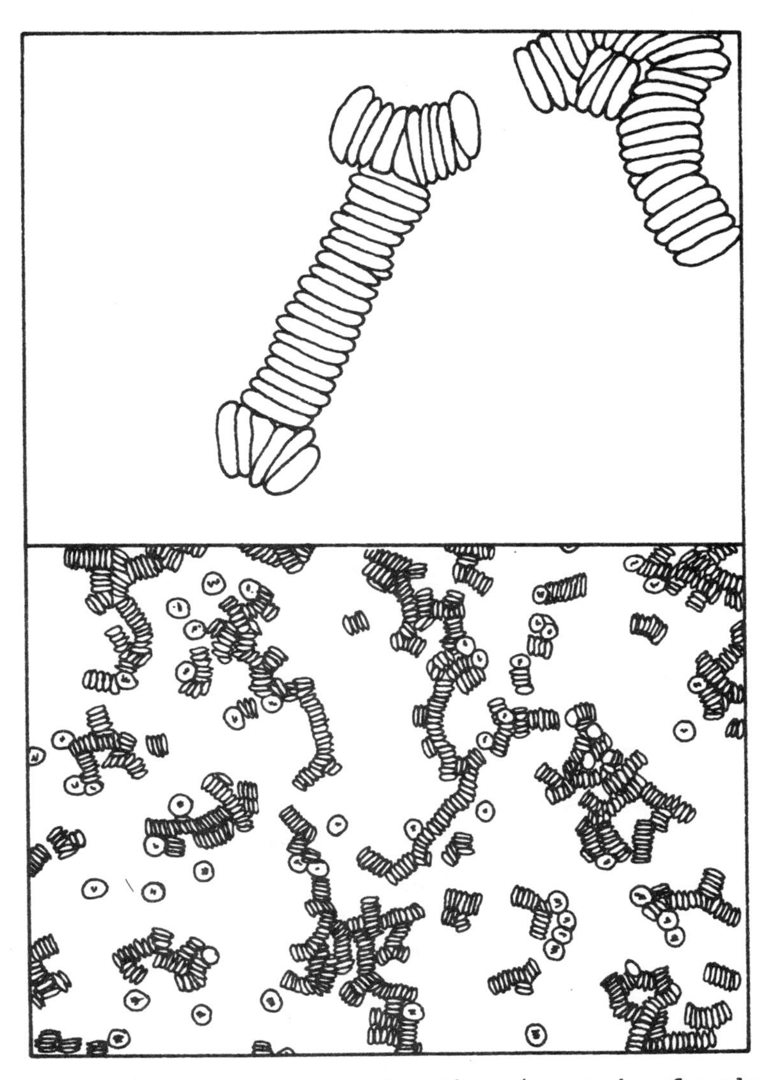

FIG. 3.6. Drawings prepared from photomicrographs of rouleaux of human erythrocytes, showing two separate aggregates (upper) and networks of rouleaux (lower). [From Goldsmith and Mason (1967).]

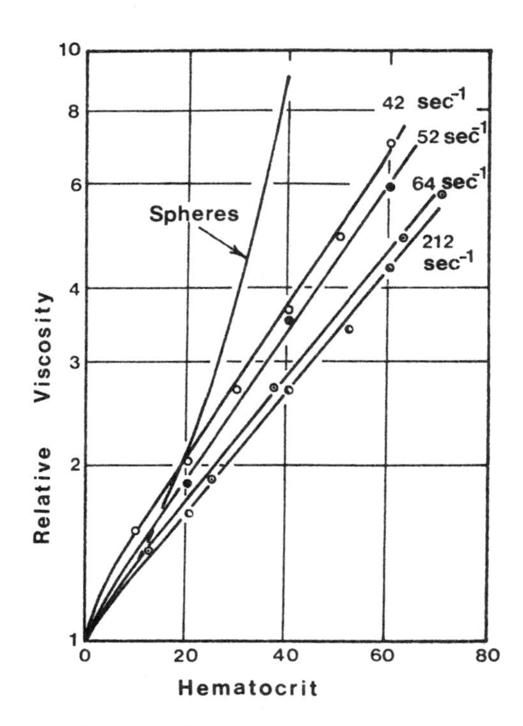

FIG. 3.7. Influence of hematocrit on the relative viscosity of blood at various rates of shear. [From Whitmore (1968), p. 79.]

hematocrit on semilogarithmic paper. For the case of rigid spheres, viscosity is seen to rise more steeply than for RBCs, which are quite deformable. In fact, as Figure 3.8 indicates, erythrocytes hardened by treatment with aldehyde show viscosity-concentration behavior similar to that of rigid spheres. The effect of the RBC membrane's flexibility in reducing viscosity over what it would otherwise be, by partial accommodation to shear stresses, is clear. RBC deformability is, of course, crucial to flow through capillaries—however, this is really a different question.

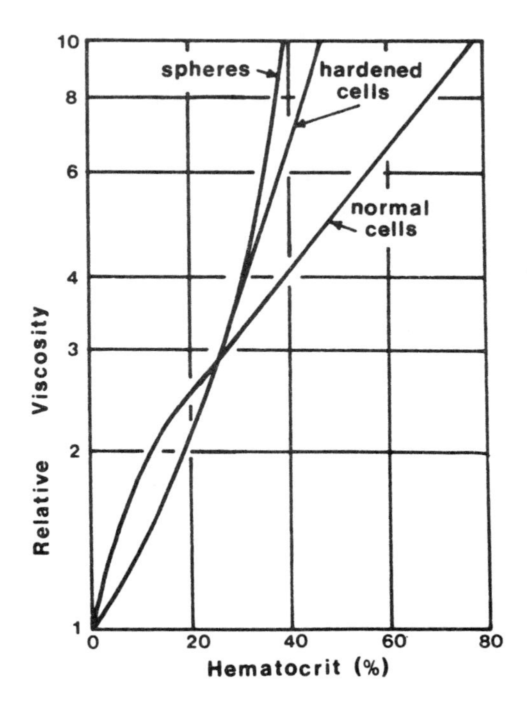

FIG. 3.8. Influence of hematocrit on the relative viscosity of normal and hardened cells suspended in saline solution (rate of shear 230 sec^{-1}). [From Whitmore (1968), p. 81.]

D. Effect of Temperature

The effect of temperature on the relative viscosities of both plasma and whole blood is still open to question. Several investigations have shown both modest increases and modest decreases in plasma and blood viscosities as temperature is lowered from 37°C (the usual temperature for blood viscometric measurements) to around 20°C.

E. Effect of Protein Content of Blood

Figure 3.9 shows viscosity-shear rate curves for whole blood and for suspensions of RBCs in isotonic saline (i.e., saline having the same osmotic pressure as plasma) containing roughly the normal plasma protein concentrations, except that only one protein is present in each case. It seems clear that the globulins are most responsible for raising blood viscosity, especially at low shear rates. Albumin probably tends to moderate this effect somewhat (note that the whole blood curve lies between the globulin and albumin curves). The fibrinogen curve lies below that for whole blood, but it should be noted that the concentration level is only 0.6 wt%. Since the viscosity of the fibrinogen-containing saline is considerably above

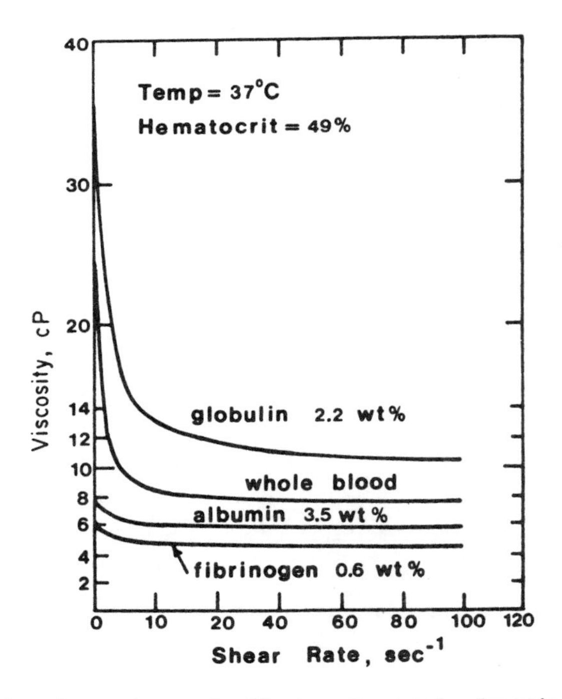

FIG. 3.9. Comparison of effects of protein fractions on viscosity of red cell suspensions. [From A. L. Copley, ed., *Symposium on Biorheology*, Wiley-Interscience, New York, 1965.]

what one would measure for pure saline, it is clear that fibrinogen does exert a strong viscosity-enhancing effect. Fibrinogen is, more importantly, known to be a key causative element in the existence of a yield stress for blood, as we will see shortly. The behavior noted here can be related to the fact that albumins are known not to cause RBC aggregation, whereas globulins and fibrinogen do cause aggregation. Many disease states related to blood flow abnormalities have been correlated with aberrations in the amounts and types of globulins in the blood.

It should again be noted in this figure that nearly constant viscosity values are reached at shear rates above approximately 30-50 sec^{-1}.

F. *The Yield Stress of Blood*

When low shear rate data for whole blood (which, as we have just observed, depend very strongly on protein content) are plotted as $\tau_y^{1/2}$ versus $\dot{\gamma}^{1/2}$, curves similar to that shown in Figure 3.10 result. Such plots clearly demonstrate the existence of a yield stress for blood (albeit a fairly low one).

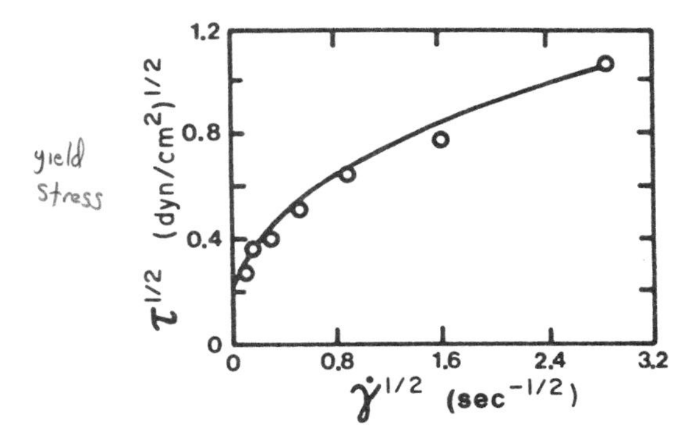

FIG. 3.10. Low shear rate data plotted to demonstrate the presence of a yield stress. [From Middleman (1972), p. 83.]

Data of several studies have uncovered the facts that the yield stress τ_y is a strong function of fibrinogen concentration and hematocrit. Figures 3.11 and 3.12 show typical results. In Figure 3.11, albumins and globulins were held at normal levels. In Figure 3.12, all protein concentrations were normal (e.g., fibrinogen was 0.25 g/100 ml). Such data may be represented quite accurately by the formula

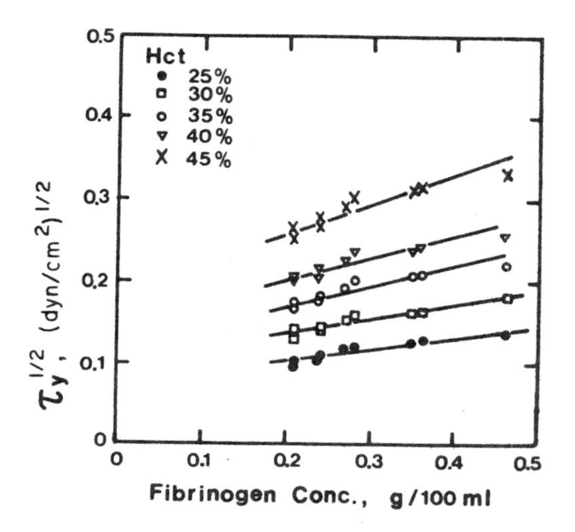

FIG. 3.11. Yield shear stress versus fibrinogen concentration. [From Merrill et al. (1965a).]

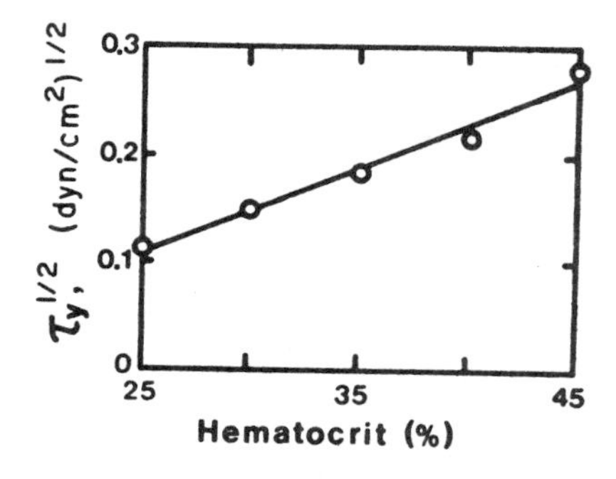

FIG. 3.12. Dependence of yield stress on hematocrit. [From Merrill et al. (1965a).]

$$\tau_y^{1/2} = (H - 0.10)(C_F + 0.5)$$

where C_F is the fibrinogen content in grams per 100 ml, H is the hematocrit expressed as a fraction (e.g., 0.48), and τ_y is the yield stress in dynes per square centimeter. Other investigators have presented formulas, based on fitting data, that have different forms (usually more complex ones). However, as comparison shows, the equation given here is a remarkably good fit. This correlation applies only for $0.21 < C_F < 0.46$ and $H > 0.10$ (below this the yield stress disappears).

Surprisingly, globulins, which tend to increase blood viscosity markedly (as discussed earlier), do not in themselves cause a yield stress to occur. Fibrinogen must also be present before a measurable yield stress occurs. In fact, it has been shown that when fibrinogen (only) is removed from blood, the yield stress vanishes.

G. The Casson Equation

As stated earlier, blood viscosity data generally fit what is called the Casson model, for which a τ-$\dot{\gamma}$ curve was given in Figure 3.4. The best fit of data to the Casson equation gives

$$\tau^{1/2} = \tau_y^{1/2} + s\dot{\gamma}^{1/2}$$

where the yield stress is given by the previous equation, and s, which is equivalent to the square root of the asymptotic "Newtonian" viscosity of blood at high shear rates, is given by the formula

$$s = \left[\frac{\mu_0}{(1 - H)^{a\alpha-1}}\right]^{1/2}$$

where μ_0 is the plasma viscosity, H is the hematocrit expressed as a fraction, and $a\alpha$ is a parameter that depends on protein composition. Figure 3.13 indicates the quality of fit of the equation to data for three blood samples of significantly different hematocrit. The

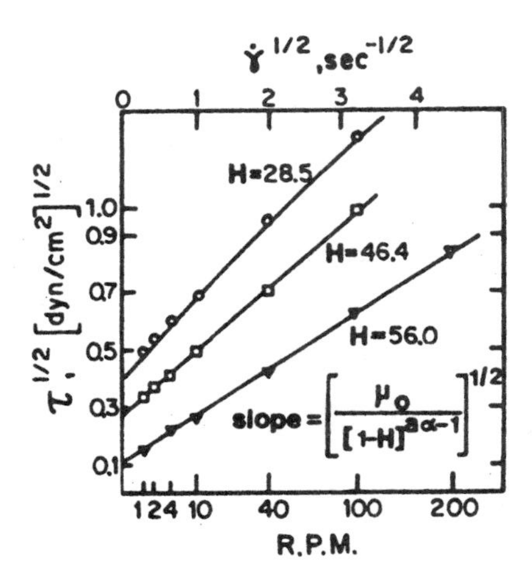

FIG. 3.13. Rheological properties of normal whole blood (Casson plot). [From Merrill et al. (1965b).]

slopes of such lines, when plotted according to the scheme of Figure 3.14, yield a value for the parameter $a\alpha$.

H. *Effect of Tube Diameter in Blood Flow Through Tubes*

As briefly mentioned earlier, blood viscosity measurements in cylindrical tube viscometers have uncovered a dependence of apparent viscosity on the tube diameter: the so-called Fahraeus-Lindqvist effect. Figure 3.15 presents some data illustrating this effect. It should be stressed that the Fahraeus-Lindqvist effect occurs only at high shear rates; therefore, the viscosity values in these figures are asymptotic with respect to shear rate dependence. As tube diameter increases all of the curves shown approach a horizontal, or asymptotic, condition.

This interesting effect is thought to be related to the existence of a cell-free layer adjacent to the tube wall, often called the "plasma skimming" layer. The existence of cell-free layers in flowing blood has been conclusively shown by high-speed photography

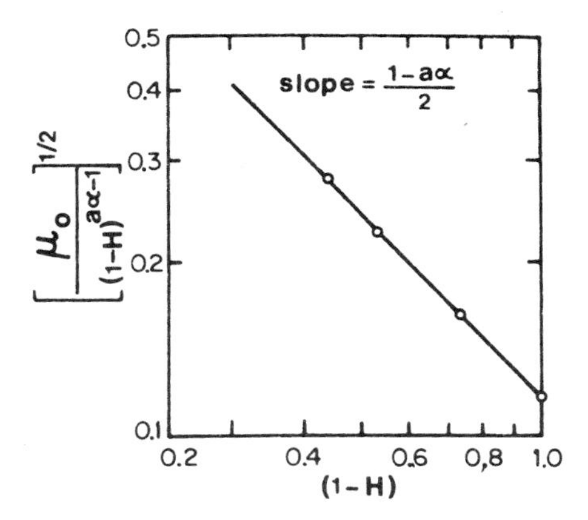

FIG. 3.14. Casson plot for normal blood. [From Merrill et al. (1965b).]

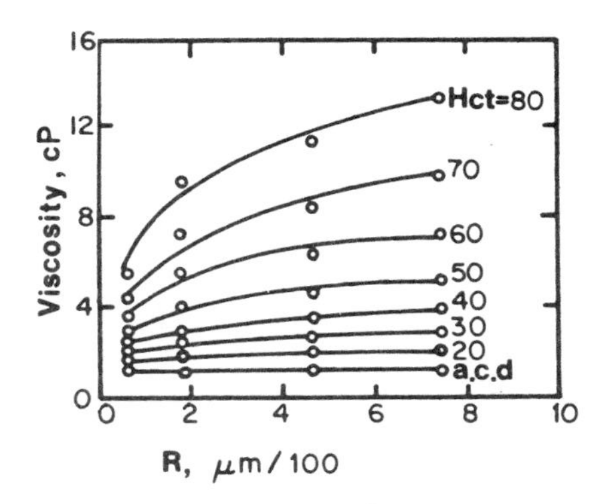

FIG. 3.15. Viscosity data of Haynes. [From Middleman (1972), p. 92.]

of actual flow in mammalian vessels and in glass tubes. There also occurs simultaneously an associated "axial accumulation" of cells near the center of the tube, that is, a concentration of cells higher than that in the feed to the tube. It is easy to deduce how the effective viscosity will be affected by axial accumulation. The hematocrit of fluid near the wall will be reduced while that of the core fluid will be increased. Since the velocity gradient is so much larger near the wall than at the center, the effect of lower viscosity at the periphery will greatly outweigh the effect of increased viscosity near the axis. Hence, the effective viscosity of blood will be less than if no axial accumulation occurred. Obviously, in very small diameter tubes the cell-free layer volume is a larger fraction of the total cross section than in a tube of larger diameter. Hence, the anomalous lowering of blood viscosity is most pronounced for slender tubes (see Figure 3.15).

Why does the shift of cells from the wall region to the core occur? This is a widely debated issue, but a relatively simple explanation is available. Any particle of significant size that is in a fluid stream in which a velocity gradient exists will rotate end over end, often with a helical trajectory, because of velocity differences (Magnus effect), as shown in Figure 3.16. As a result, the path of the particle is modified by a "Bernoulli force" (like that on a spinning tennis ball), which causes the particle to swerve toward the center. The movement of particles inward is dynamically balanced when the axial concentration is high enough, and collisions frequent enough, so that the tendency for outward movement becomes the same. This axial accumulation effect is so pronounced that if blood is drawn, using a hypodermic needle, from a small side branch of a blood vessel, or collected from capillaries, the hematocrit is about 25% less than the average hematocrit in the body as a whole.

Figure 3.17 demonstrates that the velocity profile, surprisingly, is not appreciably altered by the axial shift of blood cells.

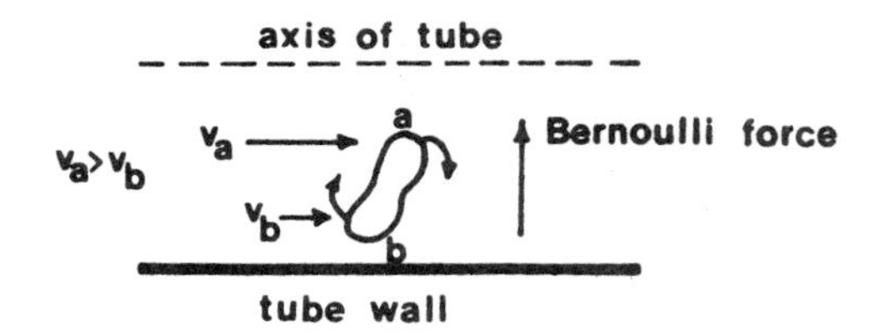

FIG. 3.16. Diagram of force causing axial accumulation of red cells in a flowing stream. [From Ruch and Patton (1965), p. 530.]

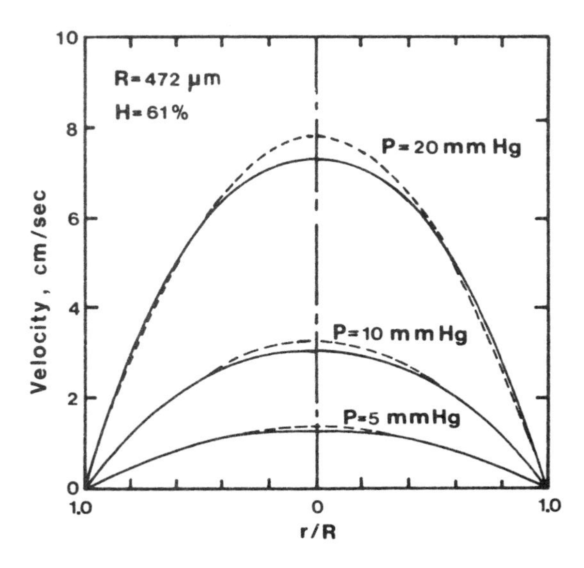

FIG. 3.17. Velocity profile of blood (hematocrit value, 61%) flowing in a tube (radius 472 μm) at three different values of the pressure gradient (P). Broken line is parabola that would apply if there were no axial accumulation. [From Haynes (1957).]

Axial accumulation does not seem to increase steadily with flow rate, as one might think (all forces becoming more intense), but rather seems to reach a saturation value, or upper limit, at a relatively low flow rate.

I. Cell-Free Marginal Layer Model

Haynes (1960) has presented a model for characterizing the Fahraeus-Lindqvist effect which assumes laminar Poiseuille flow in both the "core" region and the cell-free, or "plasma" region. The Navier-Stokes equations for these regions reduce to

$$-\frac{\Delta P}{L} = \frac{1}{r}\frac{d}{dr}\left(\mu_c r \frac{dv_c}{dr}\right), \quad 0 \leq r \leq R - \delta$$

$$-\frac{\Delta P}{L} = \frac{1}{r}\frac{d}{dr}\left(\mu_p r \frac{dv_p}{dr}\right), \qquad R - \delta \le r \le R$$

where δ is the plasma layer thickness. The boundary conditions are

$$\frac{dv_c}{dr} = 0 \quad \text{at} \quad r = 0$$

$$v_c = v_p \quad \text{at } r = R - \delta$$

$$v_p = 0 \quad \text{at } r = R$$

$$\mu_c \frac{dv_c}{dr} = \mu_p \frac{dv_p}{dr} \quad \text{at } r = R - \delta$$

The last boundary condition says merely that the shear stress is continuous in the fluid. This problem may be solved to give

$$Q = \frac{\pi R^4 \Delta P}{8L\mu_p}\left[1 - \left(1 - \frac{\delta}{R}\right)^4 \left(1 - \frac{\mu_p}{\mu_c}\right)\right]$$

By comparison to Poiseuille's law for a homogeneous fluid

$$Q = \frac{\pi R^4 \Delta P}{8L\mu}$$

one may conclude that, if Poiseuille's law is used to calculate the viscosity of blood, one will obtain an "apparent" viscosity value equal to

$$\mu_{app} = \mu_p\left[1 - \left(1 - \frac{\delta}{R}\right)^4 \left(1 - \frac{\mu_p}{\mu_c}\right)\right]^{-1}$$

In the limit of $\delta/R \to 0$, $\mu_{app} \to \mu_c$ as one would expect. When δ/R is finite but reasonably small compared to unity, the result just obtained can be written

$$\mu_{app} \cong \mu_c \Big/ \left[1 + 4\frac{\delta}{R}\left(\frac{\mu_c}{\mu_p} - 1\right)\right]$$

If one assumes that $\delta \neq f(R)$, as experiments have shown, then by plotting $1/\mu$ versus $1/R$ and measuring the intercept $1/\mu_c$ and the slope $[4\delta(\mu_c/\mu_p - 1)/\mu_c]$, one may determine a value for δ. This procedure can be repeated for blood samples of different hematocrits, and one can thereby establish the δ versus H (hematocrit) relationship depicted in Figure 3.20. For a normal hematocrit, δ is about 3 μm, a value that agrees well with actual photographic evidence.

J. The Sigma Effect

A different explanation of the Fahraeus-Lindqvist phenomenon which has wide acceptance is that it is caused by the "sigma effect." This theory rests on the premise that, when dealing with small tubes, blood can no longer be regarded as a continuum and that application of traditional continuum-based formulas (like Poiseuille's law) is not justified. Suppose a blood vessel is so small that there is room for only five red blood cells abreast. A smooth velocity profile will not exist; rather, a set of five relatively concentric laminae can be envisioned to exist (see Figure 3.18). Hence, to integrate the velocity distribution via differential calculus and thereby derive an expression for the total flow rate Q is invalid. Rather, it is necessary to perform a summation (sigma = summation) of five velocity terms.

The "sigma" theory model assumes that the concentric laminae are completely unsheared internally; that is, no velocity gradients exist laterally inside the laminae. However, the velocities of adjacent laminae are different (so that in principle an infinite shear rate exists in the planes of contact). The velocity profile thus has a "stepwise" nature. Also, it is anticipated that the thicknesses of the laminae are at least on the order of the dimensions of the suspended cells.

In deriving Poiseuille's law, integration of a smooth velocity profile v(r) is involved, i.e.,

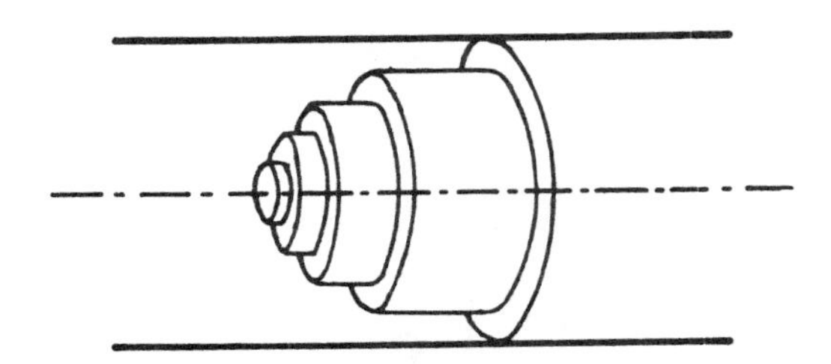

FIG. 3.18. Discontinuous model of the flow of a fluid in a cylindrical tube. [From Whitmore (1968), p. 113.]

$$Q = 2\pi \int_0^R v(r) r \, dr$$

This can be shown to be equivalent to

$$Q = \pi \int_0^R d[v(r) r^2] - \pi \int_0^R r^2 \frac{dv}{dr} \, dr$$

For any flow in which v = 0 at r = R (no "slip" at the wall), the first integral on the right side will be identically zero. Also, from the parabolic velocity function v(r) one can derive

$$\frac{dv}{dr} = \frac{-\Delta P \, r}{2\mu L}$$

Upon substitution of this into the second integral, one obtains

$$Q = \frac{\Delta P \, \pi}{2\mu L} \int_0^R r^3 \, dr$$

To generalize this equation from the case of a smooth parabolic velocity profile to a stepwise profile, let us assume the fluid flows in N concentric laminae, each of thickness ε, so that $R = N\varepsilon$ and $r = n\varepsilon$, where n = 1, 2, 3, ..., N. We now wish to rewrite the integral of r^3 as a summation, letting $r = n\varepsilon$ and noting that $dr = \varepsilon \, \Delta n = \varepsilon$ (since Δn, the difference in n values between two adjacent laminae, is always unity). Hence

$$Q = \frac{\Delta P \ \pi}{2\mu L} \sum_{i=1}^{N} (n\varepsilon)^3 \varepsilon$$

Since it is a mathematical identity that

$$\sum_{i=1}^{N} n^3 = \frac{N^2(N + 1)^2}{4}$$

one can show that

$$\sum (n\varepsilon)^3 \varepsilon = \varepsilon^4 \sum n^3 = \frac{\varepsilon^4 N^2 (N + 1)^2}{4}$$

Substitution of $N = R/\varepsilon$ and rearrangement permits deriving the final expression for Q:

$$Q = \frac{\pi \ \Delta P \ R^4}{8\mu L} \left(1 + \frac{\varepsilon}{R}\right)^2$$

Thus, an apparent viscosity given by the formula

$$\mu_{app} = \frac{\mu}{(1 + \varepsilon/R)^2}$$

is indicated by this theory. Here, μ is the viscosity value one would measure in sufficiently large tubes, that is, for ε/R values close to zero. Figure 3.19 shows a successful application of this last equation to data on ox blood, for which the quantity ε was taken to be roughly equal to the diameter of ox red blood cells, about 6 μm.

One should note from the equation for Q that for $\varepsilon/R \to 0$ (i.e., infinitely thin laminae) this formula reduces to Poiseuille's law, as it should. Also, comparison of these results with the results obtained previously for the cell-free layer theory shows that the two theories are equivalent <u>if</u>

$$\delta = \frac{\varepsilon \mu_p}{2(\mu_c - \mu_p)}$$

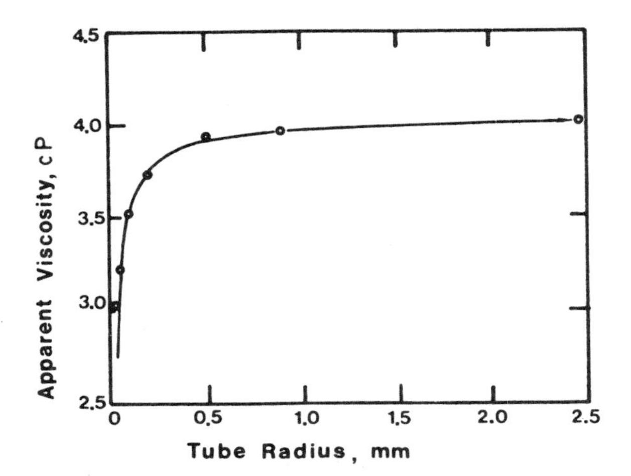

FIG. 3.19. Fahraeus-Lindqvist effect of size of tube on viscosity for ox blood (H = 40%): ⊙ data, — theory. Values calculated from sigma theory for ε value of 6.0 μm. [From Ruch and Patton (1965), p. 530.]

Figure 3.20 shows the value of ε as a function of hematocrit as determined from values of δ derived as previously described plus the use of the last equation. This figure strictly applies only to data on ox blood having a plasma viscosity of 1.093 cP [the data on which the Haynes (1960) analysis was based]. For human blood a different but very similar relationship would be expected.

Both the cell-free layer and sigma theories thus yield equations of the same form, and the only real difference is that one uses a parameter δ and the other a parameter ε. As Haynes states: "Neither theory grossly offends one's physical intuition, and it seems probable that both postulated mechanisms are present, although it is difficult to decide their relative importance."

K. *Blockage Effects*

A third explanation for the Fahraeus-Lindqvist effect has also been frequently cited. This revolves about the idea that, for small-diameter tubes, some type of blocking process occurs near the tube

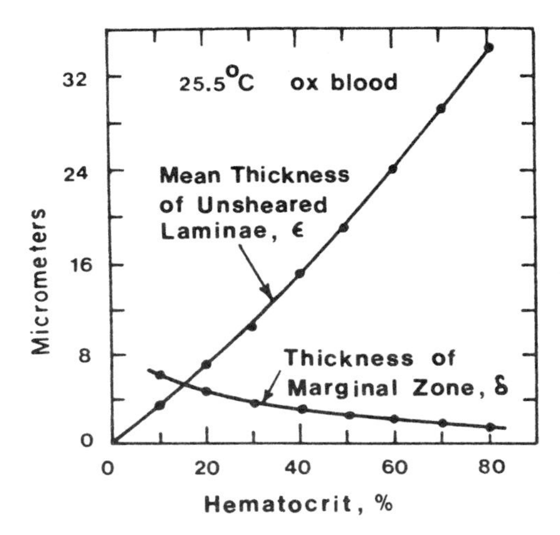

FIG. 3.20. Parameters of the cell-free layer and sigma theories. [From Haynes (1960).]

entrance which causes cells to be hindered from entering. The average hematocrit of the outlet blood would be less than that of the feed and, clearly, the viscosity of blood in the tube would be lower than that of the feed blood. This concept has been experimentally confirmed, as Figure 3.21 shows. (The entrance rejection effect is unrelated to the cell-free layer phenomenon.) It is not clear, however, whether this process, by itself, explains the Fahraeus-Lindqvist effect.

L. The Effect of Yield Stress on Blood Flow

Let us estimate the pressure drop required to keep blood flowing steadily in cylindrical tubes, such as tube viscometers and the capillaries of the systemic circulation. Assuming Poiseuille flow we know that the shear stress varies linearly with radial distance from a zero value at the tube's center to a maximum value at the wall (τ_w). The imposed pressure drop must be great enough so that $\tau_w > \tau_y$. The wall shear stress for this situation is given by

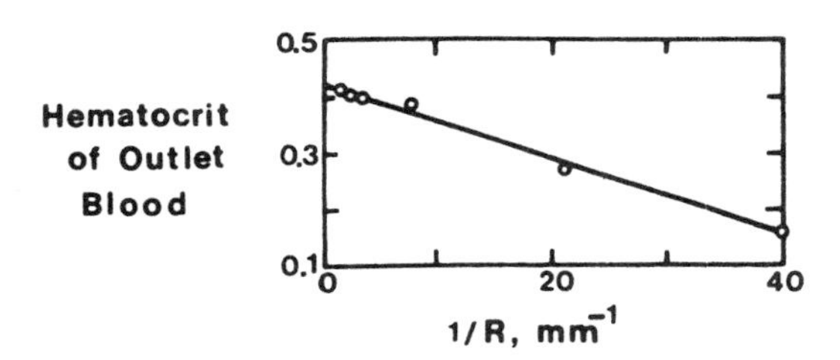

FIG. 3.21. Hematocrit of blood leaving a cylindrical glass tube. Inlet blood pool hematocrit is 0.43. [From Middleman (1972), p. 95.]

$$\tau_w = \frac{\Delta P\ R}{2L}$$

Let us assume that $\tau_y = 0.07\ \text{dyn/cm}^2$ for blood and that the dimensions of a typical tube viscometer are L = 20 cm and R = 0.1 cm. Then

$$\Delta P = \frac{\tau_y 2L}{R} = 28\ \frac{\text{dyn}}{\text{cm}^2} = 0.021\ \text{mm Hg}$$

The required pressure difference is clearly very small. For a systemic capillary of R = 5 μm and L = 1 mm (typical values), the ΔP required to overcome the yield stress can be calculated to be 0.021 mm Hg (the same value as above, since the L/R ratio is the same as before). Inasmuch as the actual physiological ΔP is roughly 16 mm Hg across a capillary (25 in/9 out), it is clear that the pressure needed to counteract the yield stress is quite small compared to the normal pressure driving force for flow. Thus, the importance of the yield stress phenomenon in real situations is negligible.

It should be mentioned that our analysis here is somewhat simplified in the sense that certain assumptions have been implicitly made (e.g., that the fluid can be considered Newtonian, and that the Fahraeus-Lindqvist effect can be neglected). However, accounting for these factors would probably make little difference.

IV. PROBLEMS ASSOCIATED WITH EXTRACORPOREAL BLOOD FLOW

When blood is treated outside the body, as in artificial kidney units and oxygenators, severe problems with hemolysis of red blood cells (rupture), blood clotting, and protein denaturation can occur. In fact, the greatest practical difficulties in using artificial organs usually involve these three problems. Such effects also can occur when synthetic materials are internally implanted (e.g., artificial heart valves) but are normally much less serious.

Hemolysis results from many factors, but primarily from excessive shear stresses in the fluid, abrupt pressure and velocity changes, turbulence, roughness of synthetic surfaces, and contact with hypo-osmotic fluids (this causes water to swell the RBCs, thereby bursting them). Since hemolysis releases free hemoglobin, which is toxic at concentrations above roughly 160 mg/100 ml, its occurrence must be minimized.

Clotting of blood, which is usually initiated by the same kinds of fluid mechanical and surface factors that create hemolysis, is triggered by platelet rupture. However, the surface factor is more important here. The development of "antithrombogenic" biomaterials has been the object of tremendous research efforts. Some materials that exhibit reasonably good antithrombogenic properties are Teflon, Dacron, and silicone rubber. Clotting in extracorporeal devices can also be controlled quite well by adding an anticoagulant, such as heparin, to the blood.

Denaturation of plasma proteins can also be caused by high local shear stresses, foreign surfaces, etc. Denaturation occurs when a protein that has a delicate structure, held together by weak hydrogen bonds, is wrenched badly out of shape. When this happens, reestablishment of the original configuration of the protein may be impossible. If the protein is an enzyme, its specific ability to catalyze reactions will be lost. Most plasma proteins are highly coiled and convoluted (unlike the long fibrous proteins that one finds in tendons, hair, etc.) and are thus fairly susceptible to denaturation.

When blood is handled outside the body it is therefore very important that all flow channels be suitably open and regular, that flow be laminar (but not too slow), and that all surfaces be inert and smooth.

PROBLEMS

1. Estimate the amount of iron (in grams) contained in the blood of a "standard" man. Compare your answer to the value given in Table 2.2.

2. For normal blood (fibrinogen content 0.3 g/100 ml, hematocrit around 45%), estimate the yield stress in dynes per square centimeter.

3. A Couette viscometer consisting of a 4.00-cm-diameter stationary inner cylinder and a 4.2-cm outer rotating cylinder and having a height of 8.0 cm is being used to measure the viscosity of blood. If the angular velocity is 60 rpm, what is the approximate shear rate in the blood? Can you estimate the torque required to rotate the outer cylinder?

4. For a cell-free marginal layer value of $\delta \cong 3\ \mu m$ (from Figure 3.20 at H = 40%), calculate the apparent viscosity for blood flowing in a 100-μm-diameter tube. Take μ_p to be 1.093 cP and μ_c to be around 3.7 cP [values from Haynes (1960)].

5. Using a "mean thickness of unsheared laminae" value of $\varepsilon \cong 15\ \mu m$ (H = 40%), determine μ_{app} for ox blood flowing in a 100-μm-diameter tube. Again take $\mu_p = 1.093$ cP and $\mu_c = 3.7$ cP. Compare your answer to that of the preceding problem. How many laminae are there?

6. Derive the "cell-free marginal layer model" equations

$$Q = \frac{\pi R^4 \Delta P}{8L\mu_p}\left[1 - \left(1 - \frac{\delta}{R}\right)^4 \left(1 - \frac{\mu_p}{\mu_c}\right)\right]$$

and

$$\mu_{app} = \mu_p\left[1 - \left(1 - \frac{\delta}{R}\right)^4 \left(1 - \frac{\mu_p}{\mu_c}\right)\right]^{-1}$$

starting with the differential equations and boundary conditions given in the text.

7. *Effect of Axial Accumulation on Apparent Viscosity of Blood.* Consider the following to be a model for blood flow through a small vessel (1 mm diameter, 20 mm long)

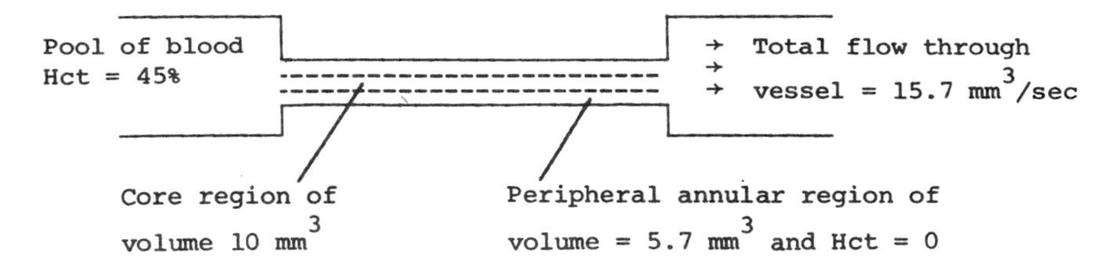

The velocity profile in the vessel is nearly parabolic in shape. In the core region the average flow rate is 12 mm^3/sec and in the peripheral region the average flow rate is 3.7 mm^3/sec. Perform a mass balance on the red blood cells, and determine the hematocrit of the core region. Next, determine the hematocrit in the vessel as a whole. What does your answer suggest about the apparent viscosity of the blood in the vessel (relative to blood of Hct = 45%)?

REFERENCES

Charm, S., and Kurland, G. S., Viscometry of human blood for shear rates of 0-100,000 sec^{-1}, *Nature*, 206, 617 (1965).

Chien, S., Usami, S., Taylor, H., Liniberg, J. S., and Gregerson, M., Effects of hematocrit and plasma proteins on human blood rheology at low shear rates, *J. Appl. Physiol.*, 21, 81 (1966).

Copley, A. L., and Stainsby, G., eds., *Flow Properties of Blood*, Pergamon, Oxford, 1960.

Fahraeus, R., and Lindqvist, T., The viscosity of blood in narrow capillary tubes, *Am. J. Physiol.*, 96, 562 (1931).

Ganong, W. F., *Review of Medical Physiology*, 5th ed., Lange Med. Publ., Los Altos, California, 1971.

Goldsmith, H. L., and Mason, S. G., The microrheology of dispersions, in *Rheology* (F. R. Eirich, ed.), Vol. 4, Academic, New York, 1967.

Haynes, R. F., *The Rheology of Blood*, Ph.D. thesis, Univ. of Western Ontario, 1957.

Haynes, R. F., and Burton, A. C., Role of the non-Newtonian behaviour of blood in hemodynamics, *Am. J. Physiol.*, 197, 943 (1959).

Haynes, R. F., Physical basis of the dependence of blood viscosity on tube radius, *Am. J. Physiol.*, 198, 1193 (1960).

Merrill, E. W., Margetts, W. G., Cokelet, G., Britten, A., Salzman, E., Pennell, R., and Melin, M., Influence of plasma proteins on the rheology of human blood, *Proceedings of the Fourth International Congress on Rheology*, (A. L. Copley, ed.), Wiley-Interscience, New York, 1965a, pp. 601-611.

Merrill, E. W., Margetts, W. G., Cokelet, G. R., and Gilliland, E. R., The Casson equation and rheology of blood near zero shear, *Proceedings of the Fourth International Congress on Rheology*, op. cit., 1965b, pp. 135-143.

Middleman, S., *Cardiovascular Transport Phenomena*, Wiley-Interscience, New York, 1972.

Ponder, E., *Hemolysis and Related Phenomena*, Churchill, London, 1948.

Ruch, T. C., and Patton, H. D., *Physiology and Biophysics*, 19th ed., Saunders, Philadelphia, Pennsylvania, 1965.

Whitmore, R. L., *Rheology of the Circulation*, Pergamon, Oxford, 1968.

Chapter 4

THE DYNAMICS OF THE CIRCULATORY SYSTEM

In this chapter we discuss the general structure and fluid dynamics of the circulatory system, and present quantitative examples relating to certain aspects of the circulation. These examples will include computation of the work of the heart, determination of hydrostatic effects in the body, and calculations of the interconversion of pressure and kinetic energy in the arteries, capillaries, and veins.

I. GENERAL STRUCTURE, VOLUMES, AND FLOW RATES

Figures 2.2, 2.3, 2.7, and 2.8 (Chapter 2) illustrate schematically and anatomically the overall structure of the circulatory system. Table 4.1 indicates the distribution of blood volume

TABLE 4.1

Approximate Estimates of Blood Distribution in Vascular Bed of a Hypothetical Man, Age 30, Weight 63 kg, Height 178 cm, Blood Volume (Assumed) 5.2 liters[a]

Pulmonary	Volume (ml)	Systemic	Volume (ml)
Pulmonary arteries	400	Aorta	100
Pulmonary capillaries	60	Systemic arteries	450
Venules	140	Systemic capillaries	300
Pulmonary veins	700	Venules	200
		Systemic veins	2050
Total pulmonary system	1300	Total systemic vessels	3100
Heart 250 ml		Unaccounted 550 ml	
(Probably extra blood in reservoirs of liver and spleen)			

[a]From Burton (1965), p. 64.

throughout the system. One should note that (a) the pulmonary circulation contains about 40% as much blood as the systemic circulation, and (b) the venous blood pool (140 + 700 + 200 + 2050 = 3090 ml) is very much larger than the arterial pool (400 + 100 + 450 = 950 ml).

Of more interest to us here than the blood volumes in various regions are the blood flow rates in different locations. Data for flows on an organ-by-organ basis and data for flows on a "type of blood vessel" basis (such as found in Table 4.4) are both available. On an organ basis, blood flows in percentages of total cardiac output at rest are as shown in Table 4.2. Note that the most active organs are the ones most highly perfused.

TABLE 4.2

Blood Flow to Different Organs and Tissues Under Basal Conditions[a]

	%	ml/min
Brain	14	700
Heart	3	150
Bronchial	3	150
Kidneys	22	1100
Liver	27	1350
Portal	(21)	(1050)
Arterial	(6)	(300)
Muscle (inactive state)	15	750
Bone	5	250
Skin (cool weather)	6	300
Thyroid gland	1	50
Adrenal glands	0.5	25
Other tissues	3.5	175
Total	100.0	5000

[a] From Guyton (1971), p. 279.

Data on a "vessel" basis have been obtained in most complete form for the systemic circulation of a dog. Table 4.3 shows typical figures. These data indicate that the numbers of vessels and the total cross-sectional area for flow increase along the arterial system, reach a maximum for the capillaries, and decrease steadily along the venous system. Vessel diameters and blood velocities go from large to small to large in proceeding from the aorta to the venae cavae. Hence, flow areas and mean velocities vary in opposite manners in the circulatory system, as one would expect. Note that, in the dog,

TABLE 4.3

Systemic Circulation of a Dog[a]

Structure	Diameter (cm)	Number	Total cross-sectional area (cm^2)	Length (cm)	Total volume (cc)	Blood velocity (cm/sec)	Tube Reynolds number[b]
Aorta	1.0	1	0.8	40	30	50	1670
Large arteries	0.3	40	3.0	20	60	23	230
Main arterial branches	0.1	600	5.0	10	50	8	27
Terminal branches	0.06	1800	5.0	1	5	6	12
Arterioles	0.002	40×10^6	125	0.2	25	0.3	0.02
Capillaries	0.0008	12×10^8	600	0.1	60	0.07	0.002
Venules	0.003	80×10^6	570	0.2	110	0.07	0.007
Terminal veins	0.15	1800	30	1	30	1.3	6.5
Main venous branches	0.24	600	27	10	270	1.5	12
Large veins	0.6	40	11	20	220	3.6	72
Vena cavae	1.25	1	1.2	40	50	33.0	1375

[a] From Whitmore (1968), p. 92.

[b] Assuming viscosity of blood is 0.03 P.

the Reynolds numbers at all points are in the laminar range ($Re < 2100$).

Similar but less extensive data are available for humans. A few of these are given in Table 4.4.

Flow velocities on the arterial side vary considerably between maximum values, at the height of the systolic (blood ejection) phase of the heart's cycle, and minimum values, during the quietest part of the diastolic (or relaxation) phase of the heart cycle. The data quoted for the dog refer to the time-averaged velocities in the arterial system. In Table 4.4, the arterial values correspond to peak flow conditions. The reason for this is to illustrate what the absolute maximum Reynolds numbers in the body are. One can see that, during the systole, flow rates exceeding laminar values occur in the ascending aorta. Reynolds numbers are not high enough for fully developed turbulence ($Re \cong 10{,}000$ or more), but some degree of tur-

TABLE 4.4

Systemic Circulation of Man[a]

Structure	Diameter (cm)	Blood velocity (cm/sec)	Tube Reynolds[b] number
Ascending aorta	2.0-3.2	63[c]	3600-5800
Descending aorta	1.6-2.0	27[c]	1200-1500
Large arteries	0.2-0.6	20-50[c]	110-850
Capillaries	0.0005-0.001	0.05-0.1[d]	0.0007-0.003
Large veins	0.5-1.0	15-20[d]	210-570
Venae cavae	2.0	11-16[d]	630-900

[a]From Whitmore (1968), p. 93.

[b]Assuming viscosity of blood is 0.035 P.

[c]Mean peak value.

[d]Mean velocity over indefinite period of time.

bulence definitely exists. Even in the descending aorta, some nonlaminar flow surely also occurs, since the critical Reynolds number for unsteady flow in branching, tapered, elastic tubes is, in many regions, probably less than the 2100 value which pertains to steady flow in straight, uniform, rigid ducts. Locally high Reynolds numbers and turbulence are also known to exist in and around the heart valves, the first major branches in the arterial system, and similar locations. During heavy exercise, when the cardiac output may be four or five times the resting value, turbulence will surely exist longer in time and further in distance down the arterial system.

Note that, because the pressure and velocity pulses are damped out in the arterial tree (as we will see shortly), the numbers for the capillaries and venous side are given as steady flow mean values.

II. CAPILLARY BLOOD FLOW

Blood flow rates and residence times may be computed for vessels such as capillaries in a straightforward manner, using the elementary methods shown below.

Let us assume that capillary diameters are 8 μm, the number of systemic capillaries in the body, $\underline{n}$, is 10^9 (1 billion), and cardiac output is 5 liters/min.

What is the linear velocity of blood flow in the capillaries? The answer is easily determined:

$$v = \frac{Q}{n\pi r^2} = \frac{5000 \text{ cc}}{\text{min}} \cdot \frac{1}{10^9 (3.14)(4 \times 10^{-4})^2 \text{ cm}^2}$$

$$= 9.95 \text{ cm/min, or } 0.166 \text{ cm/sec}$$

Assuming each capillary is 1 mm long, the blood's "residence time" is

$$t = \frac{1 \text{ mm}}{1.66 \text{ mm/sec}} = 0.6 \text{ sec}$$

Obviously, mass transfer in the capillaries must be extremely efficient, since so little time is available for exchange to occur.

The need of the body for a large number of capillaries can be suggested by computing how long a time would be required for only 1 cc of blood to flow through a single capillary at normal flow rates. The time needed would be

$$t = \frac{1 \text{ cc}}{(5000/10^9) \text{ cc/min}} = 2 \times 10^5 \text{ min} = 139 \text{ days}$$

Conversely, the actual flow rate through a capillary would equal less than one-hundredth of a cubic centimeter per day.

III. RATES OF SHEAR IN THE CIRCULATION

Whitmore (1968) has computed shear rate values for both dog and man based on the assumption of Poiseuille flow. His results are given in Table 4.5.

While flow rates and Reynolds numbers in the smaller vessels are very low, as the preceding tables have shown, it is clear that the shear rates (velocity gradients) are by no means also low, primarily because the vessel diameters are so tiny. All values cited in Table 4.5 are based on mean velocities, except for the ascending aorta figure. The columns marked "Mean" give space-averaged shear rates across the whole velocity profile. For parabolic Poiseuille velocity profiles, the shear stress increases linearly with radial distance from the center (where it is zero). It is easily shown that the "mean" shear rate is exactly two-thirds of the maximum shear rate at the wall, as the tabular values suggest.

Recalling from Chapter 3 that the non-Newtonian viscosity characteristics of blood (i.e., variation of viscosity with shear

TABLE 4.5

Rates of Shear in the Circulation[a,b]

	Man		Dog	
Structure	At the wall (sec^{-1})	Mean (sec^{-1})	At the wall (sec^{-1})	Mean (sec^{-1})
Ascending aorta	190[c]	130	400	270
Descending aorta	120	80		
Large arteries	700	470	600	400
Capillaries	800	530	700	450
Large veins	200	130	50	35
Venae cavae	60	40	200	140

[a]From Whitmore (1968), p. 96.

[b]Assuming parabolic velocity profile.

[c]At peak velocity of flow.

rate) are confined to shear rates of less than about 50 sec^{-1}, it is clear that under the actual physiological conditions of the human body, blood may be regarded as Newtonian.

IV. PRESSURE PROFILES IN THE CIRCULATORY SYSTEM

Figure 4.1 gives a reasonable picture of the pressures in the systemic and pulmonary circulations as a function of distance. Typical pulse shapes (pressure versus time for a single heart cycle) at various locations in the arterial vessels are shown. The figure is not accurate in suggesting that, for example, four pressure maxima and four pressure minima exist simultaneously along the aorta. Pulse propagation velocities are much too fast to permit this. In the aorta the transmission velocity of the pressure pulse is almost 5 m/sec. In the larger arterial branches it may be 10 m/sec, and in the smaller arteries nearly 40 m/sec.

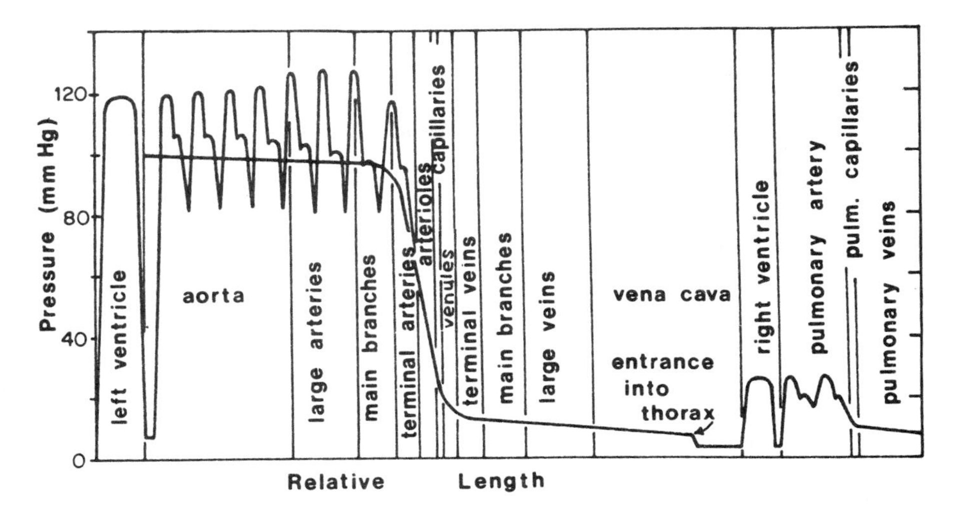

FIG. 4.1. Blood pressure in the systemic and pulmonary circulation. Note: Arterioles, capillaries, and venules are shorter than indicated. [From E. Selkurt, referred to in *Biomechanics*, Y. C. Fung, ed., ASME, New York, 1966, p. 139.]

The time-averaged mean pressures in the arterial system are given fairly accurately by [systolic + 2 × diastolic]/3.

Figure 4.2 gives a more detailed look at pressure pulses in the systemic arteries. Velocities versus time at several locations are also shown. An amplification of the pressure pulse is seen to occur. This results from (a) the effects of velocity decreases along the arterial tree because of the increasingly higher cross-sectional area (according to the Bernoulli principle, velocity decreases are accompanied by pressure rises, unless pressure losses caused by friction override), (b) decreasing arterial compliance (flexibility) along the arterial tree, (c) the reflection of the pressure waves backward from branches and from the more resistive peripheral vessels (causing a summation effect with the oncoming pulse waves), and (d) the fact that the higher pressure portions of the pulse tend to travel faster than the lower pressure parts (this causes the higher pressure segments to catch up with slower segments, thereby sharpen-

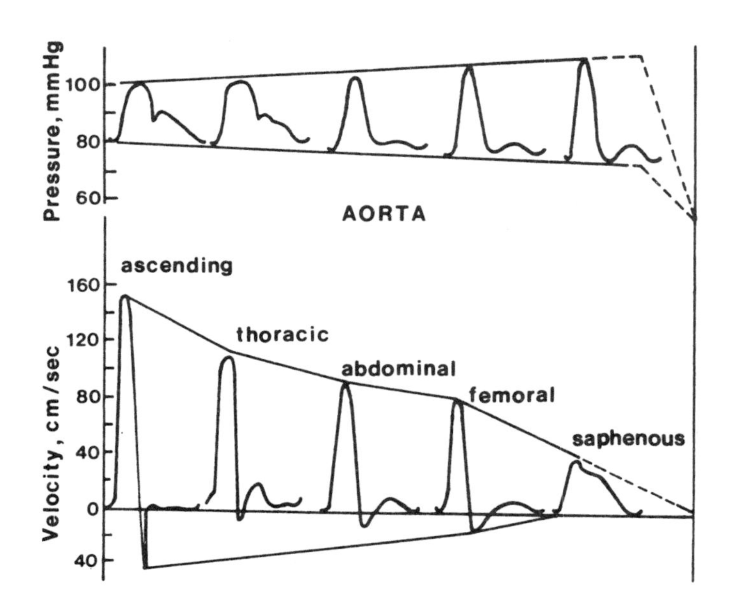

FIG. 4.2. Diagrammatic comparison of the behavior of the pressure and flow pulses in the systemic arteries during their travel peripherally. Note that the pressure pulse increases and the flow pulse decreases. [From McDonald (1960).]

ing the pulse peaks). The viscoelastic nature of the arterial walls plays an important role in all of these phenomena.

One striking feature of the velocity pulse curves is the negative velocity portions, corresponding to backflow of blood into the left ventricle as the ventricle relaxes. The sudden closing of the aortic valve soon blocks this backflow, and then squeezing of the aorta causes the velocity to return to a slightly positive state. Modeling the behavior of these pressure and velocity pulses mathematically has been the subject of much research. The simplest models begin with the analysis of pulsatile flow in rigid tubes. As one starts to take other factors into account (the viscoelasticity of the tube walls, the tapering of the tubes, the existence of branch points which cause reflections, etc.), the models become increasingly more sophisticated. A proper treatment of this whole subject area is outside the scope of the present work.

Figure 4.1 shows very clearly that the mean pressure begins to fall rapidly only when the smaller terminal arteries are reached. In fact, as Table 4.6 shows, it is the arterioles which offer most of the flow resistance. These values were computed assuming that the flow resistance equals $8\mu L/\pi R^4$ for any vessel. This gives Poiseuille's law the form $Q = \Delta P/\text{resistance}$, where Q is volumetric flow rate. Assuming constant viscosity everywhere in the circulatory system, as justified earlier, each vessel's resistance is simply proportional to its length over its radius to the fourth power (a _very_ strong dependence on radius). The relatively low resistance of the venous system is quite noteworthy. Table 4.6 refers to the systemic circulation. From Figure 4.1, however, it is obvious that the entire pulmonary circulation is also a relatively low resistance circuit. The major reason for the very large flow resistance of the systemic arterioles is that these arterioles constitute the points where flow

TABLE 4.6[a]

Relative Resistance to Flow in the Vascular Bed: Calculated from Table 4.3 and Poiseuille's Law ($R \propto L/r^4$)

Aorta	4	Venules	4
Large arteries	5	Terminal veins	0.3
Mean arterial branches	10	Main venous branches	0.7
Terminal branches	6	Large veins	0.5
Arterioles	41	Vena cavae	1.5
Capillaries	27		
Total: arterial + capillary = 93		Total venous = 7	

[a]All values are in percent. From Burton (1965), p. 89.

rates are controlled. Muscular tissue in the arterioles can vary the diameters, and hence resistances, of these vessels over a wide range. Precision of control is gained by having an inherently large mean resistance.

One final aspect of Figure 4.1 which should be noted is the location where the pressure pulses are essentially completely damped out, the arterioles. Actually it is claimed that in the pulmonary circulation, pulsatile flow persists even in the capillaries, because of the low resistance of the overall circuit. However, this certainly is not true of the systemic capillaries.

V. INTERCONVERSION OF PRESSURE AND KINETIC ENERGY IN THE CIRCULATION

To develop a better quantitative feel for the fluid mechanics of the circulatory system let us consider how the "mechanical energy components" of the blood vary throughout the circulatory system. From the well-known Bernoulli equation, we know that kinetic energy and pressure are directly interconvertible. If potential energy changes are small (let us consider a person in a horizontal position, so that this is so), then kinetic energy and pressure constitute the "total energy" (mechanical energy) of the fluid. Kinetic energy (KE) may be defined as

$$KE = \frac{1}{2\alpha}\rho\langle v\rangle^2$$

where $\langle v\rangle$ is the average fluid velocity over the cross section of the vessel, and α is a "kinetic energy correction factor" to account for the fact that the kinetic energy is really equal to $\langle v^3\rangle/\langle v\rangle$ (i.e., average of velocity cubed over the cross section divided by the average velocity). For highly turbulent flow, the velocity profile is nearly flat, $\langle v^3\rangle/\langle v\rangle \cong \langle v\rangle^2$, and $\alpha = 1$. For laminar flow and a parabolic velocity profile, $\langle v^3\rangle/\langle v\rangle = 2\langle v\rangle^2$ and hence $\alpha = 1/2$. In the transition flow region α varies between 1/2 and 1. Plots of α

versus Re are available (McCabe and Smith, 1956, p. 61). For our purposes, α will nearly always be 1/2.

When KE in, say, $g/cm\text{-}sec^2$ is multiplied by the conversion factor 7.5×10^{-4} (mm Hg)/($g/cm\text{-}sec^2$) the resultant KE is in millimeters of mercury. In this form, the KE of the fluid may be directly compared with its pressure energy level. Table 4.7 makes this comparison for blood at various points in the systemic and pulmonary circulations, for resting conditions, and for a state of elevated cardiac output.

Note that kinetic energy as part of the total fluid energy under resting conditions is significant only in the large veins and in the pulmonary artery during the systolic phase of the heart's cycle. When cardiac output increases, kinetic energy becomes much more important because pressures do not really rise very far (the arterioles automatically open up considerably, so their resistance does not increase by much), and yet velocities essentially treble (kinetic energies increase ninefold). Under conditions of heavy exercise, kinetic energy is obviously a large proportion (about half) of the total energy in the largest veins and in the pulmonary artery, during systole. It is significant in the aorta also, again during systole. In all other vessels, kinetic energy always seems to be of minor importance.

The reason for ascertaining the relative importance of kinetic energy in the circulation is to gain a sense of how much potential conversion of energy to pressure could occur if a vessel were, for some reason, to possess a local bulge (i.e., an aneurysm, caused by a weakness in the vessel wall). An aneurysm clearly would not tend to develop in areas of low kinetic energy, i.e., in the small vessels. Also, one could also estimate how much pressure loss would occur in a stenosis: a narrowing of the vessel interior caused by fatty deposits and such. Stenoses would not be expected to worsen rapidly in vessels where pressure is low, i.e., in the systemic veins or in the pulmonary system. From several standpoints, then, the vessel in which abnormalities of cross-sectional area are most

TABLE 4.7

Amount and Relative Importance of Kinetic Energy in Different Parts of the Circulation[a]

Vessel	Resting cardiac output				Cardiac output increased three times		
	Velocity (cm/sec)	Kinetic energy (mm Hg)	Pressure (mm Hg)	Kinetic energy as % of total	Kinetic energy (mm Hg)	Pressure (mm Hg)	Kinetic energy as % of total
Aorta, systolic	100	4	120	3	36	180	17
Mean	30	0.4	100	0.4	3.8	140	2.6
Arteries, systolic	30	0.35	100	0.3	3.8	120	3
Mean	10	0.04	95	Neg.[b]		100	Neg.
Capillaries	0.1	0.000004	25	Neg.	Neg.	25	Neg.
Venae cavae and atria	30	0.35	2	12	3.2	3	52
Pulmonary artery, systolic	90	3	20	13	27	25	52
Mean	25	0.23	12	2	2.1	14	13

[a]From Burton (1965), p. 103.
[b]Negligible.

likely to be most serious is the aorta. This is, indeed, borne out by the facts.

A. *Kinetic Energy Effects in Narrowed Arteries*

For normal arteries, we have seen that kinetic energy effects are usually minor. However, if for some reason (e.g., fatty deposits) the inner diameter is decreased, creating a stenosis, then kinetic energy effects are very important. If we consider an abnormal artery having a diameter one-third of normal, for which v is nine times normal, and hence the kinetic energy is 81 times normal, then the point is clear. For, if the usual kinetic energy is equivalent to 1 mm Hg, it will now be equivalent to 81 mm Hg.

Therefore, if the pressure in the artery used to be, say, 100 mm Hg at a certain point, the pressure will now be about 20 mm Hg. This lower pressure will tend to cause the vessel walls to "cave in" even more, possibly closing completely. As this begins to occur, however, frictional resistance will sharply increase, causing the flow to slow down and converting kinetic energy into pressure. The constriction will then start to reopen. In such an unstable situation the end result will be a periodic closing and opening, called flutter.

B. *Pressure Rise in an Aneurysm*

If an aneurysm of significant size occurs in an artery, the blood flow rate at the point of largest cross section may be very low. Therefore, the kinetic energy of the blood flow will be almost entirely converted to extra pressure. Under normal resting conditions this extra pressure will be small, as Table 4.7 suggests (say 4 mm Hg). However, under conditions of exercise the additional pressure may be 30-40 mm Hg, or more. This effect is not as large as the reverse effect one may find in a stenosis, but over a long time may be sufficient to make the aneurysm grow progressively worse, and ultimately burst. Aortic aneurysms the size of a fist are not rare.

VI. MECHANICAL ENERGY BALANCE

The steady-state mechanical energy balance (Bernoulli equation) for an incompressible fluid is (Bird et al., 1960, p. 212)

$$\Delta \frac{1}{2\alpha} \langle v \rangle^2 + g\, \Delta h + \frac{\Delta P}{\rho} + \hat{W} + \hat{E}_v = 0$$

where the balance is meant to apply between a fluid inlet plane and a fluid outlet plane (Δ means value at outlet minus value at inlet). The quantity h is the elevation at the center of the plane, and g is the local gravitational acceleration. $\hat{W}$ is the rate at which the system does work on its surroundings (per unit mass flow rate), and $\hat{E}_v$ is the friction loss per unit mass flow rate; α ranges from 0.5 to 1, as previously described.

A. *Horsepower of the Heart*

The Bernoulli equation may be applied to the heart, shown schematically in Figure 4.3, to determine its rate of work. Assuming (a) a cardiac output of 5 liters/min, (b) that $\Delta h \cong 0$, (c) that $\hat{E}_v \cong 0$ in the heart, and (d) that ΔKE can be neglected relative to pressure changes (this is reasonable for resting conditions, as shown in Table 4.7), then the Bernoulli equation becomes

$$\frac{\Delta P}{\rho} + \hat{W} = 0$$

or, the rate of work done by the heart is

$$-W = -\dot{m}\hat{W} = \frac{\dot{m}\Delta P}{\rho} = Q\, \Delta P$$

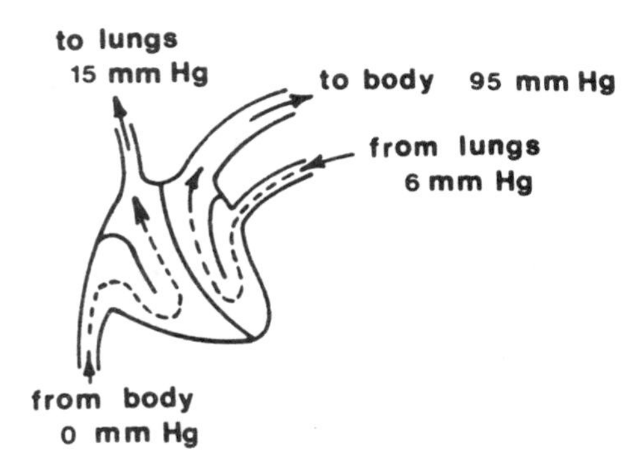

FIG. 4.3. The human heart (note: The term "body" excludes the lungs).

where $\dot{m}$ is the mass flow rate of blood and Q is the volumetric flow rate of blood. Hence,

$$-W = 5000 \text{ (ml/min) } \{(95 - 6) + (15 - 0)\} \text{ mm Hg}$$

$$= 5.20 \times 10^5 \text{ mm Hg-ml/min}$$

Converted to horsepower this becomes 0.00155 hp. Thus, it would take about 645 human hearts, at rest, to equal 1 hp. During exercise, the heart's power might increase about sixfold (flow rates increase fourfold and mean pressures rise by 50%), so that one heart is 0.0093 hp (equivalent to 108 hearts/hp).

In order to produce this much mechanical power the heart muscle actually has to convert about 10 times as much food to energy. The reason for this is that the heart muscle must be continuously maintained in an "activated" state of tension, even during the diastolic phase of its cycle. Maintenance of proper tension requires substantial energy. Hence, the heart's resting metabolic rate is equivalent to about 0.0155 hp (or about 5 W). Since 1 hp = 642 kcal/hr, this represents 9.93 kcal/hr, or 13.8% of a basal metabolic rate of 72 kcal/hr, a significant amount.

As Burton (1965) points out, the heart, pumping for a lifetime, does enough work to lift roughly 30 tons from sea level to the top of Mount Everest (∿30,000 ft), an impressive sum of work.

Figure 4.4 gives a PV (pressure versus volume) diagram for the left ventricle of the heart. The various phases of the ventricular cycle are represented. A diagram for the right ventricle would be similar in shape but with a pressure scale about one-fifth as large in value.

B. *Friction Losses in the Circulation*

If we view the circulatory system in the schematic fashion shown in Figure 4.5, and write the Bernoulli equation between two

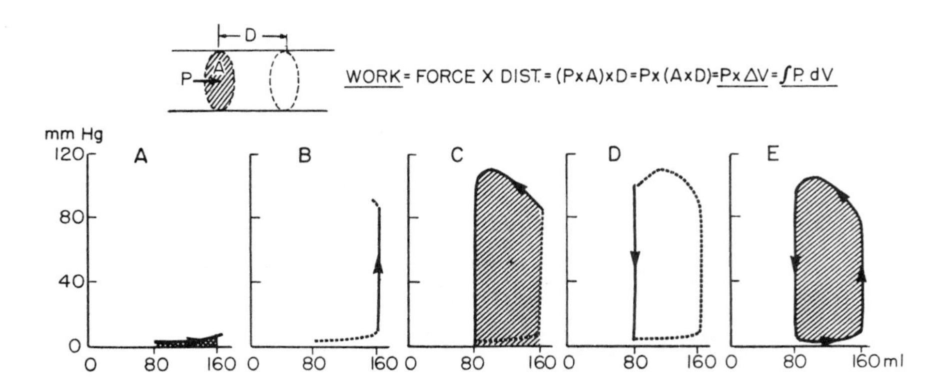

FIG. 4.4. The work diagram of the left ventricle. A, filling phase. The shaded area under the curve represents work done by the blood on the ventricle. B, isometric (or isovolumetric) contraction phase. No work is done, but elastic energy is stored in the heart muscle. C, ejection phase. The shaded area represents work done by the ventricle on the blood. D, isovolumetric relaxation phase. No work is done but stored elastic energy is given back. E, the complete cycle. The shaded area represents the net mechanical work of the ventricle in a single cycle. [From A. C. Burton, *Physiology and Biophysics of the Circulation*, 2nd ed., copyright 1972 by Yearbook Med. Publ., Chicago, Illinois. Used by permission.]

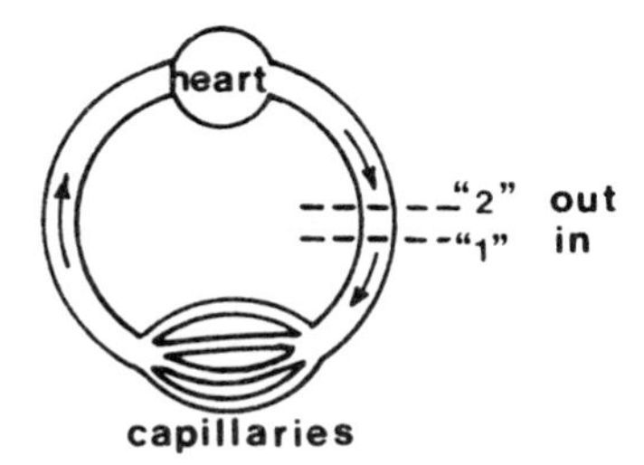

FIG. 4.5. The systemic circulation.

adjacent inlet and outlet planes ("1" and "2", respectively) so as to essentially encompass the entire circulation, then because $\Delta KE \cong 0$, $g\ \Delta h \cong 0$, and $\Delta P \cong 0$, we are left with $\hat{W} + \hat{E}_v = 0$.

This merely states that work is done by the heart (amount $-\hat{W}$) in order to overcome the frictional energy losses in the circulation (amount $\hat{E}_v$), as is obvious. Note that the heart's work and the total friction loss are equal.

C. Hydrostatics of the Circulation

At the level of the heart, the mean arterial blood pressure is about 100 mm Hg. When a person is lying down, the arterial blood pressures in the regions of the brain and of the feet are roughly 95 mm Hg.

Assuming the brain is 2 ft above the heart, and the feet are 4 ft below the heart, let us compute the arterial pressures in these areas for a person standing up.

For this situation, we may reduce the Bernoulli equation to the familiar hydrostatic equation

$$\Delta P = \rho g\ \Delta h$$

Taking $\rho = 1.056$ g/ml, we can easily show that $\Delta P = 23.7$ mm Hg/ft of length. Hence,

$$P_{feet} = 100 + 4\ (23.7) = 194.8 \text{ mm Hg}$$

$$P_{brain} = 100 - 2\ (23.7) = 52.6 \text{ mm Hg}$$

Figure 4.6 shows typical arterial and venous pressure values for horizontal and vertical body positions (based on $\rho = 1$ g/cc rather than the more exact value used above).

Note in Figure 4.6 that pressures on the venous side above the heart can be negative, relative to atmospheric pressure. Thus, one may often have "collapsed" veins in the head and neck. Fortunately, these veins take on a dumbbell type of cross section during collapse with flow channels on both sides, as shown in Figure 4.7 (note the very great differences in the scales of the abcissas in the figure).

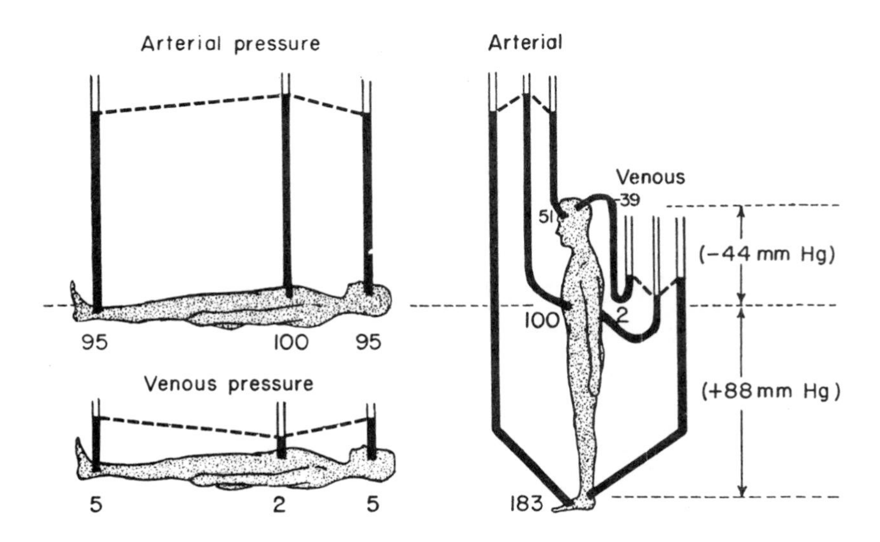

FIG. 4.6. Effects of posture on level of arterial and venous pressures. The gradient down arteries and veins due to flow (flow × resistance) is included in the diagram. The figures are estimated levels of the pressures, in millimeters of mercury, referred to the level of the right atrium as datum level. [From A. C. Burton, *Physiology and Biophysics of the Circulation*, 2nd ed., copyright 1972 by Yearbook Med. Publ., Chicago, Illinois. Used by permission.]

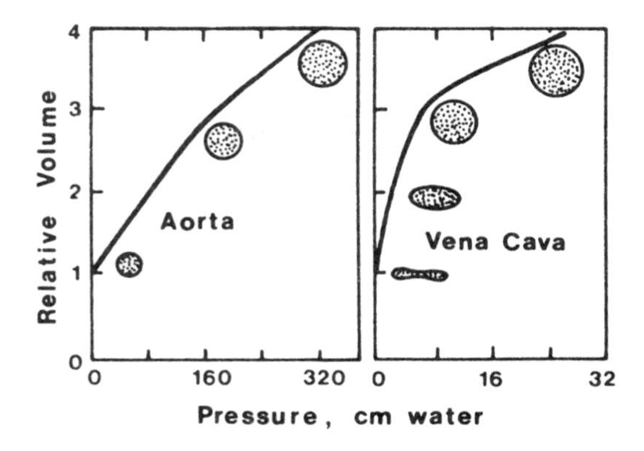

FIG. 4.7. Comparison of the distensibility of the aorta and the vena cava. The way in which the cross section of the vessels changes in the two cases is also indicated. [From Burton (1965), p. 65.]

Since the arteries are not very distensible, increases in pressure brought about by changes in posture have small effects on arterial blood volumes. However, veins, which are quite distensible, may change volume substantially. If venous vessel "tone" is poor, one may faint upon standing up suddenly, since the venous volume expands sharply, causing a decrease in the return of blood to the heart (and, therefore, to the brain).

A word should be said here about the one-way "venous valves" that exist in the larger veins of the limbs. These valves, which consist of flaps of tissue, act in conjunction with the squeezing action of adjacent leg or arm muscles to cause venous blood to be pumped back toward the heart. This prevents large elevations of venous pressures in the lower parts of the limbs because of hydrostatic effects, reduces the venous blood volumes there, and preserves good venous vessel tone (varicose veins are one result of faulty venous valves). The muscle pump mechanism is efficient enough to keep the venous pressure below 25 mm Hg in a walking adult.

PROBLEMS

1. Verify that the value shown in Table 4.3 for the Reynolds number in the aorta of a dog (value 1670) is correct for the conditions (diameter, velocity) indicated.

2. For laminar flow of a Newtonian fluid in a tube, the velocity varies with radial position as given by the formula

$$v(r) = \frac{\Delta P\ R^2}{4\mu L}\left(1 - \frac{r^2}{R^2}\right)$$

From this, derive an expression for the shear rate as a function of radial position, i.e., $\dot{\gamma}(r)$. Next, show that the ratio of the mean shear rate to the wall shear rate is exactly 2/3.

3. Using the expression for $\dot{\gamma}(r)$ developed in the preceding problem, show that the wall shear rate value given in Table 4.5 for the large arteries of a dog (value 600 sec^{-1}) is correct. Is the mean shear rate value also correct?

4. Assume that blood is flowing through an aorta of 1.0 cm diameter at an average velocity $\langle v \rangle$ of 50 cm/sec. Take α to be 1/2 and the pressure to be 100 mm Hg. If this flowing blood were then to enter a region of stenosis where the diameter of the aorta was only 0.5 cm, what would the approximate pressure in this narrowed region be?

5. Reconsider Problem 4 for the case where the flowing blood enters an aneurysmic region of diameter 1.5 cm, and determine the pressure in the aneurysm. If, for conditions of vigorous exercise, the velocity of the blood upstream of the aneurysm were four times the normal value (i.e., were 200 cm/sec), what pressure would develop in the aneurysm?

6. Use the following physiological facts (quotes from standard texts) to compute the efficiency of the human heart at rest:

(a) "The resting coronary blood flow in the human being averages approximately 225 ml/min."

(b) "Even in the normal resting state, about 65% of the oxygen in the arterial (coronary) blood is removed as the blood passes through the heart."

(c) "The total ml (STP) of oxygen bound with hemoglobin in the normal arterial blood is approximately 19.4 (per 100 ml of blood)."

(d) "Oxidizing an 'average diet' generates about 4.83 kcal for every liter of oxygen consumed."

7. Compute the mechanical work done by the human heart in one day, in lb force-ft. How far could one raise a 100-lb weight with this amount of work?

8. Estimate the work done by the left ventricle of the heart in one day, in lb force-ft, using Figure 4.4. Note that work equals $\int P\, dV$, and assume that the heart rate is 65 beats per minute. Compare this answer to that of Problem 7, and explain any difference.

9. Estimate the pressure difference between the inlet and outlet of a capillary that would be needed if blood were flowing through the capillary at a velocity of 0.2 cm/sec. Assume that (a) the capillary diameter is 8 μm (b) the capillary length is 200 μm, and (c) the apparent viscosity of blood is 2.5 cP. The friction factor for laminar flow in tubes can be expressed as $f = 16/Re$, where Re is the Reynolds number and f is defined as $f = R\,\Delta P/\rho v^2 L$. Give your answer in millimeters of mercury.

10. If a jet pilot is subjected to a force of "3 G," estimate the pressures on the arterial side of the circulation in the regions of the feet and the head. Are your answers reasonable? Discuss.

REFERENCES

Attinger, E. O., ed., *Pulsatile Blood Flow*, McGraw-Hill (Blakiston), New York, 1964.

Bird, R. B., Stewart, W. E., and Lightfoot, E. N., *Transport Phenomena*, Wiley, New York, 1960.

Burton, A. C., *Physiology and Biophysics of the Circulation*, Yearbook Med. Publ., Chicago, Illinois, 1965.

Fung, Y. C., ed., *Biomechanics*, ASME, New York, 1966.

Guyton, A. C., *Textbook of Medical Physiology*, 4th ed., Saunders, Philadelphia, Pennsylvania, 1971.

McCabe, W. L., and Smith, J. C., *Unit Operations of Chemical Engineering*, McGraw-Hill, New York, 1956.

McDonald, D. A., *Blood Flow in Arteries*, Arnold, London, 1960.

Whitmore, R. L., *Rheology of the Circulation*, Pergamon, Oxford, 1968.

Chapter 5

THE HUMAN THERMAL SYSTEM

The production of heat, its internal transport, and its dissipation from the human body are topics of great importance. In this chapter we discuss the magnitude and source of heat production in the body, the ways in which heat is transported internally from one region of the body to another, and the various means by which heat is lost to the external environment. We shall quantify the current state of knowledge where possible, and solve a few representative problems.

I. HEAT PRODUCTION

As cited in Chapter 2, the basal metabolic rate of an average person is about 72 kcal/hr. Basal means, physiologically, a state in which the subject is lying at rest, awake, under prescribed conditions (air temperature between 65° and 80°F, no recent food intake or exercise, etc.). Basal metabolic rates are usually determined in large "human calorimeters."

Figure 5.1 indicates the typical dependence of basal metabolic rate (BMR) on age and sex, in kilocalories per hour per square meter of body surface area (body area, rather than weight, gives a better correlation, as discussed earlier). The dependence of BMR on weight for various species is depicted in Figure 5.2. Table 5.1 shows energy expenditures for a typical man for various activities. It should be mentioned that food values are usually given in "large" Calories, equal to 1000 of the calories used in this text.

Guyton states that about 20% of the basal heat is produced in the liver, 15% in the brain, 12% in the heart, and the remainder elsewhere. Wissler gives similar figures: trunk 60% (mainly in liver and heart), brain 20%, and extremities 20%. The organs that are most active mechanically and chemically, and which therefore produce the most heat (liver, heart, brain), generally run 1° or 2°F higher in temperature than the surrounding tissues. In general,

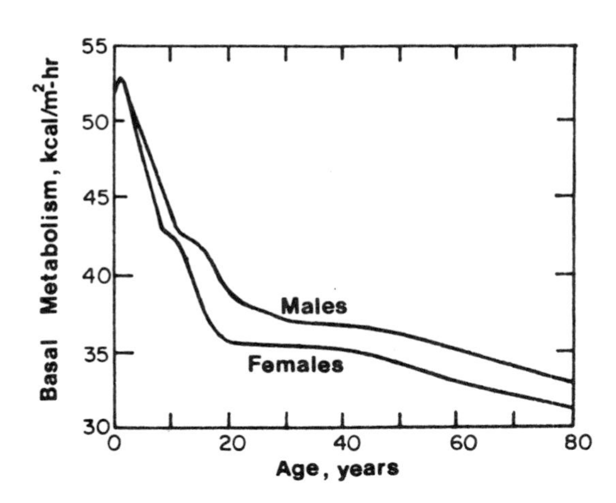

FIG. 5.1. Normal basal metabolic rates at different ages for each sex. [From Guyton (1971), p. 828.]

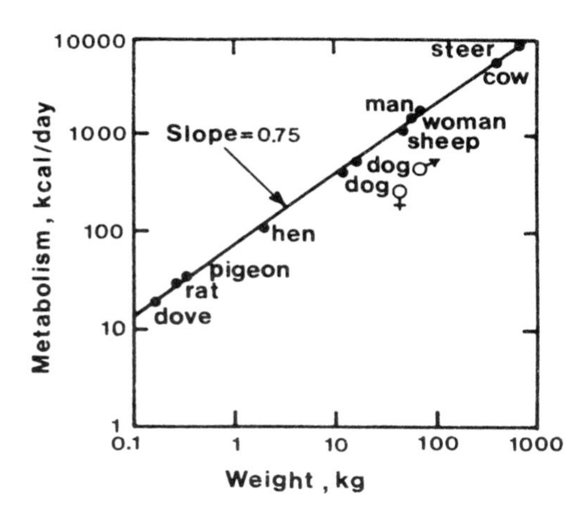

FIG. 5.2. Logarithm of metabolism plotted against logarithm of weight. [From Ruch and Paton (1965), p. 1045.]

therefore, the body "core" is usually significantly warmer than the body's extremities and surfaces, as depicted in Figure 5.3. Normal muscular activity can raise heat production to 125% or so of the BMR, but at maximum activity this figure may be as high as 1500-2000% of the BMR.

The heat produced in the body is derived from the breakdown, synthesis, and utilization of food. Figure 5.4 indicates how heat and external work are generated in the body. Starting with 100 units of food energy, ΔH (enthalpy relative to end products), we see that 5% is ultimately lost in the form of increased entropy of the end products relative to reactants. Since $\Delta G = \Delta H - T\,\Delta S$, therefore, 95% remains as potentially available free energy. The body utilizes almost all food by a scheme that involves the formation of a compound called adenosine triphosphate (ATP), which we discuss later, and the subsequent use of this ATP to supply energy for muscle contraction, chemical synthesis, etc. The many chemical reactions required to create ATP produce substantial heat generation, with the result that only about 45% of the original energy of the food re-

TABLE 5.1

Data for Different Common Activities[a]

Type of activity	Metabolic rate per unit body surface area ($kcal/m^2 hr$)	Estimated mechanical efficiency	Estimated relative velocity in still air (m/sec)
Seated, quiet	50	0	0
Seated, drafting	60	0	0-0.1
Seated, typing	70	0	0-0.1
Standing at attention	65	0	0
Standing, washing dishes	80	0-0.05	0-0.2
Shoemaker	100	0-0.10	0-0.2
Sweeping a bare floor (38 strokes/ min)	100	0-0.05	0.2-0.5
Seated, heavy leg and arm movements (metalworker at a bench)	110	0-0.15	0.1-0.3
Walking about, moderate lifting or pushing (carpenter, metalworker, industrial painter)	140	0-0.10	0-0.9
Pick and shovel work, stonemason work	220	0-0.20	0-0.9
Walking on the level with the velocity (mph):			
2.0	100	0	0.9
2.5	120	0	1.1
3.0	130	0	1.3
3.5	160	0	1.6
4.0	190	0	1.8
5.0	290	0	2.2

[a]From Fanger et al. (1968).

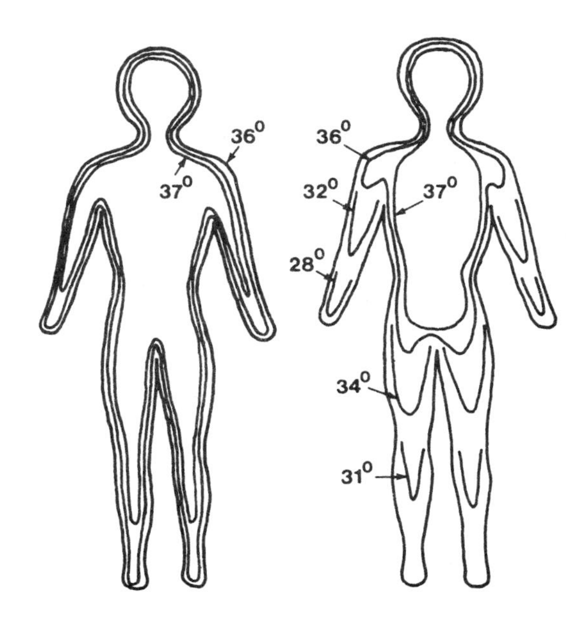

FIG. 5.3. Isotherms (surfaces connecting points of equal temperature) in the body. Left, isotherms in a warm environment; right, in a cold environment. The innermost isotherm may be considered as the boundary of the body "core"; the core includes most of the body in hot environments. When heat must be conserved, the core contracts to the proportions indicated on the right. In severe cold exposure, the combined effect of vasoconstriction and countercurrent heat exchange results in the pattern of isotherms shown in the limbs, the distal portions of which become part of the body "shell" and fall nearly to environmental temperatures. [From Ruch and Patton (1965), p. 1057.]

mains captured in the ATP. As the body's general energy source, ATP is then used to power all necessary functions, such as keeping the body repaired, synthesizing chemicals, fueling the heart and lung muscles, driving nerve impulses, etc. As Figure 5.4 indicates, a maximum of 25% of the original food's energy is ultimately convertible into external work (e.g., lifting weights). All processes except for external work entail a degradation of chemical energy into heat. Hence, if no external work is being performed, all food energy ultimately is converted into about 5% entropy and 95% heat.

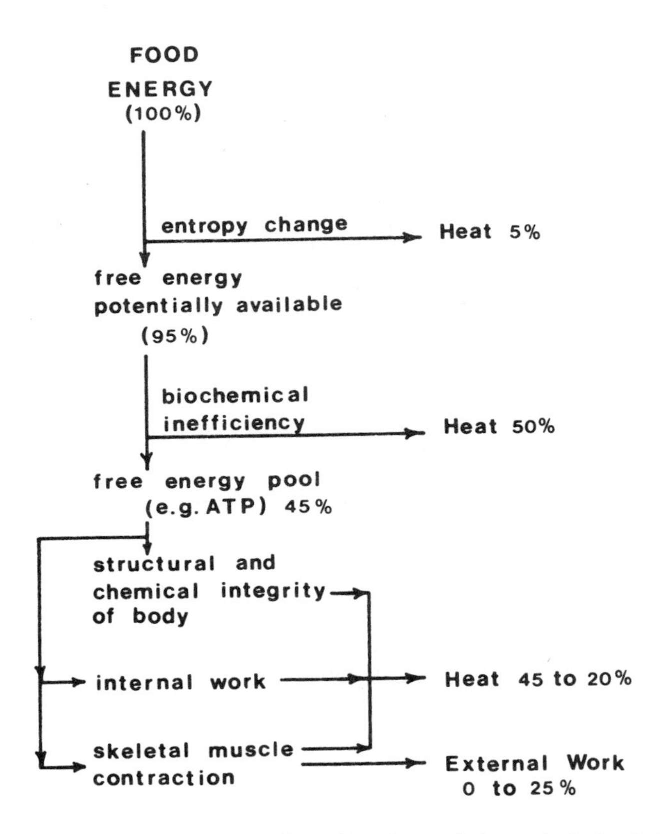

FIG. 5.4. Summary of the distribution of ingested food energy within the body and its transfer to the environment. [From Ruch and Patton (1965), p. 1034.]

II. BRIEF DESCRIPTION OF THE BIOCHEMISTRY OF DIGESTION

In order to understand how ATP is formed some knowledge of the biochemistry of digestion is required. Basically, all foods can be divided into carbohydrates, fats (or lipids), and proteins. Carbohydrates, which are polymers of monosaccharides (sugars), have the approximate formula $[C(H_2O)]_n$. The most important sugars are those having six carbon atoms (hexoses), such as glucose. Carbohydrates, especially polysaccharides such as starch, comprise a main part of the diet. Upon ingestion, hydrolysis of carbohydrates, catalyzed by enzymes, takes place, especially in the intestine. The diagram below shows the general breakdown process:

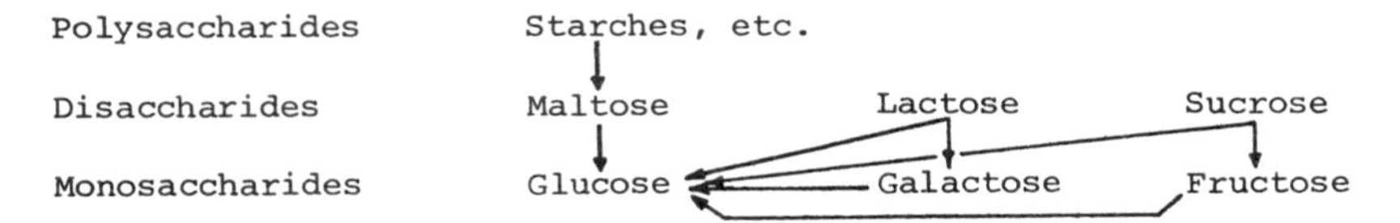

Lactose (milk sugar) and sucrose are broken down to monosaccharides and then rearranged, by the liver, to the isomeric glucose form. Hence, all carbohydrates are essentially reduced to glucose.

Lipids generally consist of fatty acids, fats, phospholipids, and glycolipids. Fatty acids are long-chain organic compounds with carboxylic acid groups at the end, e.g., palmitic acid

$$CH_3—(CH_2)_{14}—COOH$$

Fats are simply esters of fatty acids with glycerol and are termed mono-, di-, or triglycerides, depending on structure. An example of a triglyceride is tristearin, an ester of stearic acid and glycerol

$$\begin{array}{l} CH_3—(CH_2)_{16}—COO—CH_2 \\ \qquad\qquad\qquad\qquad\qquad\quad | \\ CH_3—(CH_2)_{16}—COO—CH \\ \qquad\qquad\qquad\qquad\qquad\quad | \\ CH_3—(CH_2)_{16}—COO—CH_2 \end{array}$$

Phospholipids (i.e., lipids containing one or more phosphate groups), glycolipids (lipids and glucose bound together), and sterols (e.g., cholesterol) are other important types of compounds. Hydrolysis of lipids is catalyzed by enzymes and occurs mainly in the intestines (after the bile emulsifies the lipids). One generally ends up with free fatty acids, glycerol, and some mono- or diglycerides.

Proteins are polymers of amino acids, which have the basic structure shown in Chapter 2. Some 21 amino acids occur in the body to a significant extent. The peptide linkage binding the amino acids together in proteins is hydrolyzed in the stomach and the intestines under the action of enzymes such as pepsin and trypsin.

The basic scheme of digestion is thus the enzyme-catalyzed hydrolysis of carbohydrates, lipids, and proteins to yield glucose, free fatty acids, glycerol, amino acids, and other minor species. The three basic types of foods (carbohydrates, lipids, proteins) exhibit differing energy values and ratios of oxygen consumed to carbon dioxide produced. The following three reactions for glucose ($C_6H_{12}O_6$, mol wt = 180), triolein ($C_{57}H_{104}O_6$, mol wt = 885) and hydroxylysine ($C_6H_{14}O_3N_2$, mol wt = 162) are typical of the oxidations of these types of foods:

$$C_6H_{12}O_6 + 6\ O_2 = 6\ H_2O + 6\ CO_2 + 673\ \text{kcal}$$

$$C_{57}H_{104}O_6 + 80\ O_2 = 57\ CO_2 + 52\ H_2O + 7900\ \text{kcal}$$

$$C_6H_{14}O_3N_2 + 6\tfrac{1}{2}\ O_2 = CO(NH_2)_2 + 5\ CO_2 + 5\ H_2O + 850\ \text{kcal}$$

By simple stoichiometry, one can calculate the quantities shown in Table 5.2 [referred to standard temperature and pressure (STP), $0^\circ C$ and 1 atm]. Of course, these compounds are only three of many in the diet. When an average diet is considered, the values become somewhat different, e.g. (again, at STP), those shown in Table 5.3. The energy values cited here are "bomb calorimeter" values. In reality, the energy value of protein is about 4.2 kcal/g, since in a bomb calorimeter complete oxidation to NH_3 and CO_2 occurs, whereas in the body oxidation proceeds to urea and CO_2 only.

These figures point out the high energy value, high O_2 consumption, and high CO_2 production (per gram) of fats relative to carbohydrates and proteins. An overall respiratory quotient (ratio of CO_2 produced to O_2 used) of 0.82 is typical of an average diet.

TABLE 5.2

Metabolism of Specific Compounds

	Glucose	Triolein	Hydroxylysine
Liters O_2 used/g	0.75	2.03	0.90
Liters CO_2 produced/g	0.75	1.44	0.69
Respiratory quotient	1.00	0.71	0.77
kcal/g	3.74	8.93	5.25

TABLE 5.3

Metabolism of Different Classes of Foods

	Carbohydrate	Lipid	Protein
Liters O_2 used/g	0.81	1.96	0.94
Liters CO_2 produced/g	0.81	1.39	0.75
Respiratory quotient	1.00	0.71	0.80
kcal/g	4.1	9.3	5.4

The end goal of foodstuff breakdown is to provide simple raw materials which the cells of the body can use to synthesize "high energy" compounds from lower energy compounds. The most important such high energy molecule is adenosine triphosphate (ATP), which has the structure shown in Figure 5.5.

This compound, synthesized from adenosine diphosphate (ADP), has an energy 8 kcal/mole greater than ADP, and it is this energy which is released in a controlled manner when needed by the body. The biochemistry of the metabolic pathways involved in all these

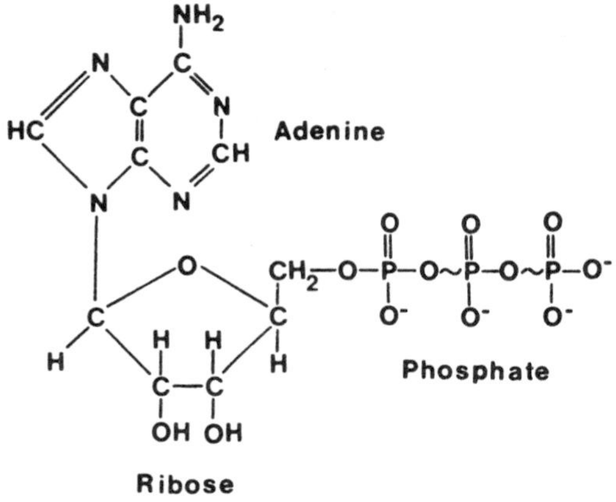

FIG. 5.5. The structure of ATP.

phenomena is outside the scope of our discussion; however, it should be mentioned that about 36 moles of ATP can be made from ADP via oxidation of 1 mole of glucose. Since glucose has a free energy value of 686 kcal/mole, the "efficiency" of energy storage in ATP is $(36)(8)/686 = 0.42$, or 42%.

III. LOSS OF HEAT TO THE ENVIRONMENT

Table 5.4 indicates that at steady state, the heat produced by the human body must be balanced by the heat lost to the external environment. This table points out that heat production in excess of usual basal amounts can be produced by muscular activity (including shivering, an automatic response of the body to colder than normal body temperature) and by chemical or hormonal action. However, we shall not specifically discuss production apart from that generated via basal and muscular activities.

Heat loss occurs by all of the usual heat transfer modes. Under normal conditions, heat losses from a seated nude body in still air

TABLE 5.4

Balance of Heat Production and Heat Losses

Production	Losses
Basal metabolism	Radiation
Voluntary muscular activity	Evaporation from skin
Involuntary muscular activity (shivering)	Evaporation from respiratory tract
Effects of hormones (thyroxin, adrenaline) on cellular metabolism	Sensible losses via respiration
Effects of temperature on metabolic rate	Convection
	Conduction

are proportioned roughly as follows: radiation, 60%; evaporation, 25%, convection, 12%; and conduction, 3%. Certain modes of heat loss can be much larger, however, in many situations (e.g., convective losses dominate when the air velocity is high).

Before considering in more detail how heat is lost from the body, it would be interesting to compute how rapidly the body's temperature would rise in the absence of any heat loss (as would happen if one were in a room having walls at body temperature and containing air saturated at body temperature).

Example 5.1: Body Temperature Rise with No Heat Loss. From Table 2.1 let us assume a body weight of 68 kg, a heat capacity of 0.86 kcal/kg-°C, and a basal heat production rate of 72 kcal/hr. then find that

$$\frac{dT}{dt} = \frac{Q}{mC_p} = \frac{(72)}{(68)(0.86)} \frac{°C}{hr} = 1.2°C/hr$$

This rate of rise, equivalent to 2.22°F/hr, would cause the body to go from 98.6°F to 106°F, which is a severely critical level, in about 3.3 hr. When one is experiencing the onset of a solid fever, a temperature rise of about 2°F/hr is indeed found, as suggested by the computation just given.

A. *Radiative Heat Losses from the Body*

All objects continually radiate energy in accordance with the Stefan-Boltzmann law, i.e., proportionately with surface area, emissivity, and fourth power of the absolute temperature. When one's surroundings are hotter than one's body (or outer clothing surface, to be more exact), a net heat gain via radiation occurs. When the surroundings are cooler, net heat loss occurs. The amount of incident radiation that is captured by a body depends on its area, the incident flux, and the body's absorptivity. It is common to estimate the absorptivity of a body as equal to its emissivity at the temperature of the surroundings, although this is strictly true only when the body is in radiative equilibrium with the surroundings.

The loss of heat by radiation from the body has been characterized by the equation

$$Q_r = K_r A_r e_s (T_s - T_r) \tag{5.1}$$

where T_s is the surface temperature of the body or clothes and T_r is the temperature of solid surroundings (not necessarily equal to the air temperature). Note that a driving force of $(T_s^4 - T_r^4)$ is not used here, as one would have expected. The reason for this is that $(T_s^4 - T_r^4)$ can be expanded into two factors, i.e.,

$$(T_s^4 - T_r^4) = (T_s^3 + T_s^2 T_r + T_s T_r^2 + T_r^3)(T_s - T_r) \tag{5.2}$$

the first factor of which is nearly constant over a normal range of conditions (since the T's are absolute they change very little) and which is therefore simply incorporated into the transfer coefficient K_r.

A_r is the area of the body which is effective in radiating heat and amounts to about 1.4 m^2 for a nude body having a total surface area of 1.8 m^2. The inner surfaces of the arms and legs are two areas that are not effective in radiation heat loss (they radiate back to the body).

The emissivity (which is approximately equal to the absorptivity) of the body is e_s. For incident infrared radiation, the absorptivity of human skin is very high, about 0.97, and is independent of color. For visible light, the skin has an absorptivity of about 0.65-0.82, depending on whether it is white or dark, respectively.

Ruch and Patton (1965) cite an average value of the coefficient K_r of about 7 kcal/hr-m^2-°C. Using this value, we can make the following sample calculation.

Example 5.2: Estimation of Radiative Heat Loss from the Body. Let us assume a surface temperature T_s of 33°C (91.4°F); surroundings at 29°C (84.2°F); A_r = 1.4 m^2; e_s = 0.97; and K_r = 7 kcal/hr-m^2-°C. From the equation cited above we determine that

$$Q_r = (7)(1.4)(0.97)(33 - 29) = 38.0 \text{ kcal/hr}$$

This magnitude is roughly 53% of an average person's BMR.

Fanger et al. (1968) present a somewhat more detailed equation for radiative heat losses:

$$Q_r = A_r e_s \sigma (T_{cl}^4 - T_r^4) \tag{5.3}$$

where σ is the Stefan-Boltzmann constant, and the fourth powers on the temperatures have been retained. These authors also explain how A_r may be split into three factors

$$A_r = f_{eff} f_{cl} A_N \tag{5.4}$$

where A_N is the total nude body area, f_{cl} accounts for increases in the body's surface area due to clothing, and f_{eff} accounts for the fraction of surface area effective in radiation. Values of f_{cl} for several typical types of clothing are shown in Table 5.5. Generally, f_{eff} values have been found experimentally to be about 0.75 for standing positions and 0.65 for seated positions.

The equation of Fanger et al. is equivalent to that given earlier, if

$$K_r = \sigma(T_s^3 + T_s^2T_r + T_sT_r^2 + T_r^3) \tag{5.5}$$

Using T_s = 306°K (33°C), T_r = 302°K (29°C), and $\sigma = 4.8 \times 10^{-8}$ kcal/m^2-hr-°K^4, Equation 5.5 predicts a K_r of 5.4 kcal/hr-m^2-°C, which is similar to the value cited earlier.

TABLE 5.5

Resistance and Surface Area Factors for Various Clothing Ensembles[a]

Clothing ensemble	I_{cl} (clo)	f_{cl}
Nude	0	1.0
Light working ensemble	0.6	1.1
U.S. Army fatigues, man's	0.7	1.1
Typical American business suit	0.7-1.0	1.1-1.15
Light outdoor sportswear	0.9	1.15
Heavy traditional European business suit	1.2	1.15-1.20
U.S. Army standard cold-wet uniform	1.5-2.0	1.3-1.4
Heavy wool pile ensemble (polar weather suit)	3.4	1.3-1.5

[a]From Fanger et al. (1968).

Table 5.6 reports additional data from the literature based on the simplified equation $Q_r = K'_r A_N (T_s - T_r)$. That is, all "unknowns" (e_s, fraction of total area effective in radiating) are lumped into the coefficient K'_r.

B. *Convective Heat Losses from the Body*

Convective heat losses from the body are strongly dependent on air velocities (or water velocities, if such is the environment). The simplest equation for characterizing convective losses is

$$Q_c = K_c A_c (T_s - T_a) \tag{5.8}$$

TABLE 5.6

Radiation Heat Transfer Coefficients for Nude Humans

Basis: $Q_r = K'_r A_N (T_s - T_r)$ (5.6)

K'_r (kcal/m^2-hr-°C)	Authors	Conditions
4.50–4.77	Colin et al. (1970)	Range of postures
4.7	Cited by Sibbons (1970)	
4.5	Gagge et al. (1964)	Seated posture

Note: One can easily show that K_r and K'_r are related by

$$K'_r = K_r (A_r/A_N) e_s \tag{5.7}$$

Based on $K_r = 7$, $(A_r/A_N) = 0.70$, and $e_s = 0.97$, the value of K'_r is 4.75. Hence, the K'_r values cited above are consistent with Ruch and Patton's (1965) K_r value of 7.

where A_c is the effective area for convective transport (not necessarily equal to A_r), T_a is the ambient temperature, and K_c is a convective heat transfer coefficient. A_c is generally about 80% of the total surface area, for a nude body (but can be dramatically lowered by curling up, for example).

Fanger et al. (1968) recommend as the starting equation for quantifying convective heat transfer the relation

$$Q_c = K_c A_N f_{cl} f_{eff} (T_s - T_a) \tag{5.9}$$

that is, A_c is written more specifically as $A_N f_{cl} f_{eff}$.

One must distinguish between "free convection" heat transfer and "forced convection" heat transfer. Pure free convection occurs under stagnant conditions when the velocity of the ambient toward the person is zero. In this case a local velocity pattern is nevertheless induced near the surface of the person because of density gradients; e.g., a warm person standing in a cool room will create upward air motion near the body's surface, which facilitates heat transfer from the body. Forced convection heat transfer occurs when the ambient is approaching the body with a definite (and usually steady) velocity. Obviously, the break point between these two modes of convection is not sharp; a gradual transition zone (range of low approach velocities) exists where both effects are important.

Tables 5.7 and 5.8 present free and forced convection heat transfer correlations from the literature. These correlations require units of v of meters per second and yield K_c in kcal/m^2-hr-°C.

For free convection with a laminar boundary layer, theory predicts

$$Nu = \text{const}(Gr\ Pr)^{0.25} \tag{5.10}$$

where Nu, Gr, and Pr are the Nusselt, Grashof, and Prandtl numbers, respectively, as defined in Table 5.9. The theoretical form for forced convection correlations is

$$Nu = \text{const}\ Re^m\ Pr^n \tag{5.11}$$

TABLE 5.7

Coefficients for Free Convection Heat Transfer from Nude Persons to Air

Coefficient[a]	Authors	Conditions
2.12	Buettner (1934)	
2.3	Colin and Houdas (1967)	Standing
1.95	Colin and Houdas (1967)	Seated
3.0	Winslow et al. (1939)	
$2.05\ \Delta T^{0.25}$	Nielsen and Pedersen[b] (1952)	Seated or standing

[a] $\Delta T = T_s - T_a$, in degrees centigrade. Coefficient K_c in $kcal/m^2$-hr-°C.

[b] Tests performed with a manikin.

where Re is the Reynolds number. Table 5.9 lists a few standard correlations for free and forced convection heat transfer from simple geometric bodies (spheres and cylinders).

Whether free or forced, convection controls in any given situation can be decided by calculating both the free and forced convection coefficients, and using the larger value. The point at which both coefficients are the same commonly occurs at rather low air velocities, e.g., only a few tenths of a meter per second.

It is interesting to check the correlations given in Table 5.8 against what is implied by the correlations in Table 5.9. This we do in Example 5.3.

Example 5.3: Prediction of Forced Convection Heat Losses from Humans Using Literature Correlations for Cylinders. Let us consider the human body to be roughly cylindrical. The equivalent diameter of this cylinder can be computed for a man 5 ft 8 in. (1.73 m) tall who has a total body surface area of 1.8 m^2:

TABLE 5.8

Coefficients for Forced Convection Heat Transfer from Nude Persons to Air[a]

Coefficient[a]	Authors	Conditions
$5.6v^{0.67}$	Colin and Houdas (1967)	Standing, cross flow
$3.66v^{0.643}$	Tamari and Leonard (1972)[b]	Standing, cross flow
$7.5v^{0.5}$	Nelson et al. (1947)	Standing, cross flow
$6.4v^{0.67}$	Colin and Houdas (1967)	Seated, vertical flow
$7.5v^{0.67}$	Colin and Houdas (1967)	Reclining, parallel flow
$10.4v^{0.5}$	Winslow et al. (1939)	Reclining, parallel flow
$2.54v^{0.72}$	Tamari and Leonard (1972)[b]	Standing, parallel flow
$6.3v^{0.5}$	Buettner (1934)	Reclining, parallel flow

[a] v is approach velocity in meters per second. Coefficient K_c in kcal/m^2-hr-°C.

[b] Experiments done on scale-model human form.

$$\text{Area} = \pi DL + 2\frac{\pi D^2}{4} = 1.73\pi D + \frac{\pi D^2}{2} = 1.8$$

Solving for D by trial and error gives D = 0.305 m = 30.5 cm. The "equivalent diameter" of the person is 30.5 cm, or about 12.0 in. This seems reasonable as an overall average for head, neck, trunk, arms, and legs.

Assuming the ambient is air at 70°F, for which Pr = 0.72, $\mu/\rho = 1.6 \times 10^{-5}$ m^2/sec, and $k = 2.2 \times 10^{-2}$ kcal/m-hr-°C, we have

TABLE 5.9

Free and Forced Convection Heat Transfer Correlations[a]

Forced convection	Free convection
Sphere	Sphere
$Nu = 2 + 0.6\ Re^{1/2}\ Pr^{1/3}$	$Nu = 2 + 0.56\ (Gr\ Pr)^{1/4}$
Long cylinder	Long horizontal cylinder
$Nu \cong 0.6\ Re^{1/2}\ Pr^{1/3}$ for $10 < Re < 10^5$	$Nu = 0.525\ (Gr\ Pr)^{1/4}$
	Vertical cylinder or thin plate
	$Nu = 0.59\ (Gr\ Pr)^{1/4}$
	The above are generally limited to Gr Pr greater than 10^4 and less than 10^9

[a] $Gr = (D^3\rho^2 g\beta\ \Delta T/\mu^2)$, where β is the coefficient of volume expansion of the fluid, $-(1/\rho)(\partial\rho/\partial T)_p$, and ΔT is the surface temperature minus the temperature of the fluid far from the surface. $Nu = K_c D/k$, $Re = Dv\rho/\mu$, $Pr = C_p\mu/k$.

from the long cylinder correlation of Table 5.9

$$\frac{K_c(0.305)}{(0.022)} = 0.6 \left[\frac{(0.305)v}{1.6 \times 10^{-5}}\right]^{1/2} (0.72)^{1/3}$$

where v is in meters per second. This yields

$$K_c = 5.4v^{1/2}$$

which is in excellent agreement with the correlations given in Table 5.8. Rapp (1970) has drawn additional very detailed comparisons between the convection coefficients measured experimentally on humans and what one would predict from various correlations on simple geometric shapes (flat plates, spheres, cylinders). In doing so, Rapp considers how a human body might be modeled as a set of connected cylinders, spheres, and so forth.

Let us now consider the question as to what air velocity would be needed for equality of free and forced convection effects, for a typical human (i.e., not a simple geometric shape). From Table 5.7, we might select 2.3 kcal/m^2-hr-°C as a likely free convection coefficient, and from Table 5.8 we might choose $5.6v^{0.67}$ as a representative forced convection coefficient. If we equate these two and solve for v, we obtain v = 0.265 m/sec (0.59 mph). Thus, below 0.265 m/sec, free convection is more important than forced convection, while above 0.265 m/sec forced convection dominates.

Example 5.4: Heat Loss via Forced Convection. For a velocity of 1 mph (0.447 m/sec), let us compute the magnitude of convective heat losses from a nude person. For v = 0.447, the correlation $5.6v^{0.67}$ yields $K_c = 3.27$ (note that this is larger than the free convection coefficient of 2.3; hence, even had we not performed the preceding calculation, we would immediately realize that at this velocity forced convection controls). The corresponding heat loss, assuming $T_s = 33°C$ and $T_a = 29°C$ (as before), and using an effective heat loss area for convection of 80% of the total area, is

$$Q_c \doteq 3.27(0.8)(1.8)(33 - 29) = 18.8 \text{ kcal/hr}$$

or about 26% of the BMR. For a higher wind velocity (1 mph is pretty mild) the loss would, of course, be much larger.

Finally, we wish to make note of some additional literature data that are of importance, the convective coefficients for humans in a water medium shown in Table 5.10. Note that the values are perhaps 10-20 times those for air. This difference is due mainly to the large thermal conductivity of water as compared to air.

TABLE 5.10

Convective Heat Transfer Coefficient in Water[a]

Authors	Experimental conditions	Transfer coefficient (kcal/m^2-hr-°C)
Lefevre (1929)	Stirred water at 5°C	57.6
	12°C	54
	18°C	54
	24°C	54
	30°C	57.6
Goldman et al. (1966)	Still water	39.63
	Stirred water	50.45
Boutelier et al. (unpublished data)	Still water	37.6
	Water agitated by shivering	52.2

[a]From Colin et al. (1970).

C. *Evaporative Heat Losses from the Body*

Evaporative heat losses occur by several mechanisms: (a) heat loss by diffusion of water through the skin, (b) heat loss by sweat secretion, and (c) heat loss by evaporation of water into inspired air. Associated with this last process is an additional heat loss arising from sensible heat transfer into inspired air.

D. *Heat Loss by Diffusion of Water Through Skin*

Water diffusion through the human skin is part of the "insensible" perspiration which is not subject to thermoregulatory control. This diffusion totals about 350 ml/day in an average person (see

Table 2.7), and is assumed to be proportional to the difference between the vapor pressure of water at skin temperature and the partial pressure of water vapor in the ambient air. The diffusional resistance of the skin's layers is fairly large, and the diffusional resistance of clothing can usually be neglected by comparison.

Inouye et al. (1953) have shown that for sedentary persons under normal conditions, the diffusional heat loss is given by

$$Q_d = 0.35A_N(P_s - P_a) \tag{5.12}$$

where P_s and P_a are in millimeters of mercury. The vapor pressure of water over the range of roughly 27°- 37°C can be represented well by the formula

$$P_s = 1.92T_s - 25.3 \text{ mm Hg} \tag{5.13}$$

This allows one easily to relate Q_d to skin temperature. Supposing that T_s = 33°C and P_a = 0 ("dry" air), then P_s = 38.1 mm Hg and Q_d = 24.0 kcal/hr, for a person of $A_N = 1.8 \text{ m}^2$. This represents the evaporative heat loss associated with 1055 ml of water per day (44 ml/hr), since the latent heat of vaporization of water is about 570 kcal/kg at 33°C. Obviously, room air is rarely bone dry, and a more typical value of 350 ml/day water diffusion is more likely. Even at 350 ml/day, Q_d would equal about 8 kcal/hr, or 11% of the BMR, a significant amount. The diffusion process is assumed to be independent of sweat secretion, i.e., the wetted area of skin due to sweat secretion under normal conditions is assumed to be a very small proportion of the total area, and does not significantly affect the diffusion area.

E. Heat Loss by Sweat Secretion

When activity levels rise above the basal state, additional heat is produced in the body, and therefore the need to cast off more heat from the body arises. One of the automatic mechanisms for increasing heat loss is the sweating response, which provides secretion of a dilute electrolyte solution from numerous glands to the skin's surface. Evaporation from the wetted surface then occurs, removing about 570 cal/g of water evaporated. Table 2.7 gives typical values of the amounts of sweat generated under different weather and exercise conditions. One can see that the maximum amounts are quite large—up to 5 or more liters each day. When one sweats copiously, not all of the sweat is effective in removing heat from the body since much of it may run off as liquid (this depends strongly on the ambient conditions).

The evaporation process can be controlled either by the rate at which sweat is supplied to the skin or by the rate at which the evaporation occurs from the wetted surface. For example, when the surrounding air is dry and moving well, all sweat reaching the surface will be evaporated as fast as it arrives. Then the evaporative heat loss in kilocalories per hour is

$$Q_e = 570\dot{m}_w \tag{5.14}$$

where $\dot{m}_w$ is the rate of water excretion by the sweat glands in kilograms per hour. When the air is stagnant and moist,

$$Q_e = K_e A_W (P_s - P_a) \tag{5.15}$$

where A_W is the wetted surface area, P_s and P_a are water partial pressures corresponding to the surface and ambient conditions, and K_e is an evaporation transfer coefficient.

Table 5.11 presents correlations for K_e which have been experimentally determined by several investigators. Note that the dependence of K_e on air velocity is essentially the same as that of the convective coefficient K_c (theoretical considerations show that the dependence should, in fact, be the same).

Example 5.5: Heat Loss via Evaporation of Sweat. The amount of cooling that can be achieved by evaporation of water from the skin can be estimated for some typical conditions. Let us assume air is

TABLE 5.11

Coefficients for Forced Convection Evaporation Heat Transfer from Nude Persons in Air[a,b]

Coefficient	Authors	Conditions
$12.70v^{0.634}$	Clifford et al. (1959)	v > 0.58 m/sec, standing, cross flow
$9.66v^{0.25}$	Clifford et al. (1959)	v < 0.51 m/sec
$10.17v^{0.37}$	Nelson et al. (1947)	0.15 < v < 3.05 m/sec
$18.4v^{0.37}$	Machle and Hatch (1947)	
$11.6v^{0.4}$	Wyndham and Atkins (1960)	
$19.1v^{0.66}$	Fourt and Powell[c]	
$13.2v^{0.6}$	Fourt and Powell[c]	

K_e in kcal/m^2-hr-mm Hg.

[a]For free convection, Clifford et al. (1959) give a coefficient $K_e = 3.37(T_s - T_a)^{0.258}$, for $1 < \Delta T < 20^\circ C$.

[b]Rapp (1970) discusses how theoretical analyses indicate that K_e/K_c should equal approximately 2.2.

[c]Based on studies with simple geometric models, as cited by Colin and Houdas (1967).

moving at 1 mph (0.45 m/sec) and is at 70°F with a relative humidity of 30%. Then, since the vapor pressure of water at 70°F and 1 atm equals 18.8 mm Hg, $P_a = 0.3(18.8) = 5.65$ mm Hg. The vapor pressure of water at the temperature of skin (say 33°C) is about 38.8 mm Hg. bitrarily using $K_e = 12.7v^{0.634}$ gives a K_e of 7.6 kcal/hr-m^2-mm Hg. We next assume a fairly large wetted area, say 1.5 m^2, corresponding to conditions of moderately strenuous activity, Then,

$$Q_e = 7.6(1.5)(38.8 - 5.65) = 378 \text{ kcal/hr}$$

This is a substantial heat loss compared to basal conditions, and very important for a person during exercise, when the metabolic rate may be 500 kcal/hr or more. A higher wind velocity would, of course, greatly increase evaporation.

F. Heat Loss Associated with Respiration

When air is inspired, heat and water vapor are transferred to it by convection and evaporation from the surface lining the respiratory tract. By the time it has reached the deepest parts of the lungs the air is at deep body temperature and saturated with water vapor. As the air moves outward through the respiratory tract some heat is transferred back to the body and water is condensed, but the expired air still contains significantly more heat and water than the inspired air. Thus, respiration results in a latent heat loss and a sensible heat loss from the body.

The rate of latent heat loss can be described by the equation

$$Q_{el} = \dot{m}_a(Y_o - Y_i)\lambda \tag{5.16}$$

where $\dot{m}_a$ is the kilograms of air breathed in and out per hour (dry basis), Y_o and Y_i are expired and inspired air water contents (in kilograms of water per kilogram of dry air), and λ is the latent heat of vaporization of water at the expired air temperature (kilocalories per kilogram).

The pulmonary ventilation rate $\dot{m}_a$ is primarily a function of metabolic rate and follows pretty well the relationship

$$\dot{m}_a = 0.006M \tag{5.17}$$

where M is the metabolic rate in kilocalories per hour. Although air breathed in comes to equilibrium with the lung tissues and is therefore saturated with water vapor at the temperature of the deep lung regions (about 37°C), further temperature and humidity changes can occur as the air is expired through the upper respiratory tract. Since conditions in these upper passages will be affected by the condition of the inspired air, then the expired air properties depend to some extent on the properties of the ambient air. Fanger et al. (1968) mention that the difference between the humidities of the expired and inspired air has been found to follow the relationship

$$Y_o = 0.029 + 0.20Y_i \tag{5.18}$$

for normal conditions. That is, if the entering air is very dry ($Y_i \cong 0$), the expired air will be less humid than if the inspired air were humid. McCutchan and Taylor (1951) have determined that the temperature of the expired air is dependent on that of the inspired air in the following fashion (in degrees centigrade):

$$T_o = 32.6 + 0.066T_i + 32Y_i \tag{5.19}$$

The proportionate relation of T_o to T_i is not unexpected. We see, however, that the inspired air humidity plays a role. For example, with very dry air ($Y_i = 0$), evaporation of water from the upper respiratory passages occurs, cooling these passages. The air, upon being expelled, is thus somewhat cooler than it would be, had the ambient air been humid.

Besides the evaporative, latent heat loss associated with respiration, there is a sensible heat loss (when $T_o > T_i$) or heat gain (when $T_i > T_o$) which may be described by the equation

$$Q_{sl} = \dot{m}_a C_p (T_o - T_i) \tag{5.20}$$

Actually this formula accounts only for sensible heat loss to the dry air. To be more accurate one should include sensible heat effects associated with water vapor, both the water vapor carried in with the inspired air and any additional water vapor picked up and conveyed out with the expired air. However, even at the body core temperature of about 37°C the saturation partial pressure of water is only

47 mm Hg, so that the maximum amount of water in air anywhere in the respiratory tracts or lungs is only 47/760 or 0.06, i.e., 6 mole %. Thus Equation 5.20 must be accurate to within roughly 6% or less.

To assess the importance of heat losses associated with respiration, let us perform a few simple computations.

Example 5.6: Heat Loss via Respiration. We will assume that 6 liters/min of bone-dry 20°C air are inspired (e.g., 12 breaths per minute at 500 ml tidal volume per breath) and the air expired is saturated with water vapor and is at 37°C. Known physical properties are

$C_{p,air}$ at 20°C = 0.25 cal/g-°C

λ_{H_2O} at 37°C = 577 cal/g

Vapor pressure of water at 37°C = 47 mm Hg

Using the ideal gas law, the dry air flow in grams per minute can be determined as follows:

$$\dot{m}_a = (6 \text{ liters/min})(\text{g-mol}/22.4 \text{ liters})(273°\text{K}/293°\text{K})(28.9 \text{ g/g-mol})$$

$$= 7.2 \text{ g/min dry air}$$

The amount of water in the expired air is

$$\dot{m}_w = \frac{7.2}{28.9}\left(\frac{47}{760 - 47}\right)(18) = 0.295 \text{ g/min}$$

The sensible heat loss associated with raising the dry air from 20° to 37°C is therefore

$$Q_{sensible} = 7.2(0.25)(37 - 20) = 30.4 \text{ cal/min}$$

while the latent heat loss derived from water evaporation is

$$Q_{latent} = 0.295(577) = 170 \text{ cal/min}$$

Note that the latent heat loss is far more significant.

The total loss, 200 cal/min, is equivalent to a rejection of 12.0 kcal/hr. This is nearly 17% of the BMR, an appreciable quantity. During exertion one's respiration increases, which provides even greater heat loss by this mode. The overall rise in the metabolic heat production rate is proportionately even greater, however, and additional heat loss modes (e.g., sweating) are needed.

An interesting point to note here is the "panting" behavior of furry animals in response to a warm environment. This has the purpose of increasing heat rejection (animals do not have a sweating mechanism) without producing hyperventilation. That is, the panting is a shallow breathing that moves fresh air into and out of the upper respiratory tract only, a region where no O_2/CO_2 exchange occurs.

G. Direct Conduction to Objects

Heat loss by this mode is generally very minor, perhaps 3% of the total heat loss for a seated person. One reason for this is that, after one has been in contact with an object for some time, the object heats up and does not thereafter provide much of a heat "sink." In fact, the object then may act more as insulation, as it prevents heat loss by other modes.

Another minor heat loss or heat gain mode which might be mentioned in passing is that associated with the ingestion of solids or liquids which are hotter or colder than the body. The reader might wish to make rough computations of how important the effects would be.

H. Heat Conduction Through Clothing

Much of the preceding material concerns various types of heat transfer from uncovered skin. The equations presented also generally apply to cases where the outermost surface, instead of being skin, is clothing of some sort. If one simply lets T_s be the temperature of the clothing surface, e_s its emissivity, A_w the area of clothing through which sweat transfer occurs, etc., the transfer equations remain valid. A primary effect of clothing is to offer a heat transfer resistance between the skin and ambient, so that the surface temperature T_s can be much lower than the skin temperature, while maintaining the skin temperature comfortably warm. Thus, all driving forces $(T_s - T_a)$ become much lower and heat losses are reduced. Obviously, clothing with a higher resistance leads to lower T_s values without sacrificing skin temperature. Clothing can also act as a barrier to water, thereby reducing the wetted outer area. This, combined with a lowering of the $(P_s - P_a)$ driving force (lower $T_s \rightarrow$ lower P_s), can reduce evaporative heat losses substantially. However, if the clothing traps sweat well, it will become wet underneath and conduct heat more readily. This loss of resistance will cause T_s to rise, and thereby tend to enhance heat transfer. Thus, clothing that is highly impermeable to sweat transfer is not generally desirable.

When one has both uncovered skin areas (e.g., head, neck, arms) and clothed areas (e.g, chest, waist, hips) as is usual, one really must calculate the heat losses for both areas separately and add them. This is necessary because the surface conditions (T_s, P_s) will vary between skin and clothes.

The dry heat transfer from the skin to the outer surface of the clothed body is quite a complicated phenomenon involving internal convection and radiation processes in intervening air spaces, and the conduction through the cloth itself. One can characterize heat transfer from skin to clothes by the relation

$$Q_{cl} = \frac{A_N(T_s - T_{cl})}{R_{cl}} \tag{5.21}$$

where R_{cl} is an overall clothing resistance. To simplify calculations Gagge et al. (1964), noting for an average business suit and underclothing that $R_{cl} \cong 0.18$, decided to define a dimensionless resistance $I_{cl} = R_{cl}/0.18$. Hence for average business attire, $I_{cl} \cong 1$ clo unit (clo indicates relative magnitude; it is dimensionless). The dry heat transfer from skin to the outer surface of the clothed body can hereafter be expressed by the following formula

$$Q_{cl} = A_N \frac{T_s - T_{cl}}{0.18 I_{cl}} \text{ (kcal/hr)} \tag{5.22}$$

The value of I_{cl} for a clothing ensemble can be found using a heated manikin clothed in the actual clothing. Unfortunately, I_{cl} is only available in the literature for relatively few clothing ensembles, and I_{cl} values for some of these are listed in Table 5.5.

It might be remarked that the effective I_{cl} value for a person seated in a padded chair (or lying down) might be substantially larger than the I_{cl} value for a standing person in the same clothing ensemble.

For high air velocities the dynamic pressure of the air current can create an airstream through the clothing, depending on the permeability of the cloth material. It is natural to treat this ventilation heat loss together with I_{cl}, i.e., to measure the I_{cl} values for different clothing ensembles as a function of the velocity. However, for the low velocities usually encountered in indoor environments, it can be assumed that the ventilation heat loss is negligible.

I. *Overall Heat Loss from the Surface of the Body*

Utilizing all that has been described above we can quantify the total heat loss from the surface of a clothed or nude person, assuming the surface to be at temperature T_s and wetted over an area A_w. In succeeding sections we will discuss the broad topic of internal heat transport within the body, i.e., how the inner, or core, temperature deep in the body is related to the skin temperature. What we have discussed so far concerns only the transport from the body's surface outward.

We can write for steady state (i.e., $dT/dt = 0$ for the body) that

$$Q = Q_r + Q_e + Q_d + Q_c + Q_{el} + Q_{sl} + Q_{cond} \qquad (5.23)$$

That is, the total heat transferred to the environment (kilocalories per hour) equals the heat lost by radiation, convection, evaporation of diffused water and sweat from the surface, evaporative and sensible heat losses associated with respiration, and direct conduction.

Q must also equal the heat generated in the body by metabolism, which is related to M, the metabolic rate measured in terms of the energy extracted from food, and external work performed, by

$$Q = M - W = M - \eta M = M(1 - \eta)$$

where η is the efficiency of doing external work. That is, for $\eta = 0.25$ (which is about maximum efficiency), the body is converting 100 units of food energy into 75 units of heat and 25 units of external work. Efficiencies for several kinds of activities are given in Table 5.1.

IV. POSITIVE AND NEGATIVE WORK

It is well known that walking uphill seems more strenuous than walking downhill. Several detailed studies have shown that there is indeed a dramatic measurable difference between the former, "positive" work, and the latter, "negative" work. The energy cost, measured by O_2 consumption, has in fact been determined to be roughly from three to seven times higher for positive work than for the same type of work done negatively.

If the movements involved in walking downhill are exactly the reverse of those involved in going uphill, it would seem that no difference in energy cost should exist. However, when walking uphill the main muscles involved are shortening while they are tensed. When proceeding downhill the active muscles are lengthening while they are in tension. Experiments on isolated muscles confirm that fewer muscle fibers are required to produce the same tension during lengthening, as opposed to shortening. Therefore, more energy is expended in climbing a hill than in descending a hill (the work, as force times distance, is the same in both cases for an equal elevation change, since the force in this case is the body "weight").

For positive work, the relation $Q = M - W$ holds. For negative work, this must be revised (change sign of W) to read $Q = M + W$. That is, in negative work, more heat is rejected by the body than is created by metabolism, since part of the heat results from the conversion of external work to heat. Nielsen (1970) has described experiments which prove that all of the negative work is really absorbed by the body and that $Q = M + W$ holds. However, he remarks that it is not known whether all of the work is transformed to heat or whether some is transformed into chemical energy, thereby suppressing to an extent normal metabolic conversion processes.

The reader should consult Nielsen's (1970) work for further references on this topic.

V. HEAT TRANSFER WITHIN THE BODY

The preceding discussion has centered on heat transfer from the body's surface to the surrounding environment, and involved various equations and correlations relating T_s, P_s, T_a, and P_a to several heat loss modes. In all of this, we assume that one has knowledge of the surface conditions (T_s, P_s), whether the surface be the skin of a nude person or the garments of a clothed person.

However, one often does not know the surface conditions. As shown in Figure 5.3, the skin temperature of a person varies strongly with environmental conditions. What _is_ generally known with fair accuracy is the inner core temperature T_c of the body [97°-99°F for most humans (98.6°F average) if measured orally and about 1°F higher if measured rectally].

From the body core to the environment there occurs a series of resistances, such as muscle, fat, skin, trapped air under clothing, the clothing itself, and the air film near the clothing exterior. Each region has its own temperature, lying between T_c and T_a. At steady state the heat flow through each layer is, of course, the same. In principle, one can choose to characterize the heat transfer from the body by writing

$$Q = \frac{A_{ij}}{R_{ij}}(T_i - T_j)$$

where i and j are _any_ two points (e.g., skin surface, bulk air), T_i and T_j are the temperatures at those two points, R_{ij} is the total heat transfer resistance between the points, and A_{ij} is some average or effective area characterizing the geometry of the situation. In the foregoing discussion we generally chose i and j to be the skin and bulk environmental locations. In the discussion to follow, we generally treat the i - j region between the body core and the skin surface, and develop additional heat transfer equations. Any other sets of two points could also have been chosen, but the ones we consider here are the most logical.

What we describe below can be integrated with the preceding material by recalling that, if

$$Q_{12} = \frac{A_{12}}{R_{12}}(T_1 - T_2) \text{ and } Q_{23} = \frac{A_{23}}{R_{23}}(T_2 - T_3)$$

then since $Q_{12} = Q_{23} = Q$, and because

$$(T_1 - T_3) = (T_1 - T_2) + (T_2 - T_3)$$

we can derive

$$Q = \frac{A_{13}}{R_{13}}(T_1 - T_3)$$

where

$$\frac{R_{13}}{A_{13}} = \frac{R_{12}}{A_{12}} + \frac{R_{23}}{A_{23}}$$

This demonstrates the familiar principle that two resistances in series are combined by adding them directly. Points 1, 2, and 3 might be, for example, the skin, the surface of one's clothes, and the bulk ambient. Seagrave (1971), for example, characterizes the heat loss from a clothed person by the equation

$$Q = K_{tot}A(T_{skin} - T_a)$$

where

$$\frac{1}{K_{tot}} = \frac{1}{K_{sc}} + \frac{1}{K_c + K_r}$$

The coefficients K_c and K_r account for convective and radiative heat losses from the surface of the clothing, while K_{sc} characterizes the heat conductance between the surface of the skin and the surface of the clothing (including any trapped air). Seagrave cites values of 6 kcal/m^2-hr-°C for K_{sc} and 3-5 kcal/m^2-hr-°C for K_{tot}. Use of Seagrave's equation requires knowing T_s, which, as mentioned earlier, may not be easily achieved.

A. Role of Blood Circulation in Internal Heat Transfer

All body tissues are poor conductors of heat. In fact, unperfused (i.e., not permeated with flowing blood) muscle or fat tissues have essentially the same thermal conductivity as cork. Hence, if heat transfer in the body depended on conduction, very large temperature gradients would be needed, and the ability to adapt to varying environmental conditions would be poor.

Therefore, the convective flow of blood throughout the body is very important in internal heat transfer. As mentioned by Ruch and Patton (1965), the circulation affects internal heat distribution in three major ways.

1. It minimizes temperature differences within the body. Tissues having high metabolic rates (e.g., liver tissue) are more highly perfused, and thus are kept at nearly the same temperature as less active tissues. Cooler tissues are warmed by blood coming from active organs (recall that the mean circulation time of blood in the body is about 1 min).

2. It controls effective body insulation in the skin region. Figure 5.6 indicates how warm blood flow to the neighborhood of the skin is increased by "vasodilation" when the body wishes to reject heat, and how the blood is bypassed from arteries to veins via deeper channels through "vasoconstriction," when conservation of body heat is vital. These automatic mechanisms either raise or lower the temperature gradient for heat transfer by conduction in the subskin layers (where no blood vessels exist).

3. Countercurrent heat exchange between major arteries and veins often occurs to a significant extent. If heat conservation is necessary, arterial blood flowing along the body's extremities is precooled by loss of heat to adjacent venous streams. This reduces

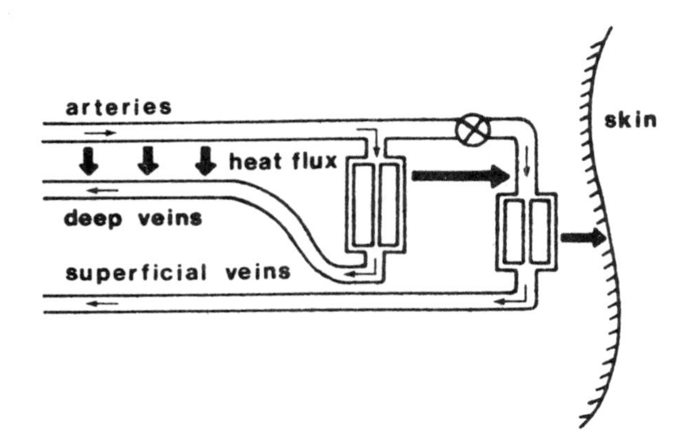

FIG. 5.6. Countercurrent heat exchange in extremities. When "valve" is open (i.e., cutaneous vasodilation), blood flow is routed through superficial capillary bed, allowing efficient transfer of heat to body surface. Blood returning through superficial veins does not exchange significant amounts of heat with deep arterial blood. When "valve" is closed (i.e., cutaneous vasoconstriction) superficial blood flow is reduced, and most blood returns via deep veins. [From Ruch and Patton (1965), p. 1057.]

the temperature of the limbs and lowers heat losses. Since most arteries lie deep, while veins occur both in superficial and deep regions, the extent of arteriovenous heat exchange depends on the route taken back to the body trunk by the venous blood. This is automatically regulated by the vasodilation-vasoconstriction mechanism. Figure 5.3 indicates how the body's internal heat distribution can vary between warm and cold ambient conditions, as determined by these three major means.

To characterize heat transfer in the nude body on an overall basis, Ruch and Patton (1965) use the definition

$$Q = \frac{A}{I_t}(T_c - T_s)$$

and determine a "mean" surface temperature T_s according to the formula

$$T_s = 0.07T_{feet} + 0.32T_{legs} + 0.18T_{chest} + 0.17T_{back}$$

$$+ 0.14T_{arms} + 0.05T_{hands} + 0.07T_{head}$$

This formula weights the temperature of each region in proportion to the fraction of surface area which it represents. The "tissue insulation" factor I_t in a typical environment is about 0.08°C-hr-m^2/kcal. Under conditions of vasodilation this value can fall by a factor of 4 (i.e., conductance rises fourfold). During a state of vasoconstriction the tissue resistance may rise to 0.20°C-hr-m^2/kcal or more. It might be mentioned here that Ruch and Patton suggest accounting for the insulating effects of clothing by simply adding a clothing resistance I_c to I_t. I_c (this is defined differently from the I_{cl} used before) for a normal clothing ensemble is said to have a value of about 0.1°C-hr-m^2/kcal. When doing this, T_s is redefined as the clothing surface temperature.

B. *A Simple Model for Heat Transfer Between Core and Skin*

To illustrate the essential features of heat transfer between successive body regions in the body, we consider the system shown in Figure 5.7. For simplicity, a rectangular geometry is assumed. Each region is considered to be characterized by some sort of average temperature T_c, T_m, or T_s (this allows temperature gradients to exist). Metabolic heat production is ignored, steady state is assumed, and the rate of blood flow from each region to the next is taken as $\dot{m}_B$ g/sec, a constant.

Heat will be transported by both conduction and convection in this situation. Warm blood flowing into a cooler region will tend

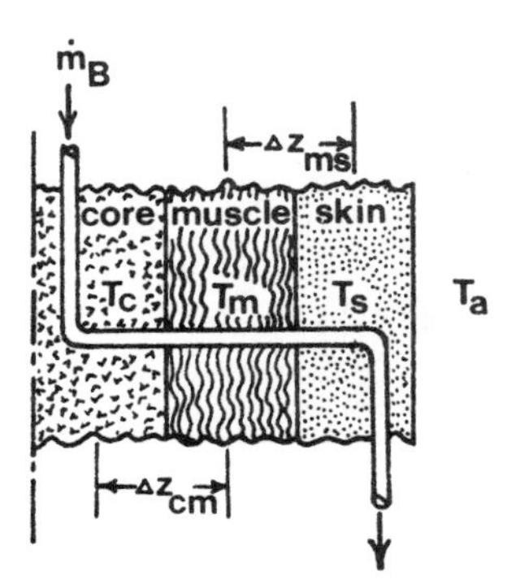

FIG. 5.7. Model system for heat transfer between core and skin. [From Seagrave (1971).]

to equilibrate with the cooler tissue. If we assume that the blood leaving any region is at the average temperature of that region (at least qualitatively correct), then we can write

$$Q = k_{cm} A \frac{(T_c - T_m)}{\Delta Z_{cm}} + \dot{m}_B C_{pB}(T_c - T_m)$$

$$Q = k_{ms} A \frac{(T_m - T_s)}{\Delta Z_{ms}} + \dot{m}_B C_{pB}(T_m - T_s)$$

where Q is the heat transfer rate toward the skin, A is the area for transfer, k_{cm} is the thermal conductivity characterizing conductive transport between core and muscle (similarly for k_{ms}), and C_{pB} is the blood heat capacity.

The system can be regarded as one containing only conductive transfer by writing the equations given above as

$$Q = k'_{cm} A \frac{(T_c - T_m)}{\Delta Z_{cm}} = k'_{ms} A \frac{(T_m - T_s)}{\Delta Z_{ms}}$$

where k'_{cm} and k'_{ms} are effective thermal conductivities

$$k'_{cm} = k_{cm} + \frac{\dot{m}_B C_{pB} \Delta Z_{cm}}{A}$$

$$k'_{ms} = k_{ms} + \frac{\dot{m}_B C_{pB} \Delta Z_{ms}}{A}$$

These effective thermal conductivities vary linearly with blood flow rate, with lower limits of k_{cm} or k_{ms}, when $\dot{m}_B = 0$. As $\dot{m}_B$ increases, convective transport is more important. As $\dot{m}_B$ decreases, or for lower ΔZ values or larger A values, conductive transport becomes more significant.

This simple model, though very approximate, nevertheless shows the basic way in which conductive and convective transport interact in the process of internal bodily heat transfer. We now consider another model of this same type, but one of greater sophistication and validity.

C. A More Detailed Model for Heat Transfer Between Core and Skin

One of the better models developed to describe heat transfer between the body core and skin is that of Keller and Seiler (1971). Their model is shown in Figure 5.8. The region of interest is that between the isothermal core and the ambient. The total thickness δ is assumed to be small enough so that rectangular coordinates can be used for the analysis. Note that the outermost portion, the skin, is considered to be so thin that its thickness is not explicitly accounted for.

The actual thickness (δ) of the peripheral region will depend on the blood perfusion rate and the tissue conductivity, and to some extent on the metabolic heat production rate. Although the tissue composition varies from well-perfused muscular tissue to poorly perfused fatty tissue (as one goes outward), this model assumes uniformity across the entire tissue space.

Let us define an effective thermal conductivity in the same fashion as before (letting q be the thermal energy flux):

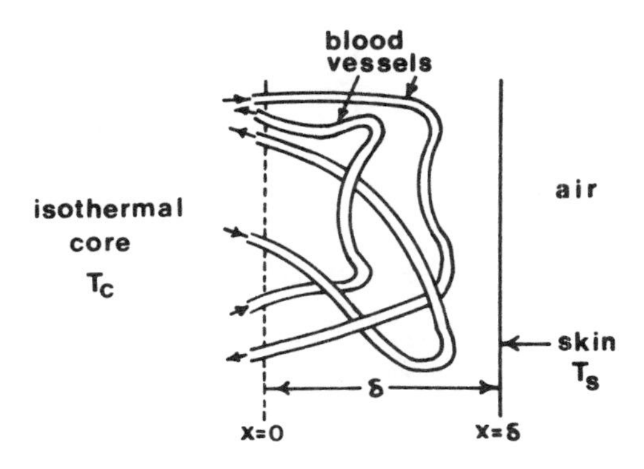

FIG. 5.8. Schematic diagram of subcutaneous tissue region emphasizing its vascularization and temperature variation. [From Keller and Seiler (1971).]

$$q\Big|_{x=\delta} = \frac{k_{eff}}{\delta}(T_c - T_s)$$

Because q will vary with x (even at steady state) _if_ metabolic heat production is important, then the definition given above requires that q be evaluated at a specific location. In this case we choose $x = \delta$ (skin). The analysis of Keller and Seiler (1971) is, in essence, directed at determining how k_{eff} depends on all of the heat transfer mechanisms operating in the tissue layer.

Figure 5.9 shows a very thin element in the tissue region, lying between x and $x + \Delta x$. We can expect for both vein and artery that the blood flow rate decreases as x increases, because of flow through capillaries. By heat transfer to the tissue, we also would anticipate a drop in temperature along the artery. Transfer of heat to the venous blood from the tissue and via capillary flow would cause venous temperature to rise in the flow direction.

Assuming that flow rate drops linearly with distance, i.e.,

$$\frac{dm_a}{dx} = -\frac{dm_v}{dx} = -g$$

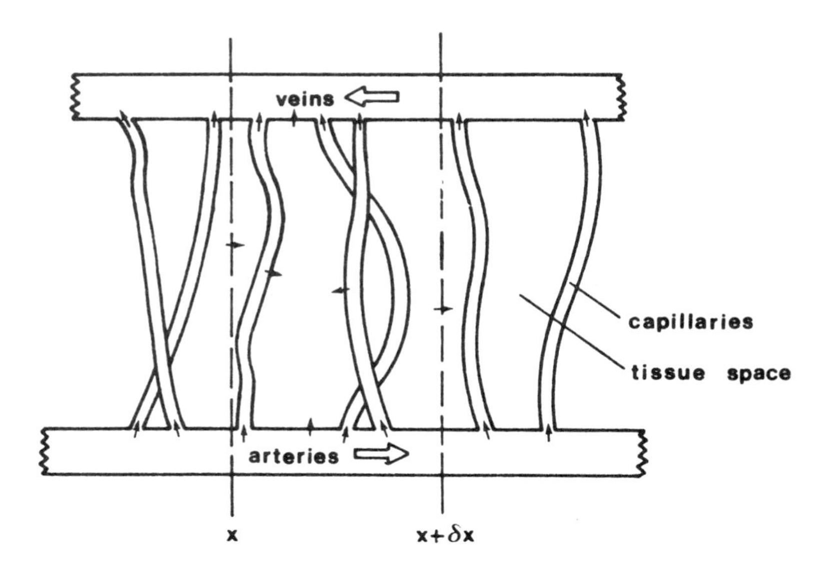

FIG. 5.9. Schematic diagram of an element in subcutaneous region. [From Keller and Seiler (1971).]

where g is the tissue perfusion rate in g/cc-sec and m is the arterial or venous flow rate in g/cm^2-sec, and that the blood entering the venous system is in equilibrium with the surrounding tissue (an important assumption), then the following equations can be derived for the model:

$$k \frac{d^2T}{dx^2} + (ha + C_p g)(T_a - T) + ha(T_v - T) + J = 0$$

$$[m_a^0 - \int_0^x g\, dx] \quad C_p \frac{dT_a}{dx} + ha(T_a - T) = 0$$

$$C_p[m_v^0 + \int_0^x g\, dx] \frac{dT_v}{dx} + (ha + C_p g)(T_v - T) = 0$$

where J is the metabolic heat generation rate, cal/cc-sec, and ha is the "heat transfer coefficient times area" factor characterizing heat transfer between artery and tissue and between vein and tissue (same ha value assumed for both). Boundary conditions are

$$T = T_a = T_c \quad \text{at } x = 0$$

$$T = T_v = T_s \quad \text{at } x = \delta$$

Since

$$q\Big|_{x=\delta} = -k \left.\frac{dT}{dx}\right|_{x=\delta}$$

the definition of k_{eff} may be rewritten as

$$k_{eff} = -\frac{\delta}{(T_c - T_s)} k \left(\frac{dT}{dx}\right)\Big|_{x=\delta}$$

1. *Solution for ha = 0 and J = 0*

When no exchange between tissue and arterial or venous blood occurs (a poor assumption), and when metabolic heat production can be neglected (often a good assumption), simple solutions are obtained:

$$T_a = T_c \quad \text{for all } x$$

$$T = T_c + (T_c - T_s)\left[\frac{e^{\lambda x} - e^{-\lambda x}}{e^{\lambda\delta} - e^{-\lambda\delta}}\right]$$

where $\lambda = (C_p g/k)^{1/2}$. A solution for $T_v(x)$ could also be derived, but was not given in Keller and Seiler's paper. Note that this case does not exclude heat transfer between tissue and capillary blood (in fact it assumes equilibration between them) but only excludes heat transfer between the tissue and arterial or venous blood.

Figure 5.10 gives temperature profiles for this limiting case for the choice of δ = 1 cm. Profiles are given for various values of λ, which represents the ratio of convective to conductive heat transport. For λ = 0, conductive transport dominates and linear profiles result. As λ becomes large, however, convective transport

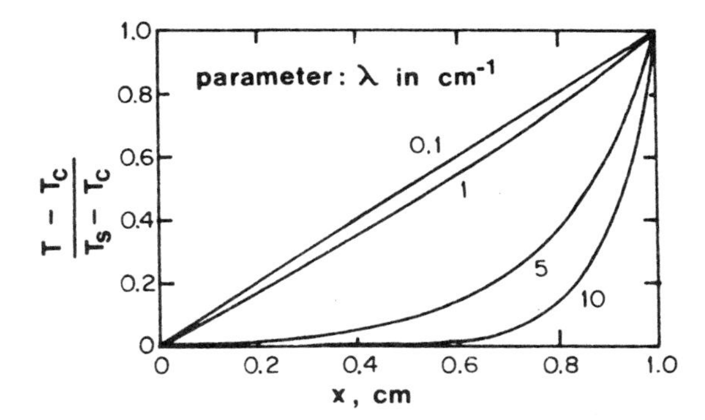

FIG. 5.10. Temperature profiles for $\delta = 1$ cm, ha = 0, and various values of λ, ratio of capillary-perfusion-induced heat transfer to conductive heat transfer. [From Keller and Seiler (1971).]

dominates, the profiles become highly curved, and a situation is approached where the variation of temperature from T_s to T_c occurs within a distance of the skin which is proportional to $1/\lambda$. For this limiting case $k_{eff} = k\lambda\delta/[\tanh(\lambda\delta)]$ and varies with $\lambda\delta$ as shown in Figure 5.11.

2. *More General Solutions*

Retaining the assumptions of g = const and J = 0, both of which are probably correct, but letting ha be nonzero, as surely must be the case, more general solutions are obtained. These are rather complex, and we omit writing them down here. However, to demonstrate the effects on tissue temperature profiles and k_{eff} that result when ha is allowed to be nonzero we present, in Figure 5.12, a few curves computed from this more general solution.

Note that a large ha variation has little effect on tissue temperature profiles. Increasing ha tends to counteract the effect of capillary perfusion until, in the extreme when ha $\rightarrow \infty$, the tem-

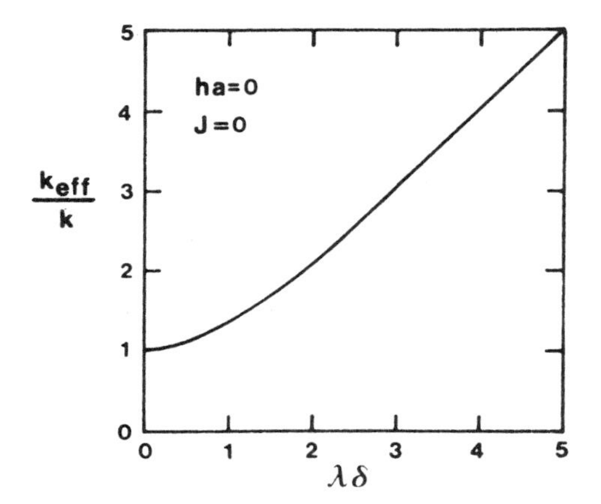

FIG. 5.11. Illustration of dependence of effective thermal conductivity on dimensionless quantity $\lambda\delta$ in the limiting case where arterial-venous heat exchange is negligible. [From Keller and Seiler (1971).]

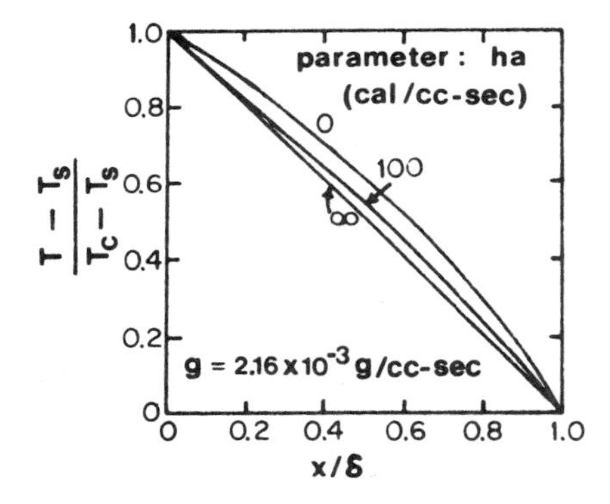

FIG. 5.12. Dimensionless temperature profiles illustrating the effect of various extents of arterial-venous heat exchange at a fixed capillary perfusion rate. [From Keller and Seiler (1971).]

perature profile is linear and $k_{eff} = k$. Figure 5.13 shows the fraction of the maximum k_{eff} increase above k which is attainable for any given amount of arterial and venous heat transfer. For $ha = C_p g$, for example, arterial precooling lowers the difference $(k_{eff} - k)$ to 65% of its maximum (obtained when ha = 0).

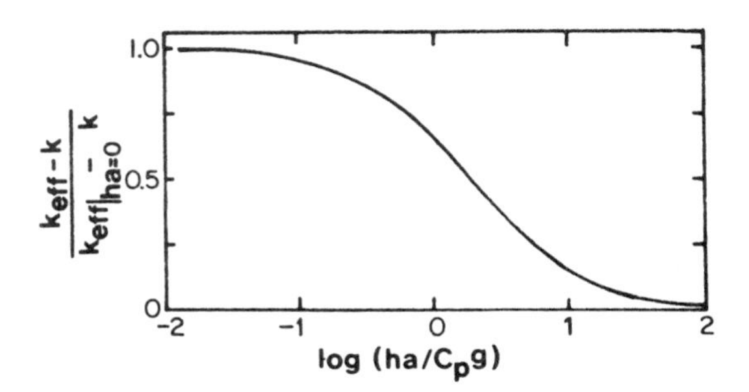

FIG. 5.13. Illustration of dependence of effective thermal conductivity on ratio of arterial-venous heat exchange rate to rate of heat transfer due to capillary perfusion. [From Keller and Seiler (1971).]

D. Pennes' Model for the Radial Temperature Distribution in the Human Arm

One of the earliest models that was developed for predicting temperature gradients in the human body was that of Pennes (1948), in which the human forearm was modeled as a cylinder. The aim of the model was to try to fit data on radial temperature profiles in arms. Pennes' model assumes:

1. A uniform metabolic heat generation rate, J_m (cal/cc-sec) in the arm.

2. The blood perfusion rate, g (g blood/cc-sec) is uniform and results in a volumetric heat transfer rate to the tissues, J_b (cal/cc-sec), according to the equation

$$J_b = gC_p(T_a - T_v)$$

where T_a is the arterial blood temperature and T_v is the venous blood temperature.

3. The temperature of blood leaving the capillaries and returning to the veins is given by

$$T_v = T + K(T_a - T)$$

where T is the tissue temperature, and K is an equilibration constant with a value between 0 and 1. Hence, one can write

$$J_b = gC_p(1 - K)(T_a - T)$$

in general. For K = 0, complete equilibration pertains, $T_v = T$, and therefore $J_b = gC_p(T_a - T)$.

4. Uniform thermal conductivity k in all arm regions.

5. No axial or angular temperature gradients.

6. Steady-state conditions.

7. Heat loss to the environment follows Newton's law of cooling, i.e.,

$$q = -k \left[\frac{dT}{dr}\right]_{r=a} = H(T_s - T_e)$$

where T_s is the surface temperature, T_e is the environment bulk temperature, and a is the arm radius.

Note that, while T_a is usually a constant, T_v (and hence J_b) normally varies with radial position, r.

A heat balance on a radial increment of the arm yields the equation

$$-k\left[\frac{d^2T}{dr^2} + \frac{1}{r}\,\frac{dT}{dr}\right] = J_m + J_b$$

This must be solved subject to the boundary condition described under assumption 7 above. For the special case of $J_m + J_b$ = const (which really only occurs when $J_m >> J_b$), the solution is

$$T = T_s - \frac{(J_m + J_b)}{4k}[a^2 + r^2]$$

in terms of T and T_s, or

$$T = T_{ax} - \frac{(J_m + J_b)}{4k} r^2$$

in terms of T_{ax} (the center line, or axis, temperature) and T. Note that

$$T_{ax} = T_s - \frac{(J_m + J_b)}{4k} a^2$$

When $J_b = gC_p(1 - K)(T_a - T)$, as shown above, the conduction equation becomes

$$\frac{d^2T}{dr^2} + \frac{1}{r}\frac{dT}{dr} + AT = B$$

where

$$A = \frac{gC_p(K - 1)}{k} \qquad B = gC_p\frac{(K - 1)T_a - J_m}{k}$$

The solution of this is

$$T = \frac{(T_s - B/A)J_0(i\sqrt{A}r) + B}{J_0(i\sqrt{A}a) \qquad A}$$

where J_0 is the Bessel function of an imaginary variable of zero order and the first kind. Pennes also derived the relation between T_s and the environmental temperature from this by substitution of the boundary condition into the result given above. The relation is

$$T_s = \frac{(Bk/\sqrt{A})[-iJ_1(i\sqrt{A}a)] + HJ_0(i\sqrt{A}a)T_e}{k\sqrt{A}[-iJ_1(i\sqrt{A}a)] + HJ_0(i\sqrt{A}a)}$$

where J_1 is the Bessel function of an imaginary variable of the first order and first kind.

Figure 5.14 shows a comparison of this model with some experimental data. The lowest curve is the theoretical result for uniform J_b, in this case for $J_b = 0$ (e.g., as would occur for zero blood flow). The only heat source is metabolism, and, from data of other investigators, J_m was set at 0.0001. The dashed curves in

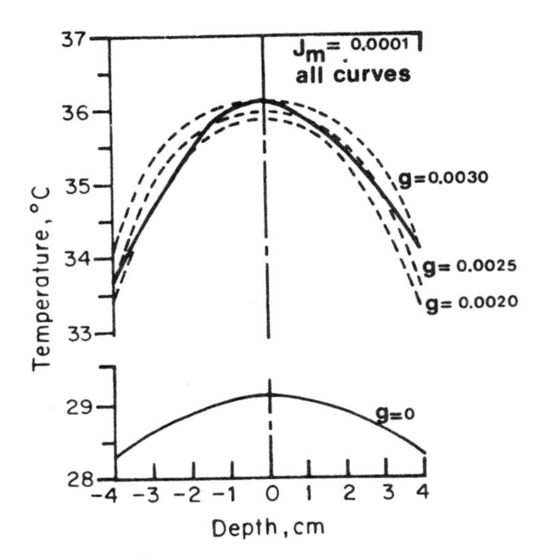

FIG. 5.14. Radial temperature profiles in the human arm from Pennes' model and experimental data. [From Pennes (1948).]

the upper portion of the figure are theoretical curves evaluated from the preceding two equations, for the case where J_b is a function of T. Full equilibration between blood and tissue was assumed (K = 0). Again a value of J_m = 0.0001 was used. T_e was experimentally measured as 26.6°C. T_a was not measured and a temperature of 36.25°C was arbitrarily assigned (with a look at the data, no doubt). The blood flow rate g was varied, as the curves show. The experimental curve (solid line) is most closely approximated when g $\cong$ 0.0002-0.0003. As discussed by Pennes, the only data available on the human forearm suggest values in the range 0.00025-0.0005. If K = 0.50 (half-equilibration), the best fit of theory with data is obtained when g $\cong$ 0.0004-0.0005. These values still seem reasonable. However, it is unlikely that K would be as high as 0.5.

Other parameters used were C_p = 1.0 cal/g-°C, H = 0.0001 cal/cm^2-sec-°C, and k = 0.0005 cal/cm-sec-°C. The experimental data were obtained by inserting a needle containing a thermocouple through the arms of several subjects. Traverses were made horizontally at a point about one-third of the way from the elbow to the wrist. The single experimental curve in Figure 5.14 represents the mean of all data for all subjects.

E. A Model for Axial Temperature Profiles in Extremities

All of the models considered thus far have been concerned with predicting radial temperature distributions. However, in extremities (arms, legs) the variation of temperature with axial length is often crucial in determining heat losses from the extremities. The phenomenon of countercurrent arterial-venous exchange which precools or prewarms arterial blood plays a central role in the conservation or rejection of body heat, as described earlier.

Mitchell and Myers (1968) have developed a simple model for countercurrent exchange in limbs, shown schematically in Figure 5.15. Their model assumes that (a) temperatures vary only axially, (b) constant transfer coefficients characterize heat transfer between artery and vein, artery and environment, and vein and environment, (c) blood flow rates are constant in the arteries and

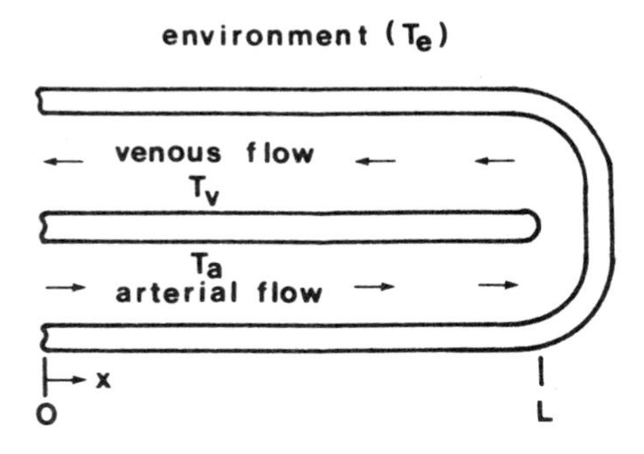

FIG. 5.15. Analytical model for countercurrent heat exchange. [From Mitchell and Myers (1968).]

veins, (d) metabolic heat generation is neglibible, (e) steady state exists, and (f) all blood and tissue properties are constant.

Differential thermal balances on their model yield the following equations:

$$\text{Arteries}\quad \dot{m}C_p \frac{dT_a}{dx} + (UA)_i(T_a - T_v) + (UA)_a(T_a - T_e) = 0$$

$$\text{Veins:}\quad \dot{m}C_p \frac{dT_v}{dx} + (UA)_i(T_a - T_v) - (UA)_v(T_v - T_e) = 0$$

which must be solved in conjunction with the boundary conditions

$$T_a = T_o \quad \text{at } x = 0$$

$$T_a = T_v \quad \text{at } x = L$$

Here T_e is environment temperature, $(UA)_i$ is the transfer coefficient times area factor characterizing heat exchange between arteries and veins, and L is the length of the extremity.

If we define dimensionless conductances as

$$N_a = \frac{(UA)_a L}{\dot{m}C_p}, \quad N_v = \frac{(UA)_v L}{\dot{m}C_p}$$

$$N_i = \frac{(UA)_i L}{\dot{m}C_p}$$

dimensionless temperatures as

$$u = \frac{T_a - T_e}{T_o - T_e}, \quad \nu = \frac{T_v - T_e}{T_o - T_e}$$

and dimensionless distance as $\xi = x/L$, then our set of equations becomes

$$\text{Arterial flow:}\quad \frac{du}{d\xi} + N_i(u - \nu) + N_a u = 0$$

$$\text{Venous flow:}\quad \frac{d\nu}{d\xi} + N_i(u - \nu) - N_v\nu = 0$$

with boundary conditions $u(0) = 1$ and $u(1) = \nu(1)$.
These are linear equations and are easily solved to give

$$u = \exp\left[\frac{(N_v - N_a)\xi}{2}\right] \frac{B \cosh A(1 - \xi) + \sinh A(1 - \xi)}{B \cosh A + \sinh A}$$

$$\nu = \exp\left[\frac{(N_v - N_a)\xi}{2}\right] \frac{B \cosh A(1 - \xi) - \sinh A(1 - \xi)}{B \cosh A + \sinh A}$$

where

$$A = \frac{1}{2}\left[(N_a + N_v)(N_a + N_v + 4N_i)\right]^{1/2}$$

$$B = \left[\frac{N_a + N_v + 4N_i}{N_a + N_v}\right]^{1/2}$$

For the type of configurations shown in Figure 5.16, where the numbers and locations of arteries and veins are quite similar, it is reasonable to assume that $N_a \cong N_v$. When this is true the solutions

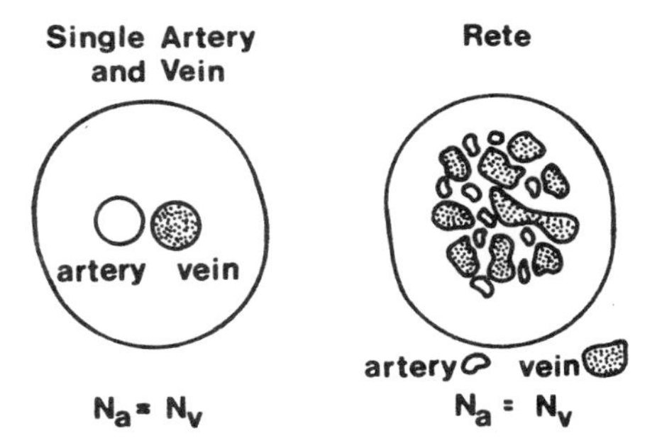

FIG. 5.16. Anatomical models for countercurrent heat exchange. [From Mitchell and Myers (1968).]

presented above become a bit simpler, as given below. Two main parameters appear which govern the heat transfer behavior: N_o, the conductance between arteries or veins and the environment, and N_i, the conductance between arteries and veins. The solutions are

$$u = \frac{B \cosh A(1 - \xi) + \sinh A(1 - \xi)}{B \cosh A + \sinh A}$$

$$\nu = \frac{B \cosh A(1 - \xi) - \sinh A(1 - \xi)}{B \cosh A + \sinh A}$$

where

$$N_o = N_a = N_v$$

$$A = N_o \left[1 + 2\frac{N_i}{N_o} \right]^{1/2}$$

$$B = \left[1 + 2\frac{N_i}{N_o} \right]^{1/2}$$

A graphical presentation of this solution is shown in Figure 5.17 for various N_o and N_i/N_o values. For low values of N_o, little cooling of the arterial or venous flows exists. When N_o is large, however, the arterial blood undergoes a significant temperature drop. It is interesting to note that substantial rewarming of the venous blood will then occur <u>if</u> N_i is relatively large, while in the other extreme, if $N_i \cong 0$, the venous blood not only fails to rewarm but continues to cool off. Mitchell and Myers (1968) have shown that the most <u>probable</u> ranges of values for N_i and N_o are

$$N_i = 0.08\text{-}0.4, \quad N_o = 0.08\text{-}4, \quad \frac{N_i}{N_o} = 1$$

Figure 5.17 encompasses these ranges. Further details of their model are omitted here. However, it should be mentioned that two of their assumptions seem to be particularly suspect. One is their assumption

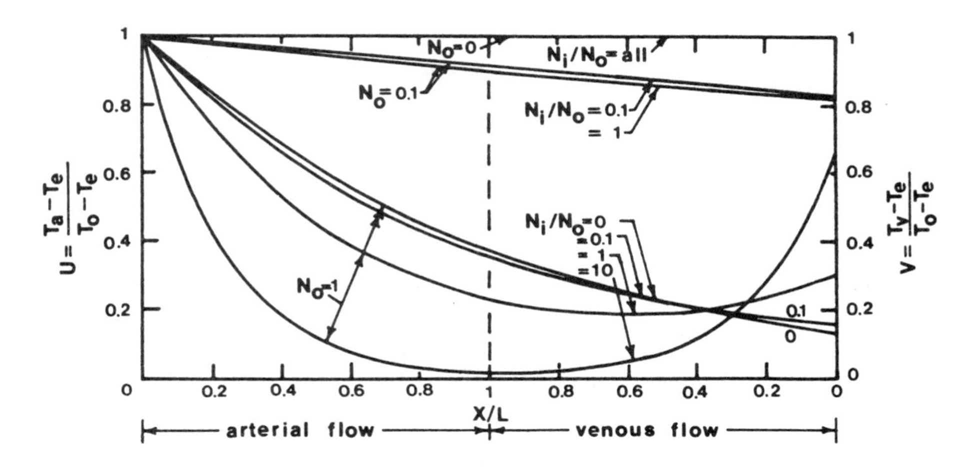

FIG. 5.17. Axial temperature profiles in the arteries and veins of the human arm. [From the model of Mitchell and Myers (1968).]

of constant blood flow rates down the arteries and back up the veins. Interconnection by capillaries would make a decrease with distance more likely [as Keller and Seiler (1971) assumed]. Second, their model essentially views the arteries and veins as being uniformly and symmetrically dispersed through the cross section of the limb. Figure 5.18, which shows an anatomical cross section through the upper arm, suggests that this is hardly the case. Nevertheless, their model is useful as a first approximation since the major phenomena are represented.

F. *Wissler's Model for the Entire Body*

Wissler (1966) has developed a series of models for the whole body. His earliest model was a direct extension of the cylindrical model of Pennes in which the body was represented by six interconnected cylindrical elements: two arms, two legs, head, and torso. Each element was assumed to be uniform in all respects (properties, blood perfusion rate, metabolic heat generation rate).

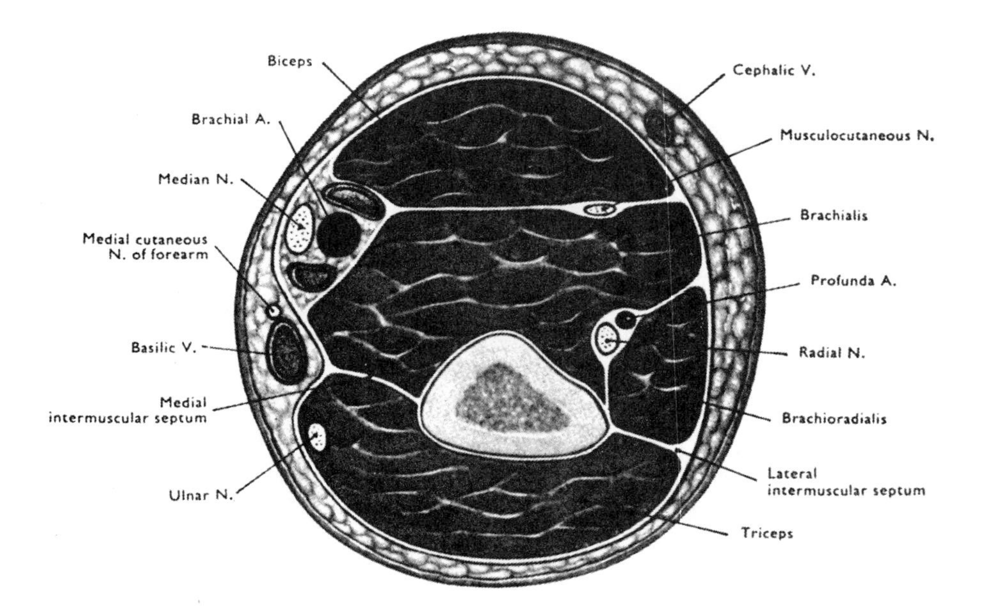

FIG. 5.18. Section through the distal third of the right arm. [From *Cunningham's Manual of Practical Anatomy*, 13th ed., Vol. 1, Oxford Univ. Press, London, 1966, p. 65.]

For the ith element, the steady-state energy balance equation is

$$k_i\left[\frac{d^2T_i}{dr^2} + \frac{1}{r}\frac{dT_i}{dr}\right] + J_{mi} + (V\rho C_p)_i(T_{ai} - T_i) = 0$$

where transfer between arteries or veins and tissue is neglected (only capillary-tissue transfer is accounted for, and equilibration is assumed). The boundary condition on this equation is

$$-k_i \left.\frac{dT_i}{dr}\right|_{r=a_i} = H_i(T_i - T_{ei})$$

where T_{ei} is the environment temperature adjacent to element i. H_i was written as $H_i = H_r + H_c + H_e$, the sum of radiative, convective, and evaporation heat transfer coefficients. Each coefficient was estimated from correlations and physiological data.

Connections between the six elements were made at a heart-and-lung junction, where all venous streams are mixed. An energy balance on this junction states that the rate of heat transport into it (venous blood) equals the rate of heat transport out of it (arterial blood) plus the rate of heat loss through the respiratory system, i.e.,

$$\sum_{i=1}^{6} \pi a_i^2 L_i (V\rho C_p)_i (T_{ha} - T_{vi}) = -Q_r$$

Countercurrent heat exchange between the large arteries and veins was accounted for approximately by separate countercurrent heat exchangers located between each element and the heart. The equation characterizing each exchanger was

$$T_{ha} - T_{ai} = \frac{(UA)_i}{\pi a_i^2 L_i (V\rho C_p)_i}(T_{ha} - T_{vi})$$

Analytical solutions for this model were obtained, and steady-state temperature profiles for various environmental conditions were presented graphically.

Wissler later extended this same model to unsteady-state situations by including terms of the form $\rho C_p(\partial T_i/\partial t)$ on the right-hand side of the heat balance equations. Of greater interest, however, is a subsequent unsteady-state model developed by Wissler in which the body was modeled using 15 cylindrical elements. This model is shown in Figure 5.19. Several factors, such as local blood flow rate variations, thermal conductivity variations, metabolic heat generation variations, heat losses via sweating, and effects of body geometry differences, were taken into account. The solutions were obtained by numerical integration using a digital computer. The basic heat balance equations for each element in this extended model had the form

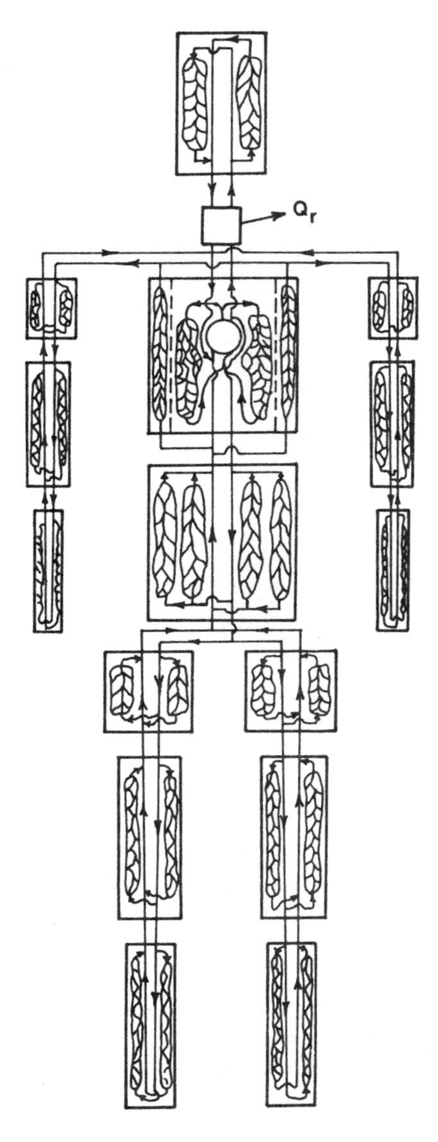

FIG. 5.19. A schematic diagram showing the geometric arrangement of the elements and the circulatory system. [From Wissler (1966).]

$$(\rho C_p)_i \frac{\partial T_i}{\partial t} = \frac{1}{r}\frac{\partial}{\partial r}\left(k_i r \frac{\partial T_i}{\partial r}\right) + J_{mi} + q_{ci}'(T_{ai} - T_i)$$

$$+ h_{ai}(T_{ai} - T_i) + h_{vi}(T_{vi} - T_i)$$

where heat transfer between arteries or veins and tissues is now accounted for. Hence, energy balances for the arterial and venous blood pools in each element are also needed. These take the forms

$$(M'C_p)_{ai} \frac{\partial T_{ai}}{\partial t} = Q_{ai}(T_{am} - T_{ai}) + 2\pi L_i \int_0^{a_i} h_{ai}(T_i - T_{ai})\, r\, dr +$$

$$H_{avi}(T_{vi} - T_{ai})$$

and

$$(M'C_p)_{vi} \frac{\partial T_{vi}}{\partial t} = Q_{vi}(T_{vn} - T_{vi}) + 2\pi L_i \int_0^{a_i} (q_{ci} + h_{vi})(T_i - T_{vi})\, r$$

$$dr + H_{avi}(T_{ai} - T_{vi})$$

Special modifications of these equations are needed for particular elements, e.g., the thoracic element where the heart and lungs are located. Appropriate initial and boundary conditions complete the theoretical system description. Wissler's (1966) papers should be consulted for details of the solution technique, and for presentations of specific results.

PROBLEMS

1. Verify the figures given in Table 5.2 for the metabolism of glucose.

2. *Drinking hot coffee.* You are cold, and your average body temperature is 96°F. If you drink a cup of hot coffee (8 oz, 140°F), how

much would this raise your body temperature, if evenly distributed? If the heat were distributed initially to only about 20% of your body mass (visceral region), what would the temperature rise of this region be? Do you feel the psychological benefits of the hot coffee are more or less important than the physiological benefits?

3. *Heat production and loss in a marathon runner.* A white male, 5 ft 8 in, 150 lb, is running on level ground at 10 mph in a marathon. The air is still, at 60°F, and has a relative humidity of 20%. The sky is sunny and clear (sun's radiant flux 1150 kcal/m^2-hr). The runner is almost nude since he is wearing only track shorts, and his skin temperature is about 30°C.

(a) Calculate the heat loss in kilocalories per hour from the runner's body due to convection. Assume 95% of his body is effective for convective heat transfer.

(b) Estimate the energy gained (in kilocalories per hour) by the runner by direct interception of the sun's radiation. Assume half of his body is effective for this and that the body's absorptivity is 0.65.

(c) Estimate the net radiant energy lost from the runner by radiative interaction with the solid surroundings (e.g., buildings), in kilocalories per hour. Assume the surroundings are at 60°F and assume that 75% of the runner's body area is effective in this radiation interchange. Use an emissivity/absorptivity value of 0.97.

(d) Compute the energy lost by sweat evaporation, assuming that 60% of the runner's body is wet.

(e) Calculate how much heat is dissipated from the runner by diffusion of water through his skin (assume that sweat secretion and evaporation does not affect heat loss by this mechanism).

(f) Determine the heat generated by the runner via metabolism, assuming his metabolic rate to be 600 kcal/hr per m^2 of body surface area. Then, using this metabolic rate, find the heat loss associated with evaporation from the respiratory tract (in kilocalories per hour). Finally, calculate the sensible heat loss in kilocalories per hour due to respiration.

(g) Using the values determined in parts (a)-(f), compare the sum of the metabolic heat production rate and the energy gained by radiation to the sum of all of the energy loss items. How well do the sums compare? Discuss the relative importance of each quantity in both sums.

4. *The dangers of hypothermia.* During the months of April and May the springtime runoff of melting snows creates excellent conditions for white water canoeing in many parts of the country. Unfortunately, if one happens to tip over and one is not wearing a "wet suit," the danger of suffering fatal hypothermia is great.

Consider the case of an average 68-kg male non-wet-suited canoeist who falls overboard into 40°F water. Assume his metabolic rate is 200 kcal/hr and that all heat losses other than convective losses (e.g., radiation, respiration) are constant at 150 kcal/hr.

We cannot calculate the rate of convective heat loss due to immersion in the water because the skin temperature T_s is unknown. However, we can write that

$$Q_c = K_c A_c (T_s - T_w) = \frac{A_N}{I_t}(T_c - T_s)$$

Assuming $I_t = 0.04°C\text{-hr-m}^2/\text{kcal}$ (wet conditions), $T_c = 37°C$, $K_c = 57\ \text{kcal/m}^2\text{-hr-°C}$ (from Table 5.10), and $A_c = A_N = 1.8\ \text{m}^2$, determine the unknown skin temperature. Then compute the convective energy loss rate.

At this rate (if it remained unchanged), how long would it take for the average body temperature to fall from 37° to 32°C, at which point unconsciousness would set in and drowning would result?

5. *Deliberately induced hypothermia by extracorporeal blood cooling.* In open-heart surgery, deliberate cooling of the body is sometimes performed in order to reduce the amount of artificial blood oxygenation that must be carried out (see Chapter 11). Assume that blood is circulated at 400 cc/min from a 70-kg man, whose body is initially at 99°F, to a heat exchanger where it is cooled to 40°F.

It then returns to the patient. How long would it take to cool the core of the body (20 kg) to 80°F? Assume that the core has a uniform temperature at all times, and that there is no appreciable heat transfer between the core and the peripheral regions. Take the metabolic rate of the core region to be 50 kcal/hr and use a blood heat capacity of 0.92 cal/g-°C.

6. *Heat and moisture loss by respiration in high altitude mountain climbing.* A severe problem encountered in expedition-type mountain climbing (at elevations of 18,000 ft or above) is that, because the air is generally cold and very dry, respiration can result in a substantial heat loss and (more importantly) extreme dehydration (climbers usually get lazy about drinking adequate water, since they must go to the trouble of melting snow).

Assume that a climber, during 12 hr/day of strenuous climbing, has a metabolic rate of 500 kcal/hr, and an average metabolic rate of 100 kcal/hr for the other 12 hr/day. Estimate his daily loss of water via respiration, assuming the ambient air is bone dry. Add to this other estimated losses of: 350 g/day (insensible perspiration); 500 g/day (sweat); 800 g/day (urine); and 100 g/day (feces). How many quarts of water will he have to drink daily?

Estimate the hourly heat loss via respiration (both evaporative and sensible heat losses) during the time he is climbing, assuming the ambient air is at 0°F.

7. *Insulating value of down clothing.* Assume a person whose skin temperature is 80°F is standing, clothed, in a moderate wind at 0°F. If the total surface area of his clothing is 2.4 m^2 and if he cannot afford to lose more than 60 kcal/hr through his clothing in order to remain comfortable, how thick must his clothing be? Assume he is wearing down-filled clothing of uniform thickness, that the function of the down is essentially to create a layer of stagnant air (therefore one really must calculate the thickness of "dead air" needed), and that the down is 60% efficient in trapping dead air. What would be the resistance of this clothing in clo units?

REFERENCES

Buettner, K., cited by Colin and Houdas (1967), *op. cit.*

Clifford, J., Kerslake, D., and Waddell, J. L., The effect of wind speed on maximum evaporative capacity of man, *J. Physiol.*, 147, 253 (1959).

Colin, J., and Houdas, Y., Experimental determination of the coefficient of heat exchange by convection of human body, *J. Appl. Physiol.*, 22, 31 (1967).

Colin, J., Timbal, J., Guieu, J., Boutelier, C., and Houdas, Y., Combined effect of radiation and convection, in the book by Hardy (1970), *op. cit.*, p. 81.

Fanger, P. O., McNall, P. E., and Nevins, R. G., Predicted and measured heat losses and thermal comfort conditions for human beings, *Symposium on Thermal Problems in Biotechnology*, ASME, New York, 1968.

Gagge, A. P., Winslow, C. E. A., and Herrington, L. P., The influence of clothing on physiological reactions of the human body to varying environmental temperatures, *Am. J. Physiol.*, 124, 30 (1938).

Gagge, A. P., Rapp, G. M., and Hardy, J. D., Mean radiant and operative temperature for high temperature sources of radiant heat, *ASHRAE Trans.*, 70, 419 (1964).

Goldman, R. F., Breckenridge, J. R., Reeves, E., and Beckmann, K. L., Wet versus dry suit approaches to water immersion protective clothing, *Aerospace Med.*, 37, 485 (1966).

Guyton, A. C., *Textbook of Medical Physiology*, 4th ed., Saunders, Philadelphia, Pennsylvania, 1971.

Hardy, J. D., ed., *Physiological and Behavioral Temperature Regulation*, Thomas, Springfield, Illinois, 1970.

Inouye, T., Hick, F. K., Tesler, S. E., and Keetan, R. W., Effect of relative humidity on heat loss of men exposed to environments of 80, 76, and 72°F, *ASHRAE Trans.*, 59, 329 (1953).

Keller, K. H., and Seiler, L., Jr., An analysis of peripheral heat transfer in man, *J. Appl. Physiol.*, 30, 779 (1971).

Lefevre, K., Chaleur animale et bio-énergétique, in *Traité de Physiologie*, Masson, Paris, 1929, pp. 353-608.

McAdams, W. H., *Heat Transmission*, 3rd ed., McGraw-Hill, New York, 1954.

McCutchan, J. W., and Taylor, C. L., Respiratory heat exchange with varying temperatures and humidity of inspired air, *J. Appl. Physiol.*, 4, 121 (1951).

Machle, W., and Hatch, T. F., Heat: Man's exchanges and physiological responses, *Physiol. Rev.*, 27, 200 (1947).

Mitchell, J. W., and Myers, G. E., An analytical model of the countercurrent heat exchange phenomenon, *Biophys. J.*, 8, 897 (1968).

Nelson, N., Eichna, L. W., Horvath, S. M., Shelley, W. B., and Hatch, T. F., Thermal exchanges of man at high temperatures, *Am. J. Physiol.*, 151, 626 (1947).

Nielsen, B., Heat production and heat transfer in negative work, in the book by Hardy (1970), *op. cit.*, p. 215.

Nielsen, M., and Pedersen, L., Studies on the heat loss by radiation and convection from the clothed human body, *Acta. Physiol. Scand.*, 27, 272 (1952).

Pennes, H. H., Analysis of tissue and arterial blood temperatures in the resting human forearm, *J. Appl. Physiol.*, 1, 93 (1948).

Rapp, G. M., Convective mass transfer and the coefficient of evaporative heat loss from human skin, in the book by Hardy (1970), *op. cit.*, p. 55.

Ruch, T. C., and Patton, H. D., *Physiology and Biophysics*, 19th ed., Saunders, Philadelphia, Pennsylvania, 1965.

Seagrave, R. C., *Biomedical Applications of Heat and Mass Transfer*, Iowa State Univ. Press, Ames, 1971.

Sibbons, J. L. H., Coefficients of evaporative heat transfer, in the book by Hardy (1970), *op. cit.*, p. 108.

Tamari, Y., and Leonard, E. F., Convective heat transfer from the human form, *J. Appl. Physiol.*, 32, 227 (1972).

Winslow, C. E. A., Gagge, A. P., and Herrington, L. P., The influence of air movement upon heat losses from the clothed human body, *Am. J. Physiol.*, 127, 505 (1939).

Winslow, C. E. A., and Herrington, L. P., *Temperature and Human Life*, Princeton Univ. Press, Princeton, New Jersey, 1949.

Wissler, E. H., A mathematical model of the human thermal system, *Chem. Eng. Prog. Symp. Ser.*, 62, No. 66, 65 (1966).

Wyndham, C. H., and Atkins, A. R., An approach to the solution of the human biothermal problem with the aid of an analog computer, in Proc. 3rd Int. Conf. Med. Electron., London, 1960.

BIBLIOGRAPHY

Brebner, D. F., Kerslake, D., and Waddell, J. L., The diffusion of water vapour through human skin, *J. Physiol.*, 132, 225 (1956).

Breckenridge, J. R., and Goldman, R. F., Solar heat load in man, *J. Appl. Physiol.*, 31, 659 (1971).

Fan, L. T., Hsu, F. T., and Hwang, C. L., A review of mathematical models of the human thermal system, *I.E.E.E. Trans. Biomed. Eng.*, 18, 218 (1971).

Guibert, A., and Taylor, C. L., Radiation area of the human body, *J. Appl. Physiol.*, 5, 24 (1952).

Kerslake, D., and Waddell, J. L., The heat exchange of wet skin, *J. Physiol.*, 141, 156 (1958).

Walker, J. E. C., and Wells, R. E., Jr., Heat and water exchange in the respiratory tract, *Am. J. Med.*, 30, 259 (1961).

Winslow, C. E. A., Herrington, L. P., and Gagge, A. P., Heat exchange and regulation in radiant environments above and below air temperature, *Am. J. Physiol.*, 131, 79 (1940).

Chapter 6

MODELING THE BODY AS COMPARTMENTS, SOURCES, AND STREAMS

One result of the recent involvement of engineers in biomedical problems is the growth of the idea that the human body may be viewed as a tremendously complex chemical plant, containing pumps, pipes, reactors, filters, etc. This approach is often oversimplified, especially with respect to all of the subtle process control mechanisms that exist in the body, and which are usually not adequately included. Nevertheless, this modeling approach has merit. Pharmacologists have for some time been actively developing and applying compartmental models of the body to the problems of determining how medications are distributed and eliminated from the body. In this chapter we wish to discuss some of the process flowsheet models that have appeared, and present the elements of compartmental analysis.

I. PROCESS FLOWSHEET MODELS

Figure 6.1 shows a flowsheet model developed by Huckaba (1971) and his colleagues. The similarity of this diagram to those for usual chemical plants is very striking. Note the solid, liquid, and gas intake and disposal streams (with "valves" representing the on-off control devices in the areas of the mouth, rectum, and urethra), the duplex pump (heart), the filters (kidneys), various mass transfer devices (lungs), and the process control unit (brain).

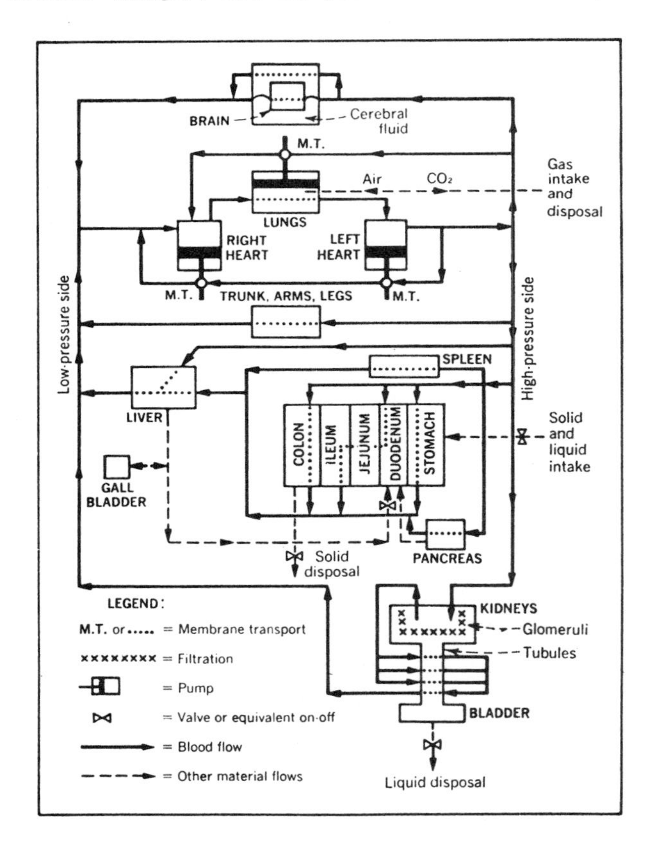

FIG. 6.1. The human body as a process flowsheet. [Reprinted by special permission from *Chemical Engineering*, January 11, 1971. Copyright 1971 by McGraw-Hill Book Company, New York.]

The piping arrangement in the gastrointestinal (GI) tract is particularly interesting.

A similar kind of flowsheet, shown in Figure 6.2, is the one developed by Hills (1971). However, this one is simplified and encompasses only the primary features of the cardiorespiratory system. Hills mentions the concept of classifying various bodily functions according to a "unit operations" scheme. He gives the following examples:

Fluid flow	Blood flow in the vessels
Absorption	O_2 and CO_2 transfer in lungs
Filtration of liquids	Plasma filtration by the kidneys, and by capillary walls (lymph formation)
Crushing and grinding	Chewing
Leaching	Digestion
Gas cleaning	Centrifugal particle removal in nasal passages; particle deposition in lungs
Pneumatic transport	Coughing, sneezing
Crystallization	Bone formation, gallstone formation
Evaporation	Water loss from lungs and skin
Convection and radiation	Heat transport from skin
Chemical reactors	All cells, tissues, organs (especially the liver)

The ultimate purpose of modeling is usually to permit mathematical descriptions to be formulated which, upon solution, yield information about a particular body function, e.g., the feedback control of respiration. It is obviously unnecessary to include specifically every single portion of the body in such models. For example, in constructing a model of respiratory control, the legs, arms, etc., per se would be omitted. Likewise, for those portions that <u>are</u> included it may also be pointless to represent them in great detail. In a model developed for characterizing drug absorption through the walls of the stomach and intestines, one would probably not model the region as stomach-duodenum-jejunum-ileum,

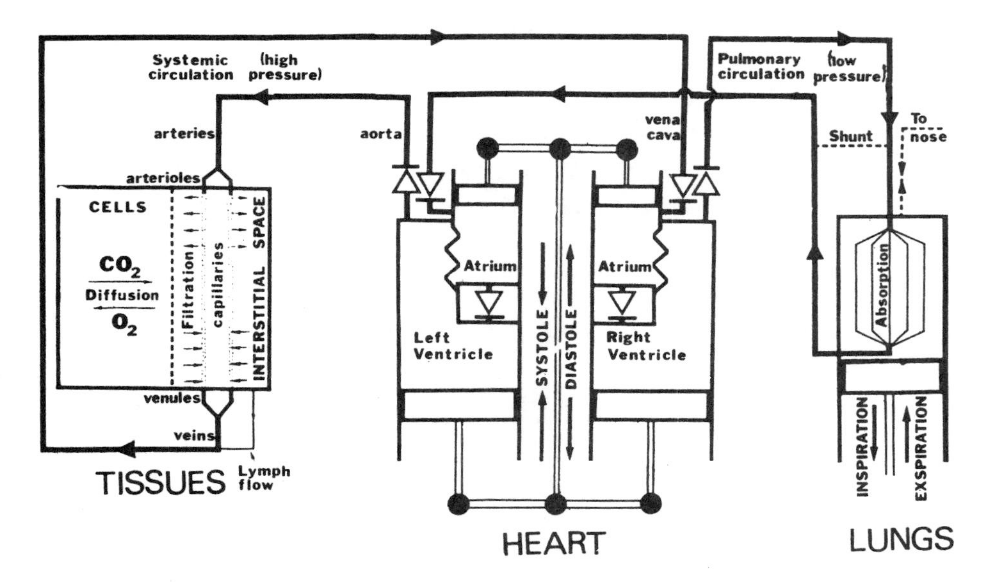

FIG. 6.2. Simplified flow diagram of the cardiorespiratory system. [From Hills (1971).]

etc., but would lump these all together in a section marked "GI tract." Hence, the scope and level of detail of every model are a strong function of its nature and purpose.

II. BASIC APPROACHES TO PHARMACOKINETIC MODELING

Two basic types of models have evolved in the pharmocokinetic literature. The type of model used in classical compartmental analysis divides the body into one or more compartments without making any particular statements regarding the specific contents of the interiors (e.g., the fluids and tissues contained therein). Such compartments are typically, but not always, used to represent fairly large regions, e.g., the entire gastrointestinal tract. Moreover, the contents of each compartment are regarded as homogeneous, although clearly this is often not a good assumption. Finally, the inputs and outputs associated with these compartments, indicated by lines with arrows, are not identified as actual fluid flows or as diffusive fluxes, but are left in general form. All that is said, usually, is that they can be zero order or first order. For many purposes, the use of large compartments without details is acceptable.

A second fundamental group of models has evolved in which the contents of each defined region are specifically stated. For example, a region may be said to consist of blood plus muscle tissue, blood plus fatty tissue, etc., as shown in Figure 6.10. Hence, each region may consist of two or more subregions. Equations must be written for each subregion in order to characterize the region as a whole. Various assumptions are made, depending on the situation at hand and the purpose of the model. Sometimes mass transfer equilibrium between the fluid (invariably blood) and the tissue(s) is assumed. Or, a finite mass transfer resistance between the subregions may be specified. Axial diffusion in any or all subregions may be neglected. Also, metabolic consumption of drug in the blood and/or tissue may be specified in some way. Clearly, these types of models are usually applied on a local scale rather than a "whole body" scale, e.g., one region with two subregions might represent the brain. And, in further contrast to the classical compartment models, the mass fluxes <u>are</u> normally defined as either actual convective (flow) or diffusive fluxes.

These latter models (called fluid/tissue models) have the potential of characterizing drug transport much more accurately, and can yield much more information, than models of the former kind. However, much more information must be supplied in order to construct these more detailed models (types and volumes of tissues and fluids, interregion mass transfer coefficients, flow rates, etc.). Also, one must ordinarily tie several such fluid/tissue models together in order to create a model for, say, the whole body. Much more computation time is needed, of course, to solve the equations for the more detailed models.

Which type of model one uses depends therefore on the situation involved (type of drug and its properties), the physiological information available, the end use of the model, the accuracy desired, and so forth. A drug that does not transfer into tissues and which is absorbed and eliminated slowly can obviously be characterized well by a single homogeneous tank, the "body." If one is dealing with drugs that transfer quickly into tissues, one might have to resort to a body model consisting of several regions, each one of which contains blood and tissue subregions.

III. EXAMPLES OF PHARMACOKINETIC MODELS

Example 6.1: A Simple Drug Distribution Model. A simple compartment type of model widely used in the field of pharmacokinetics is shown in Figure 6.3. This model consists of the drug (D), the GI tract (G), the urine (U), and all of the remainder of the body (B, body minus urine and GI tract). M represents all of the "metabolized," inactive forms of the drug. This model further assumes that

1. Transfer from one compartment to another is irreversible.
2. The rate of transfer of drug from a compartment is proportional to the amount of drug in that compartment (this is called

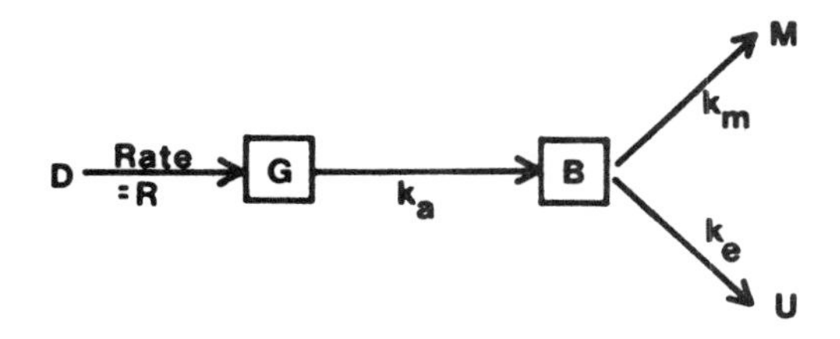

FIG. 6.3. Compartment model for drug distribution. [From Rowland and Beckett (1964).]

first-order kinetics). Hence, absorption, excretion, and metabolization are first-order processes, with rate constants k_a, k_e, and k_m, respectively.

3. The rate of release of drug from the "dosage form" is constant (while it lasts).

4. The drug is not metabolized until after absorption.

The following equations then apply (letting D, G, U, and B stand for the amount of drug in each compartment):

$$-\frac{dD}{dt} = R \text{ (a constant)} \tag{6.1}$$

$$\frac{dG}{dt} = R - k_a G \tag{6.2}$$

$$\frac{dB}{dt} = k_a G - k_e B - k_m B \tag{6.3}$$

$$\frac{dU}{dt} = k_e B$$

Integrating Equation 6.1 with the boundary condition that $D = D^0$ at time zero gives

$$D = D^0 - Rt$$

and integration of Equation 6.2, with $G = 0$ at $t = 0$, yields

$$G = \frac{R}{k_a} [1 - \exp(-k_a t)] \tag{6.4}$$

Substituting Equation 6.4 into Equation 6.3 permits one to derive the following expression for the amount of the drug in the body as a function of time:

$$B = \frac{R}{(k_e + k_m)} \left\{1 - \exp[-(k_e + k_m)t]\right\} - \frac{R}{(k_e + k_m - k_a)} \left\{\exp(-k_a t) - \exp[-(k_e + k_m)t]\right\} \tag{6.5}$$

Figure 6.4 shows a typical curve of the concentration of B (amount of B/body compartment volume) versus time for the constant-release-rate drug, and a typical curve for drugs that release in a first-order manner. Clearly, the former curve is physiologically better. Most dosage forms do, in fact, release their contents in a first-order fashion and it has only been recently that "sustained release" (i.e., constant release, or zero-order release) forms have been developed. Such improved forms ensure greater uniformity of medication, with less chance of "overshoot" (concentrations above the harmful level) and greater durations of time at or above the minimum effective level.

The various assumptions made above are common to most pharmacokinetic models. In particular, zero- or first-order behavior is almost always assumed so that the resulting equations will be linear and solvable by standard methods (e.g., Laplace transforms). Irreversible transfer, a poor assumption, is often specified, again to simplify the mathematics. One might also question the use of a

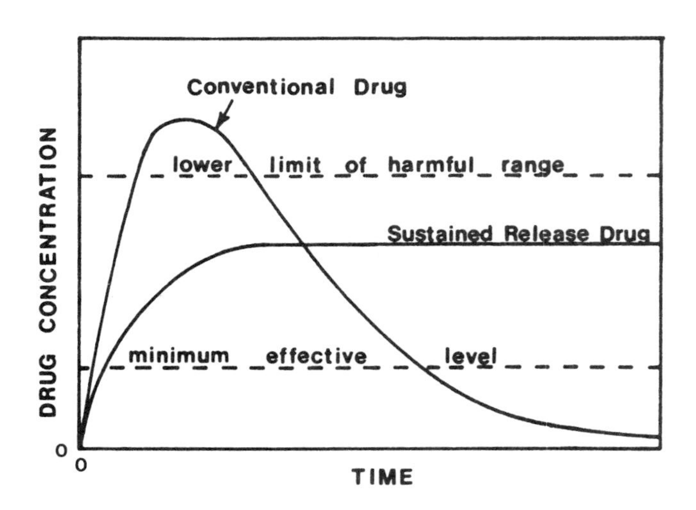

FIG. 6.4. Concentration of drug in the body as a function of time for two types of drug dosage forms. [From Rowland and Beckett (1964).]

single compartment to represent nearly all of the body. The validity of these models and assumptions rests greatly, however, on the exact situation being treated.

Example 6.2: A Simple Urea Distribution Model. Urea, an end product of protein breakdown, is present in the blood in a significant steady-state concentration, determined by the balance between the urea production rate in the body and the urea removal rate by the kidneys. In persons suffering from defective kidney function, urea tends to build up to toxic levels in the body. One way to remove this urea is by cleansing the person's blood in an artificial kidney machine (see Chapter 9). However, in doing so, the blood is often cleared of urea at a rate faster than the other body fluids [e.g., cerebrospinal fluid, (CSF)] can transfer their urea to the blood. This induces an osmotic shift of water into the brain and other regions, causing potentially dangerous swelling.

The model shown in Figure 6.5 was developed by Dedrick and associates (1968) to describe the kinetics of urea transport into or out of the cerebrospinal fluid region. The model is basically divided into two compartments: the well-perfused viscera and its associated blood, and the less perfused lean tissues (arms, legs, etc.) and their associated blood. Connected to the visceral blood is the brain region. Rather easy diffusion is assumed to occur

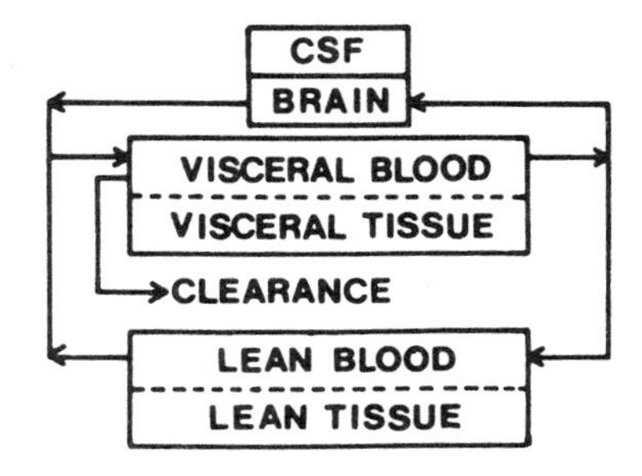

FIG. 6.5. Model for urea distribution kinetics. [From Dedrick et al. (1968).]

across the dashed-line regions, whereas much slower transport is suggested by the solid line dividing the brain-CSF compartments. The stream marked "clearance" allows for net urea removal by an artificial kidney device, or can be used (with reversed sign) to represent urea production in the body.

The model is utilized by writing differential equations, initial conditions, and boundary conditions for the various compartments and by specifying all necessary parameter values. Upon integrating the resulting set of equations, numerically or analytically, one obtains information on the amount of urea in each compartment as a function of time. The mathematical formulation of such equations is discussed shortly.

Example 6.3: A Model for Bile Transport of Drugs. As part of a project of larger scope, Bischoff and coworkers (1970a) modeled the transport of the anticancer drug methotrexate (MTX) in the biliary system. Figure 6.6 shows their model. MTX is carried to the liver by the portal vein and the hepatic artery (see Figure 2.8), and is secreted along with the bile into the bile ducts, which lead to the duodenum. If one assumes a "carrier" mechanism by which the MTX is transported into the bile, i.e.,

$$\text{MTX} + \text{S} \rightleftarrows \text{MXT-S} \quad (\text{S} = \text{carrier})$$

$$\underset{\text{(liver)}}{\text{MTX-S}} \rightarrow \underset{\text{(bile)}}{\text{MTX}}$$

where the first step is assumed to be in equilibrium (the second step being much slower), then the rate of excretion of MTX into the bile duct is given by the expression for F_0 shown in the model diagram. Flow down the bile ducts was modeled by a group of three tanks in series (this provides mixing and time delay). Blood flow rates are represented by Q, drug concentrations by C, and drug flow rates in the bile ducts by F.

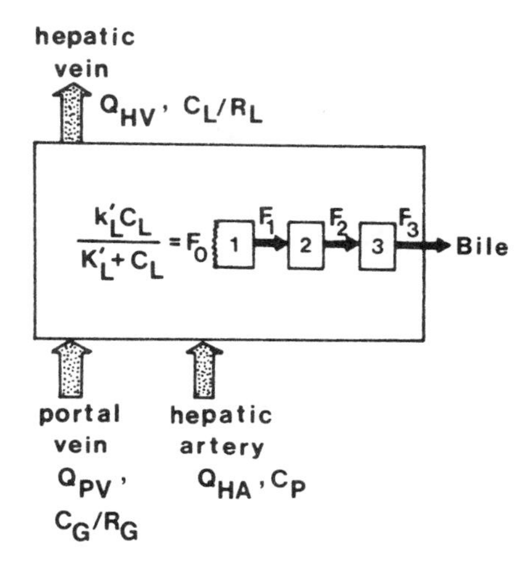

FIG. 6.6. Bile transport model. [From Bischoff et al. (1970a).]

Figure 6.7 shows a comparison of the model's predictions with data obtained by cannulating (connecting to a tube) the bile ducts of mice that had received intravenous injections of MTX. This model was solved in conjunction with a larger model, for the rest of the body, which yielded the blood plasma curve shown on this figure. Figure 6.8 is a diagram of the complete model, where the stream marked "k_L, D_L" represents the bile transport of MTX into the lumen of the duodenum (the inner portion of the tubular tract).

IV. MODELING OF LARGE MULTICOMPARTMENT SYSTEMS

Let us now consider one of the general, yet detailed, compartment models developed by Bischoff and Brown (1966) to describe the distribution of drugs in the human body. Figure 6.9 shows the macroscopic structure of the model. Note that this scheme lumps

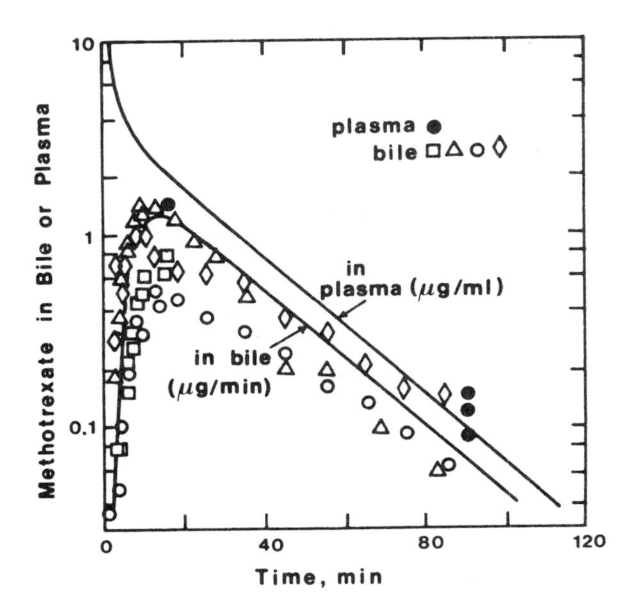

FIG. 6.7. Biliary excretion of MTX in mice. [From Bischoff et al. (1970a).]

together the head and upper extremities, and the trunk and lower extremities.

Representing the various major sections of the body as homogeneous regions makes a poor model. Each region contains several subregions such as muscle, fatty tissue, and blood. A further breakdown of tissues into intracellular spaces and interstitial spaces is also possible. One must usually assume some form of local region representation, such as the one shown in Figure 6.10. Certain drugs may or may not penetrate fatty tissue; others may enter the interstitial space but not transfer into the intracellular space. A local region model can account for such variations of behavior.

A particular, specific form of the general model with local regional subcompartments which Bischoff and Brown (1966) have inves-

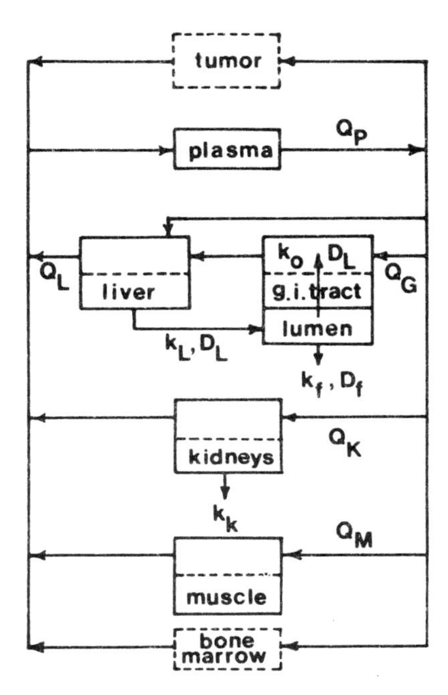

FIG. 6.8. Compartment model for distribution of methotrexate in the body. [From Bischoff et al. (1970b).]

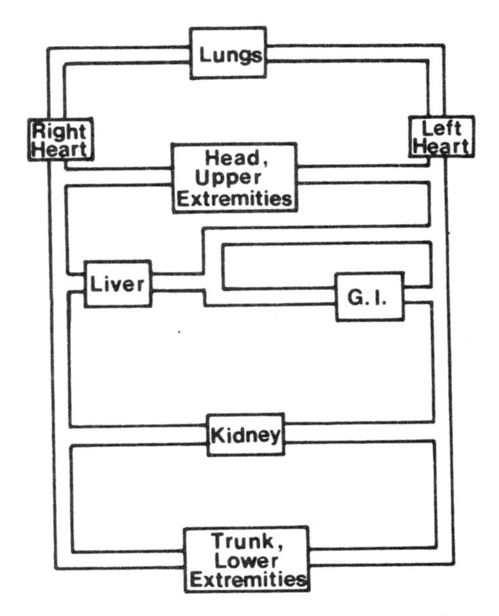

FIG. 6.9. General compartment model for the human body. [From Bischoff and Brown (1966).]

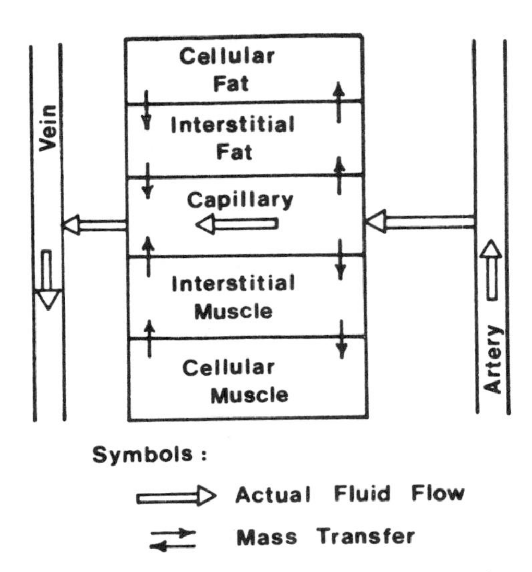

FIG. 6.10. Model for a local tissue region. [From Bischoff and Brown (1966).]

tigated is shown in Figure 6.11. Each main compartment has been divided into four compartments. Looking at the compartments representing the lungs, for example, we note that the capillary bed (total blood in lungs) has been divided into two subsections of 30- and 50-cc volume. This allows one to have a concentration gradient exist across an organ (an even better representation would be obtained using a large number of smaller sections in series, but this is too cumbersome; division into two sections is often adequate to characterize mass transfer effects). The number 288 represents the cubic centimeters of interstitial fluid volume in the lungs, while 550 stands for the intracellular fluid volume. Note that this particular model does not distinguish between muscle and fatty tissue, but lumps them together. Figure 6.11 also includes several "mixing tanks" in the fluid lines. Some means must be used to represent the blood volumes in the arteries and veins, and judiciously placed tanks serve this purpose in the model (two effects of finite blood volume between organs are holdup, or time delay, and mixing of blood coming from different sources).

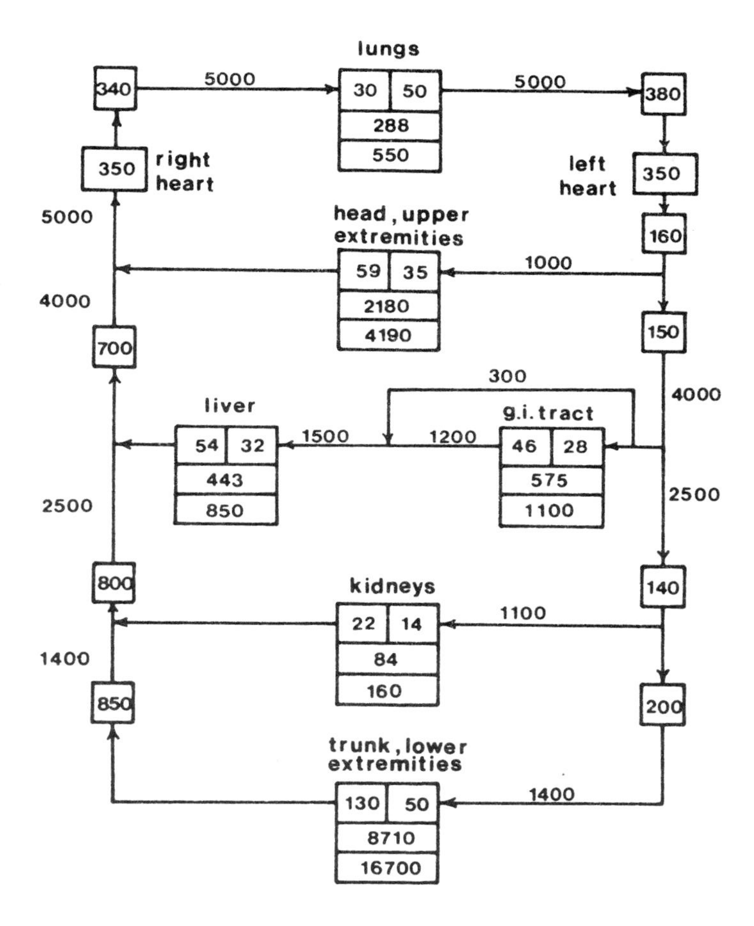

FIG. 6.11. Numerical details of a specific pharmacokinetic model of the body. Volumes are in cubic centimeters and flows in cubic centimeters per minute. [From Bischoff and Brown (1966).]

With this basic model for the human body one then proceeds to write differential mass balances for each separate compartment, no matter how small. A few of these equations are cited below:

Right heart:
$$V_1 \frac{dC_1}{dt} = (\text{venous return}) - Q_1C_1$$

Pulmonary artery:
$$V_2 \frac{dC_2}{dt} = Q_1C_1 - Q_2C_2$$

First lung capillary:
$$V_3 \frac{dC_3}{dt} = Q_2C_2 - Q_3C_3 + k_3A_3(C_5 - C_3)$$

Second lung capillary:
$$V_4 \frac{dC_4}{dt} = Q_3C_3 - Q_4C_4 + k_4A_4(C_5 - C_4)$$

Lung interstitial:
$$V_5 \frac{dC_5}{dt} = k_3A_3(C_3 - C_5) + k_4A_4(C_4 - C_5) + k_6A_6(C_6 - C_5)$$

Lung cellular:
$$V_6 \frac{dC_6}{dt} = k_6A_6(C_5 - C_6) - k_{r6}C_6$$

Pulmonary vein:
$$V_7 \frac{dC_7}{dt} = Q_4C_4 - Q_7C_7$$

The k_j are permeabilities, and the k_{ri} represent first-order reaction rate coefficients. V's are volumes, Q's are volumetric flow rates, and the A's stand for the areas available for mass transport between adjacent compartments. The equation for the "first lung capillary" states, for example, that solute accumulation (i.e., volume of the compartment times the rate of concentration change) occurs in the first lung "blood" compartment (No. 3) as a result of solute (a) being carried into the compartment with blood coming from compartment 2, (b) solute transferred from the adjacent lung interstitial compartment (No. 5) by transport across the capillary walls (note the linear driving force form of this term), minus (c) solute carried out of compartment 3 by the blood leaving that compartment.

Thirty-five equations characterize this model. While all are linear and are, in principle, easily integrated numerically (given the proper initial and boundary conditions, of course), the sheer number of equations means that much computer time is required. Two cases to which the model has been applied are discussed here. The first considers a drug, or tracer, which remains entirely in the bloodstream; all permeabilities are zero. A fast injection into the right heart (e.g., via a tube run up through a vein into this region) is assumed. Mathematically, the injection is simulated by a delta function of the form (Bischoff uses $\lambda = 100$)

$$\delta(t) = \lim_{\lambda \to \infty} \frac{2\lambda}{\sqrt{\pi}} e(-\lambda^2 t^2)$$

which gives a sharp pulse having the property that $\int_0^\infty \delta(t)\,dt = 1$. The model equations, upon numerical integration by computer, indicate the concentration of the tracer in various regions of the body as a function of time. Figure 6.12a shows some of these. Note (a) how the peaks decrease as one proceeds further from the source, and (b) how the concentrations in all regions ultimately approach a uniform value.

The second example considers a solute such as glucose which transfers well into the interstitial fluid, but very poorly into cell interiors. Figure 6.12b shows typical response curves for such a case. One can see that the basic nature of the response is similar to that of the first example, except that the peaks are somewhat less sharp. We now have solute accumulation in the interstitial fluid, as shown. The total solute injected here was predetermined so that all fluids would have a concentration of unity at large time (in Figure 6.12b, however, the intracellular fluid response is too low to graph).

One central aspect of pharmacokinetic model building is the problem of obtaining meaningful values for all of the physiological parameters involved (volumes, permeabilities, etc.). Estimating parameter values is a formidable task. A large proportion of the modeling work that has been presented in the literature sidesteps these difficulties by taking a "data fitting" approach. In this approach one simply uses enough compartments with sufficient numbers of "adjustable" parameters to permit one to "fit" available experimental data. Since one can always fit <u>any</u> data, given <u>enough</u> adjustable parameters, this approach works. However, the physiological validity of the overall model, and of all of the final parameter values, is highly uncertain at best. The resulting models are

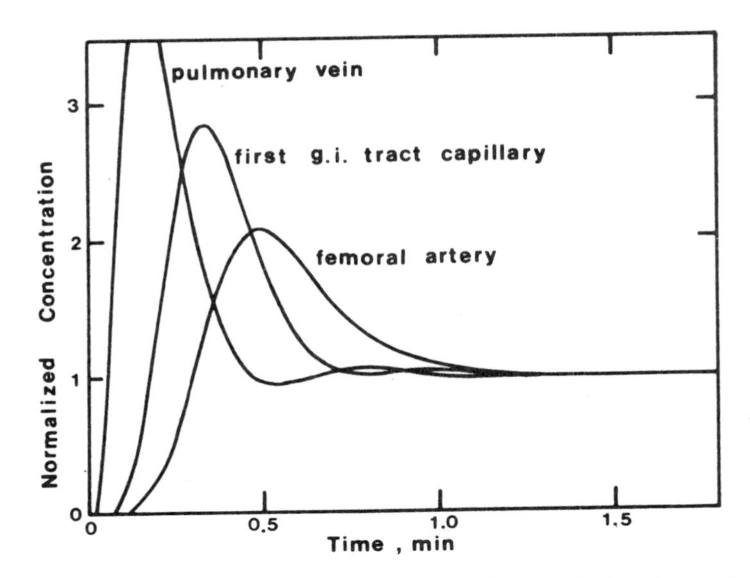

FIG. 6.12a. Tracer response curves. [From Bischoff and Brown (1966).]

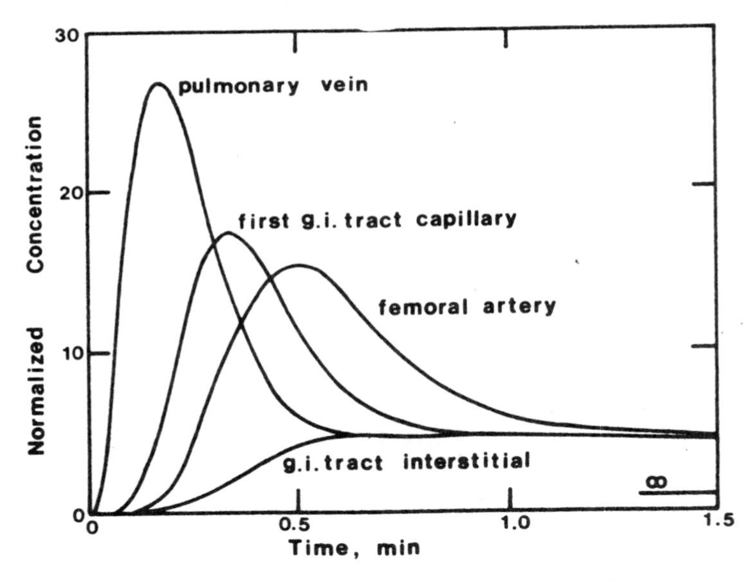

FIG. 6.12b. Response curves for glucose or similar species. [From Bischoff and Brown (1966).]

also often incapable of being extended to different situations with accuracy. To be honest, one must really take an a priori approach, i.e., formulate the best and most logical model one can, estimate parameters without bias, make predictions with the model, and then compare predictions with data. If lack of agreement is found, one can cycle back and search for erroneous assumptions or parameter values, but any changes made must be justified on some logical basis. Arbitrary refinement of parameter values to give better agreement between model and data produces no physiological insight, and is a misleading technique.

V. DISSOLUTION OF DRUGS IN SOLID FORM

Many pharmacokinetic models assume that the drug involved is liquid and is administered intravenously (thereby bypassing the GI tract absorption barrier) or is swallowed and is transported by absorption through the GI tract walls according to known kinetics (zero or first order). When dealing with drugs taken orally in solid dosage form, the complex processes of disintegration, deaggregation, and dissolution must be taken into account. As Figure 6.13 indicates, dissolution occurs not only from the small particles ultimately created by fragmentation of the dosage form, but to a small degree from the intact solid itself (while it lasts).

In practice, the complexities of solid drug dissolution are usually ignored, with the process being modeled as first or zero order. It should be realized that if subsequent steps like absorption or elimination are rate controlling (i.e., much slower), then the details of drug release need not be accurately known. Many reviews of dissolution in the literature (see the *Journal of Pharmaceutical Sciences*) will provide the reader with further discussion of this topic.

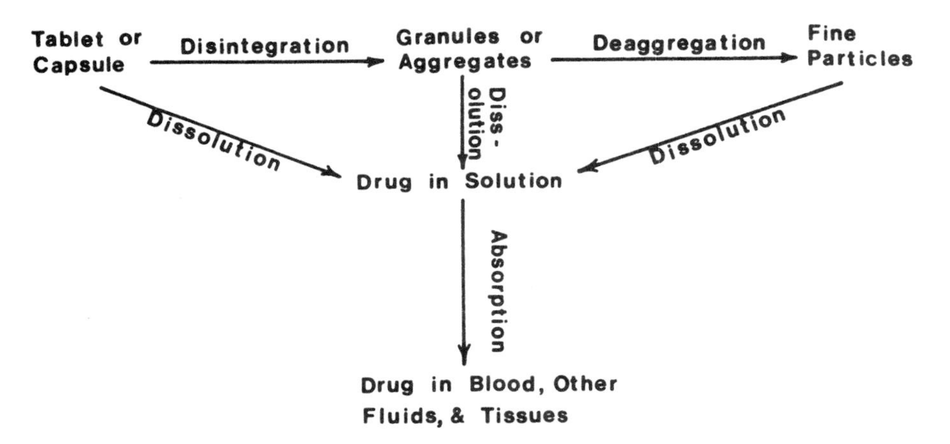

FIG. 6.13. Processes involved when a tablet or capsule is exposed to fluid following oral administration. [From Wagner (1971), p. 99.]

VI. DISTRIBUTION AND ACCESSIBILITY OF BODY WATER AND TISSUE COMPARTMENTS

It is very important, in pharmacokinetic modeling, to recognize that the total water in the human body is contained in several compartments, each of which has a different accessibility (i.e., comes to equilibrium with the blood at a different rate). Figure 6.14 shows the distribution of body water according to Edelman and Leibman (1959).

Various tracers and indicator substances have been used to determine the volumes of these compartments and the speed with which they tend to reach equilibrium with the circulating blood. Scholer and Code (1954) have shown that deuterium oxide given by intravenous injection initially distributes rapidly into a volume only about 25% as large as the final volume of distribution. About 2 hr are required for nearly complete equilibration. Other investigations suggest that between 1/2 and 2 hr are needed for good equilibration, depending on the person and the substance used.

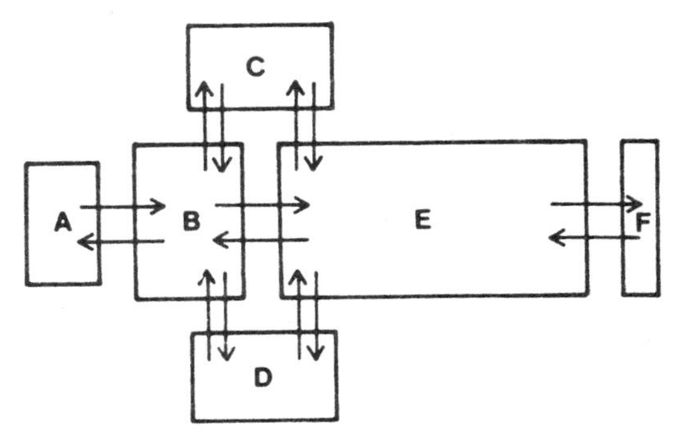

Code on figure	Water compartment	Percentage of body weight	Percent of total body water
A	Plasma	4.5	7.5
B	Interstitial-lymph	12.0	20.0
C	Dense connective tissue and cartilage	4.5	7.5
D	Inaccessible bone water	4.5	7.5
F	Transcellular	1.5	2.5
	Total extracellular water	27.0	45.0
E	Total intracellular water	33.0	55.0
	Total body water	60.0	100.0

FIG. 6.14. Body water compartments in an average normal young adult male. [Adapted from Edelman and Leibman (1959).]

Since few drugs or tracers distribute into exactly the same fluids and tissues, it is impossible to identify constant real "volumes" of tissues or fluids which apply to all substances. Even though some drugs have fluid distribution volumes essentially equal to either the total body water or total extracellular water, this agreement does not necessarily prove congruence. Drugs are known to enter some fluids and not others, to concentrate in certain local regions and not in others, to enter red blood cells or not at all, and to bind to proteins to very different extents.

Drug distribution into different types of tissues (muscle, fat) varies widely. Some substances can penetrate bone, cartilage, and other dense tissues, whereas others cannot. Lipid solubility, pH, and protein complexation are a few of many other factors which affect how a substance partitions between blood and tissue. In addition to the differing solubilities of a drug in different tissues which one would measure at equilibrium, the kinetics of distribution to various tissues are quite nonuniform. Blood flow rates to tissues range from roughly 500 to less than 2 ml/100 ml of tissue each minute. Figure 6.15 clearly shows that the distribution of a substance into tissues can vary significantly, and in particular that the distribution as equilibrium is approached is different from the distribution at earlier times.

The great range of volumes and drug accessibilities of both tissues and body water compartments can complicate pharmacokinetic analyses severely. For lack of detailed information one usually, in practice, chooses to model the body as a few large homogeneous compartments and neglects these variations. One must be careful

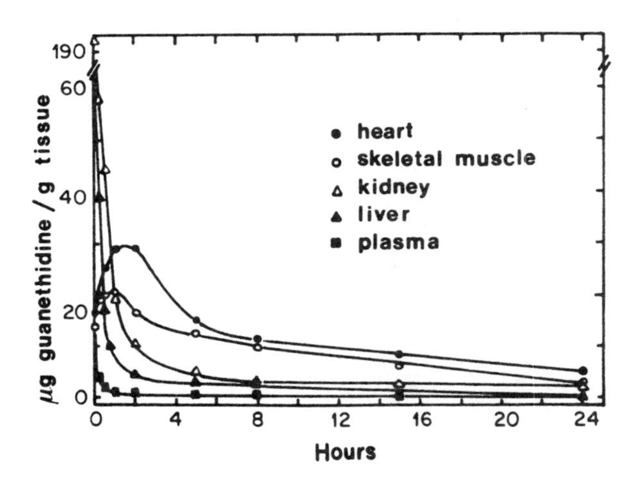

FIG. 6.15. Time course of tissue distribution of guanethidine in the rat after intravenous administration (28 mg/kg). Each value is the mean of four experiments. [From Schanker and Morrison (1965).]

therefore, after fitting data to such models and determining parameter values, not to claim great physiological significance for the parameter values.

VII. BASIS FOR ZERO-ORDER AND FIRST-ORDER CHEMICAL KINETIC BEHAVIOR IN BIOLOGICAL SYSTEMS

Chemical reactions are involved in a great many biological processes. They not only govern metabolism, but are linked to many diffusion and absorption phenomena as well. Most chemical reactions in biological systems are catalyzed by specific enzymes, and can often be represented by the Michaelis-Menten scheme

$$E + S \underset{k_{-1}}{\overset{k_1}{\rightleftarrows}} ES \overset{k_2}{\rightarrow} E + P$$

where the enzyme E is viewed as reacting with a substrate S to form a complex ES, which subsequently decomposes to give back the enzyme and yield a product P. If one assumes that the decomposition step is slow relative to the forward and backward parts of the reversible ES formation step (i.e., $k_2 << k_1, k_{-1}$), then one can consider the first step to be essentially at equilibrium and that

$$K = \frac{k_{-1}}{k_1} = \frac{(E)(S)}{(ES)} = \text{an equilibrium constant}$$

where (E) signifies concentration of E, etc. Since the total enzyme content of the system is always the same, i.e.,

$$E_o = (E) + (ES) = \text{const}$$

one can easily show that $(ES) = E_o(S)/[(S) + K]$. Now, the overall reaction rate is that of the second step, therefore

$$\text{Reaction rate} = k_2(ES) = \frac{k_2E_o(S)}{(S) + K}$$

If one plots reaction rate versus substrate concentration, as shown in Figure 6.16, it is clear that at low (S) the reaction is nearly first order, while at sufficiently high (S) it is zero order in behavior [at high (S) the process is limited by the amount of enzyme available, and this is a fixed quantity]. Of course, a transition region also exists.

Processes that do not involve chemical reaction (e.g., pure diffusion) can be analyzed in similar terms, and it can be shown how first- and zero-order types of behavior arise naturally. However, space does not permit our considering these explicitly here.

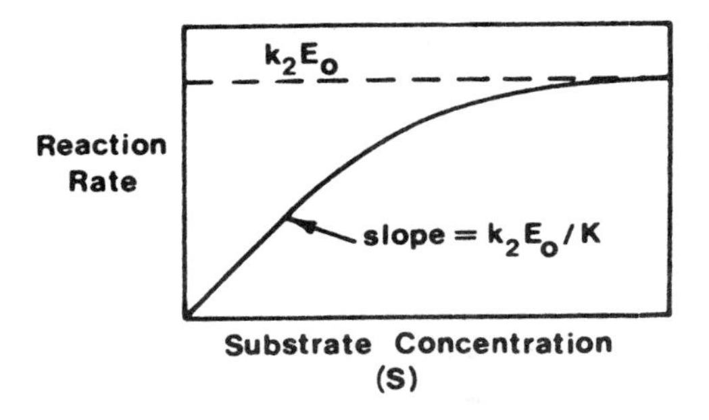

FIG. 6.16. Reaction rate dependence on substrate concentration according to Michaelis-Menten kinetics.

VIII. CONCENTRATION-TIME BEHAVIOR IN SIMPLE COMPARTMENTAL SYSTEMS

A. *The One-Compartment Open Model*

The way in which the concentration of active drug in the body is affected by the rates of absorption and elimination steps can be conveniently demonstrated by considering a simple system, such as the so-called one-compartment open model shown in Figure 6.17. This

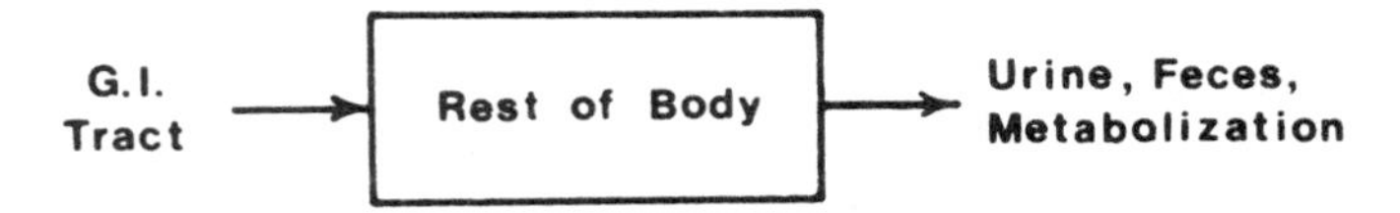

FIG. 6.17. One-compartment open model.

is similar to that of Figure 6.3 except now we are considering a drug that is readily available to the GI tract, e.g., a drug swallowed in liquid form. The drug elimination modes (metabolization, excretion in urine and feces) are combined for simplicity, since first-order irreversible kinetics are assumed for all steps.

We can model this situation as

$$A \xrightarrow{k_1} B \xrightarrow{k_2} C$$

where A is the amount of drug in the GI tract, etc. This is the same type of model as for a series chemical reaction. Notari (1971) summarizes the solutions to the differential rate laws for this system, which are

$$\frac{dA}{dt} = -k_1 A$$

$$\frac{dB}{dt} = k_1 A - k_2 B$$

$$\frac{dC}{dt} = k_2 B$$

in Table 6.1, for the initial conditions that B = C = 0 and $A = A_0$ at time zero. Here A, B, and C are amounts, not concentrations, and k_1 and k_2 are constants equal to what we normally call rate constants divided by the volumes of the compartments to which they

TABLE 6.1[a]

Summary of Conditions and Resulting Equations for the Time Dependency of Each Component in $A \xrightarrow{k_1} B \xrightarrow{k_2} C$

General case[b] $k_1 \simeq k_2$	Rapid final step $k_2 >> k_1$	Rapid initial step $k_1 >> k_2$
$A = A_o e^{-k_1 t}$	$A_o e^{-k_1 t}$	$A_o e^{-k_1 t}$
$B = A_o k_1 (e^{-k_1 t} - e^{-k_2 t})/(k_2 - k_1)$	$(A_o k_1/k_2) e^{-k_1 t}$	$A_o e^{-k_2 t}$
$C = A_o[1 + \frac{1}{k_1 - k_2}(k_2 e^{-k_1 t} - k_1 e^{-k_2 t})]$	$A_o(1 - e^{-k_1 t})$	$A_o(1 - e^{-k_2 t})$

[a] From Notari (1971).

[b] The special case where $k_1 = k_2$ has not been considered. Then $B = k_1 A_o t e^{-k_1 t}$.

refer.* When $k_1 = k_2$, both the absorption and elimination steps have the same inherent rates, and the concentration-time behavior in the system looks like that shown in Figure 6.18. On the other hand, when absorption is very rapid compared to elimination (say $k_1 = 500k_2$) the behavior shown in Figure 6.19 pertains (note that in this situation there exists the danger of reaching undesirably high drug levels). Conversely, when elimination is rapid relative to absorption (say $k_2 = 20k_1$) we would have curves like those in Figure 6.20 (note that the drug concentration in the body probably never gets large enough for a therapeutic effect to occur).

B. *Analysis of Data Using the One-Compartment Model: $k_1 > k_2$ Case*

Two methods are commonly used to determine values for k_1 and k_2 from body compartment (B) data. Both methods start with the equation (see Table 6.1)

$$C_B = \frac{B}{V_d} = \alpha(e^{-k_2 t} - e^{-k_1 t}) \tag{6.6}$$

where $\alpha = A_o k_1/V_d(k_1 - k_2)$ and V_d is the volume of distribution of drug in the body compartment. As $A \to 0$ (large times) we see that if $k_1 > k_2$, which is the most common case,

$$C_B \cong \alpha e^{-k_2 t}$$

or

$$\ln C_B \cong -k_2 t + \ln \alpha$$

*Note that if one wishes to associate a mass input or output with an actual physical flow, one can relate the rate constant k to a volumetric flow rate Q and a compartment volume V. For example, if urine is the only output from the body in the scheme depicted in Figure 6.17, one can show that $k_2 = Q_2/V_d$, where Q_2 is the flow rate of urine and V_d is the apparent volume of distribution of drug in the body compartment.

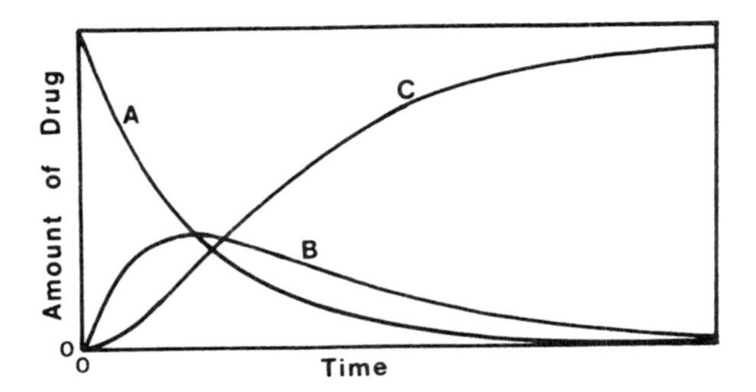

FIG. 6.18. Consecutive irreversible first-order rate processes. The amount of drug in compartments A, B, and C as a function of time for the case where $k_1 = k_2$ in $A \xrightarrow{k_1} B \xrightarrow{k_2} C$. [From Notari (1971).]

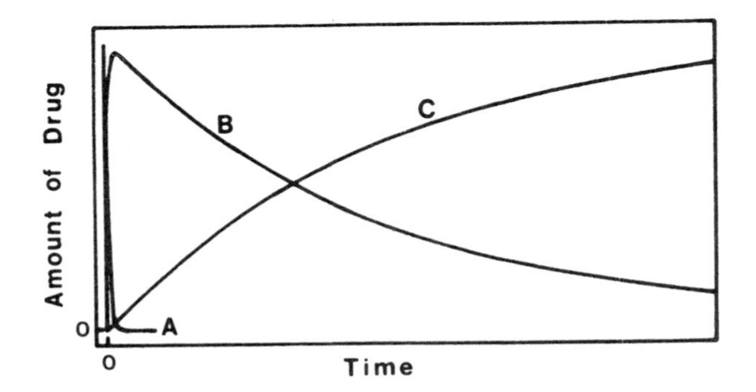

FIG. 6.19. Rapid initial step case. Drug in compartments A, B, and C as a function of time for the case where $k_1 = 500k_2$ in $A \xrightarrow{k_1} B \xrightarrow{k_2} C$. [From Notari (1971).]

Thus a plot of ln C_B versus time should be linear with a slope of $-k_2$ and an intercept of ln α. Figure 6.21 shows the result of such a plot for the case where $k_1/k_2 = 10$.

Equation 6.6 can be rearranged to give

$$e^{-k_2 t} - \frac{C_B}{\alpha} = e^{-k_1 t}$$

or

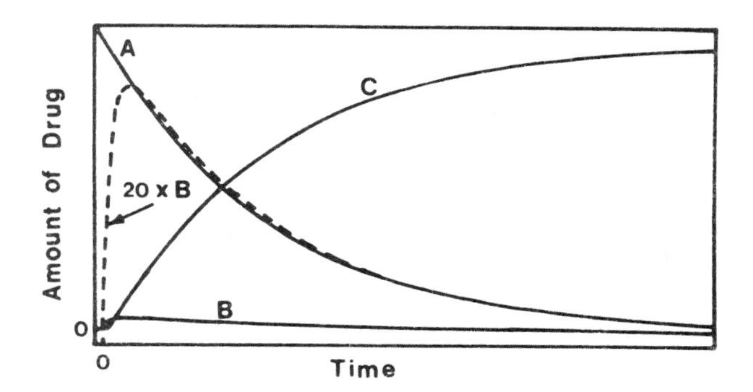

FIG. 6.20. Rapid elimination case. Drug in compartments A, B, and C as a function of time for the case where $k_2 = 20k_1$ in $A \xrightarrow{k_1} B \xrightarrow{k_2} C$. [From Notari (1971).]

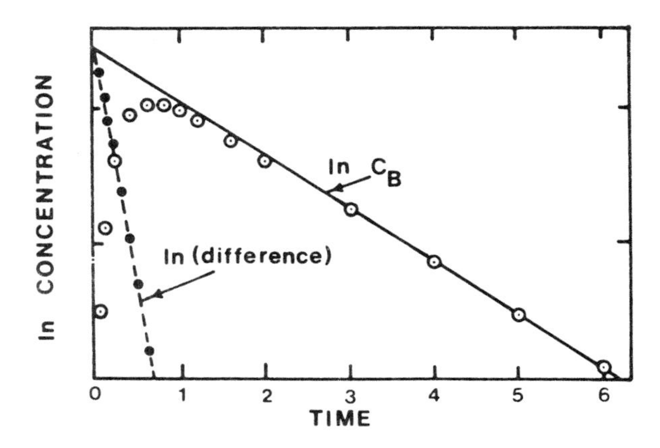

FIG. 6.21. Ln of C_B versus time for a one-compartment open model system, with $k_1 = 10k_2$. [From Notari (1971).]

$$\ln(e^{-k_2 t} - \frac{C_B}{\alpha}) = -k_1 t$$

Since k_2 and α are now known, a plot of $\ln(e^{-k_2 t} - C_B/\alpha)$ versus t will yield a linear line with slope of $-k_1$ (we will demonstrate this shortly using some actual data). Note that an accurate a priori value of A_o is not required.

A similar method, called feathering, is also common. After a straight line is fitted to the ln C_B versus t plot in the large time (low A region), this line is extrapolated back to time zero, as shown in Figure 6.21. The difference between the experimental values and the extrapolated line values is determined and plotted as ln(difference) versus time. These values can be shown to fit a straight line with slope of $-k_1$.

These two methods obviously apply only to situations where significant B values exist while $A \cong 0$. Therefore, when $k_2 > k_1$ other techniques must be used.

C. Application of the One-Compartment Model to a Sustained-Release Medication

Wiegand and Taylor (1960) studied the pharmacokinetics of the drug HT1479 [1-(o-methoxyphenyl)-4-(γ-methoxypropyl)piperazine phosphate], and interpreted their data, shown in Figure 6.22, according to the open one-compartment model. They studied the response to an orally administered solution of the drug, and to an oral sustained-release formulation (trade name Gradumet).

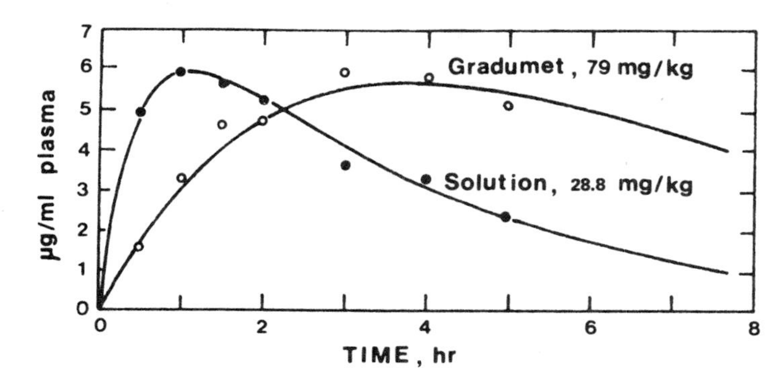

FIG. 6.22. Average plasma HT1479 concentrations from six dogs after administration of PO_4 salt of HT1479 as solution and as sustained-release tablets. Initial dose is indicated on figure. [From Wiegand and Taylor (1960).]

The sustained-release tablet, having an original amount of drug A_o, is considered to consist of a fraction f_i that is released immediately and a fraction f_r that is released in a first-order manner. The model they used was essentially the same as that shown in Figure 6.3 (note that, although several compartments are used, this is still considered to be a one-compartment model, since the body is represented by only one region). In this study, the slow-release portion of the drug was considered to be released according to first-order kinetics, with a rate constant k_r. Thus, for the amount of drug in the tablet we have

$$\frac{dA}{dt} = -k_r A$$

which integrates to give $A = A_o f_r e^{-k_r t}$ (note that $A_o f_i$ is released immediately, so that at t = 0 only $A_o f_r$ remains). For the GI tract, we have

$$\frac{dG}{dt} = A_o f_r k_r e^{-k_r t} - k_a G$$

or, integrating with the initial condition that $G = A_o f_i$ at $t = 0$,

$$G = \frac{A_o f_r k_r}{k_a - k_r}\left(e^{-k_r t} - e^{-k_a t}\right) + A_o f_i e^{-k_a t}$$

The body is characterized by the differential equation

$$\frac{dB}{dt} = k_a G - (k_e + k_m)B$$

The solution to this is

$$B = \frac{A_o f_r k_a k_r}{(k_a - k_r)(k_d - k_r)}\left[e^{-k_r t} - e^{-k_d t}\right]$$

$$+ \frac{A_o f_i k_a - [A_o f_r k_a k_r/(k_a - k_r)]}{k_d - k_a}\left(e^{-k_a t} - e^{-k_d t}\right)$$

where $k_d = k_e + k_m$. Since B represents the amount of drug in the body, the concentration of drug is obtained as $C_B = B/V_d$, where V_d is the apparent volume of distribution of the drug in the body (the body is assumed to be uniform).

Wiegand and Taylor used this model to interpret data as follows. First, k_r, f_i, and f_r were determined by carrying out separate experiments on the drug dissolving in simulated gastric juice (essentially a standard solution of HCl, NaCl, and pepsin). Values of $k_r = 0.25\ hr^{-1}$, $f_i = 0.12$, and $f_r = 0.88$ were obtained. Then the data were analyzed to yield the values $k_d = 0.28\ hr^{-1}$, $k_a = 2.0\ hr^{-1}$ and $V_d = 3.52$ liters/kg (the initial dose was on a per kilogram of weight basis also). This latter determination was actually done twice, once for the drug-in-solution case and once for the sustained-release case. Excellent agreement of the k_a, k_d, and V_d values was found. Figure 6.22 shows the experimental data, plus curves computed from the $C_B(t)$ equation derived above, using the parameter values just cited. Note that, for the solution case, $f_r = 0$, $f_i = 1$, and hence the $C_B(t)$ relation simplifies considerably. Figures 6.23 and 6.24 show the data for the solution case plotted according to the first method cited above. A curve fit to the late-time data yields $k_d \cong 0.28\ hr^{-1}$ [intercept $\alpha = A_o k_a/V_d(k_a - k_d) = 9.21$]. Plotting $\ln(e^{-k_d t} - C_B/\alpha)$ versus time gives $k_a \cong 2.0\ hr^{-1}$ as also shown. Now knowing k_a, k_d, the intercept value from the first plot, and $A_o = 28.8$ mg/kg, one can compute V_d as approximately 3.5 liters/kg.

D. *The Special Case of Intravenous Injection*

The one-compartment open model just discussed has a somewhat simpler solution for the case of an intravenous injection. Since this model views the body as a single perfectly mixed tank, the concentration of drug in the body is uniform even if only a short time has elapsed since the injection. Obviously this is only an approximation to reality but may not be a bad assumption for a drug

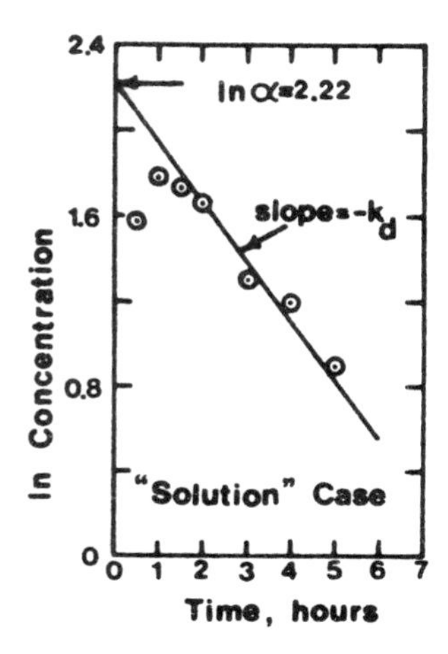

FIG. 6.23. Extraction of value of k_d from solution case data.

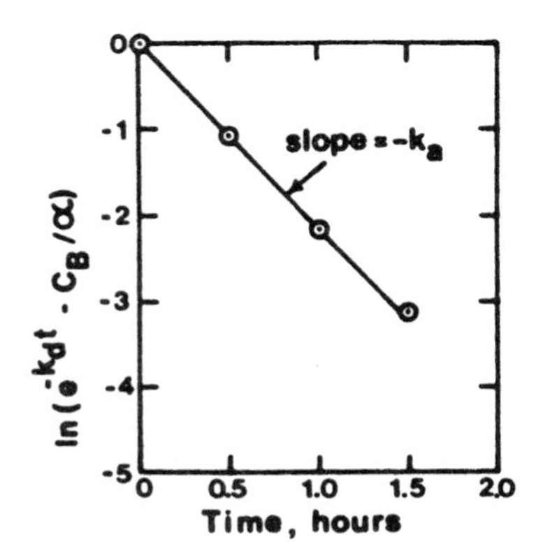

FIG. 6.24. Plot of solution case data to determine the value of k_a.

that is slowly eliminated and metabolized, and which distributes fairly uniformly among all body regions (fluids, tissues, etc.).

In this case the model becomes

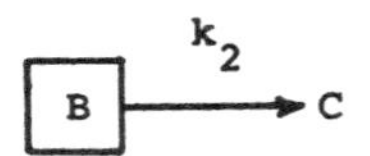

and the equation for B(t) is

$$B = B_0 e^{-k_2 t}$$

where B_0 is the amount of drug in the body at time zero. This function represents an exponential drop-off with time.

E. *The Special Case of Constant Intravenous Infusion*

If a drug is continuously administered intravenously to the body, we may model the process as follows:

$$A \xrightarrow{R} \boxed{B} \xrightarrow{k_2} C$$

where the drug A is supplied according to zero-order kinetics (i.e., constant rate, equal to R). Then, for the body

$$\frac{dB}{dt} = R - k_2 B$$

which, for B = 0 at t = 0, integrates to

$$B = \frac{R}{k_2}\left(1 - e^{-k_2 t}\right)$$

Note that as $t \to \infty$, $B \to R/k_2$. This solution is similar to our previous one for the sustained-release oral medication.

F. *The Two-Compartment Open Model*

Since most drugs tend to distribute somewhat differently between blood and tissue (and, in fact, enter various tissues such as fat and muscle to differing degrees) and since the therapeutic effect generally depends on tissue concentration, then accurate models must often divide the body compartment into <u>at least</u> two compartments, e.g., blood and tissue.

One might, for example, modify the model used earlier to take tissue-blood distribution into account, by constructing the model shown in Figure 6.25 (here P is blood plasma). Analytical solutions for P(t) will be considered later; for now let us simply illustrate some qualitative effects. Figure 6.26 shows the effects of varying the blood-tissue distribution constant from 4 to 1 to 1 to 4 on the blood's drug concentration. Note that a larger distribution into the tissues causes the blood drug concentration to be comparatively lower initially and comparatively higher later on (this assumes all elimination occurs from the blood, probably a poor assumption). Figures 6.27 and 6.28 show more interesting results, i.e., the effects of the k_{12}/k_{21} ratio on the fraction of the total dose which is in the blood and tissue subcompartments at any time.

Since this model omits a pathway for drug elimination by metabolization directly from the tissue space, it is unrealistic. Thus, it should be used for drugs that are known to be excreted, but not actually chemically altered in form.

A better model would be, for example, that shown in Figure 6.29. To be really realistic, a very complete model of the form given in Figure 6.30 could be used. One must always compromise tractability against validity, however, so the scheme of Figure 6.30 would rarely be selected. The optimum model will depend strongly on the particular drug involved.

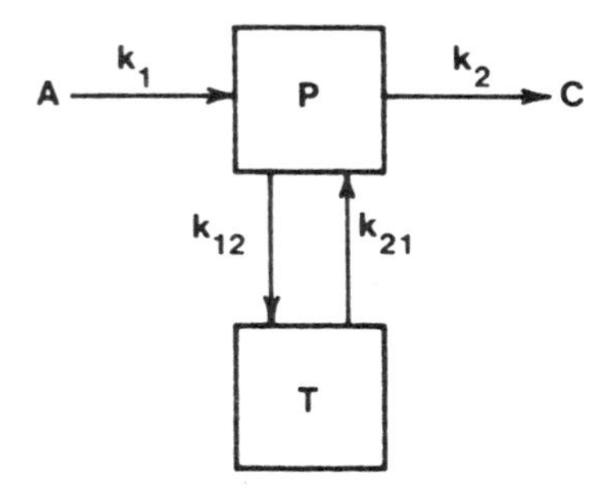

FIG. 6.25. Two-compartment open model.

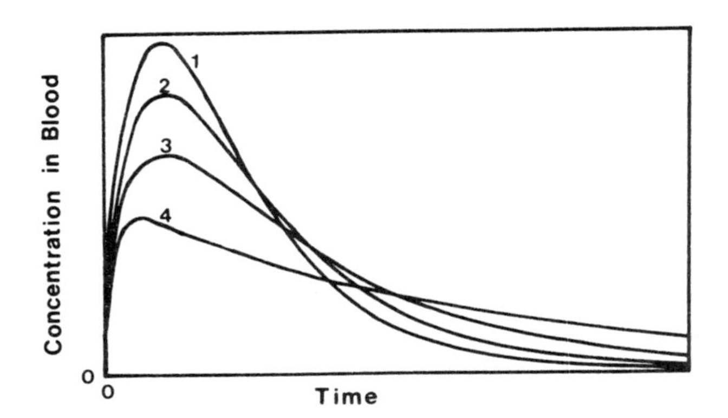

FIG. 6.26. Effect of distribution between blood and tissues on the blood level pattern. Rate constants have the values: $k_1 = k_2 = 1$ and k_{12}, k_{21} = 1, 4 in curve 1; 2, 3 in curve 2; 3, 2 in curve 3; and 4, 1 in curve 4. [From Notari (1971).]

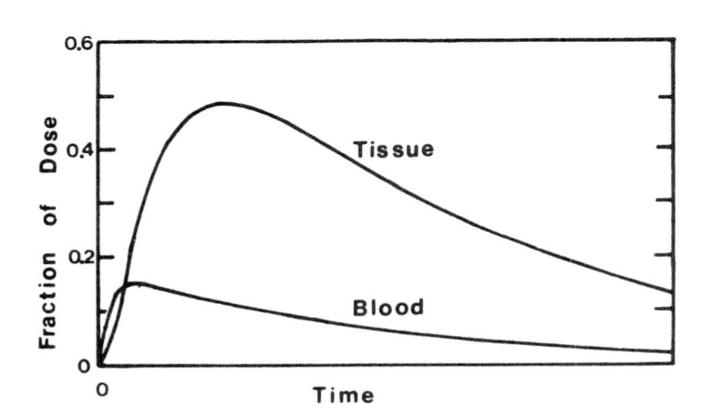

FIG. 6.27. The fraction of the total dose in the blood and tissue compartments when $k_1 = k_2 = k_{21} = 1$ and $k_{12} = 4$. [From Notari (1971).]

In any event, for the simple two-compartment model originally presented, the solution for P(t) is known to be

$$P = k_1 A_0 \left[\frac{(k_{21} - \alpha)e^{-\alpha t}}{(k_1 - \alpha)(\beta - \alpha)} + \frac{(k_{21} - \beta)e^{-\beta t}}{(k_1 - \beta)(\alpha - \beta)} + \frac{(k_{21} - k_1)e^{-k_1 t}}{(\alpha - k_1)(\beta - k_1)} \right]$$

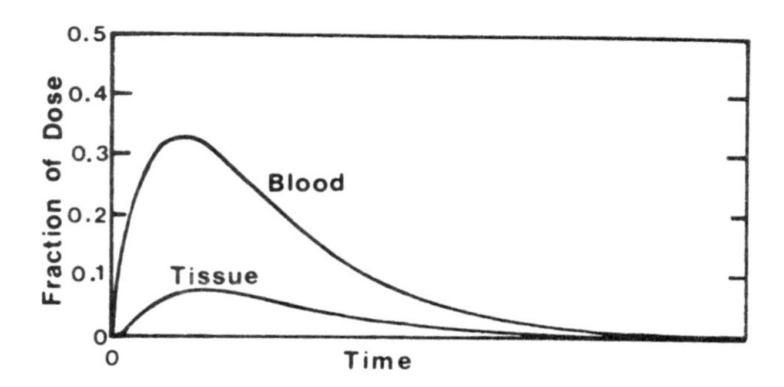

FIG. 6.28. The fraction of the total dose in the blood and tissue compartments when $k_1 = k_2 = k_{12} = 1$ and $k_{21} = 4$. [From Notari (1971).]

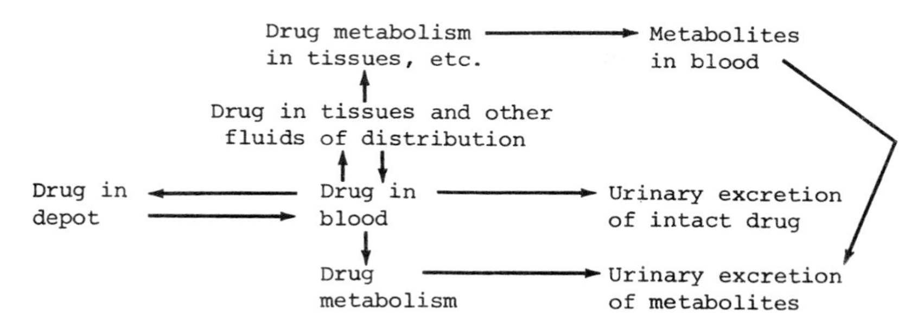

FIG. 6.29. A simple model for drug uptake, distribution, and elimination.

where

$$\alpha = \frac{1}{2}\left[a + (a^2 - b)^{1/2}\right], \quad \beta = \frac{1}{2}\left[a - (a^2 - b)^{1/2}\right]$$

$$a = k_{12} + k_2 + k_{21}, \quad b = 4k_{21}k_2$$

The solution for T(t) is the same except the leading group of constants is $k_1k_{12}A_o$ instead of k_1A_o, and the factors $(k_{21} - \alpha)$, $(k_{21} - \beta)$, and $(k_{21} - k_1)$ are missing from the numerators of the three terms. Note that the solutions have a <u>triexponential</u> form.

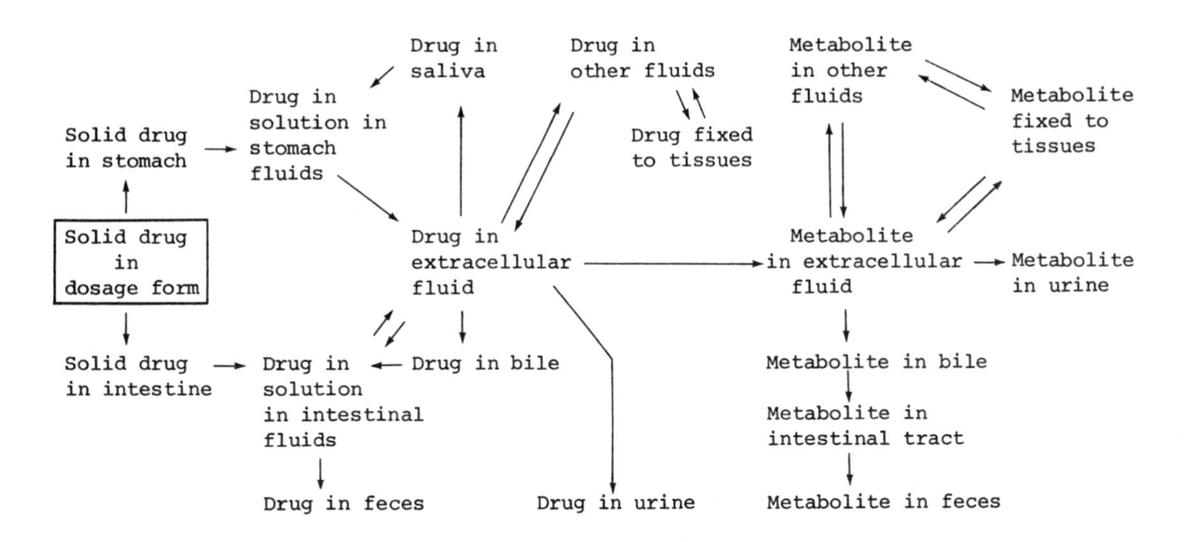

FIG. 6.30. A general and realistic model for drug absorption, distribution, metabolism, and excretion. [From Wagner (1971), p. 11.]

G. *The Case of Intravenous Injection*

Although the general solution above is to some extent unwieldy, for limiting cases, such as that of a single IV injection, more manageable expressions are obtained. For an IV injection the model becomes essentially that shown in Figure 6.31. The differential equation for the blood plasma (P) compartment is then

$$-\frac{dP}{dt} = (k_{12} + k_2)P - k_{21}T$$

For this the solution is (for a plasma <u>concentration</u> $C_o = P_o/V_p$ at $t = 0$)

$$C = Ae^{-\alpha t} - Be^{-\beta t}$$

where α and β are as previously defined, V_p is the volume of the plasma compartment, and

$$A = \frac{C_o(\alpha - k_{21})}{\alpha - \beta}$$

$$B = \frac{C_o(\beta - k_{21})}{\beta - \alpha}$$

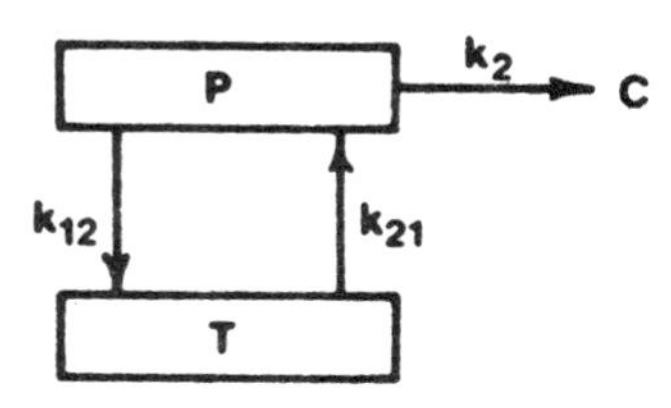

FIG. 6.31. A two-compartment model for intravenous drug injection.

Data can be analyzed for this biexponential solution according to the feathering method described previously, as shown in Figure 6.32. From the slopes α and β and intercepts A and B one can determine the various kinetic constants using the relations

$$A + B = C_o$$

$$k_{21} = \frac{C_o\alpha + A\beta - A\alpha}{C_o}$$

$$k_2 = \frac{\alpha\beta}{k_{21}}$$

$$k_{12} = \alpha + \beta - k_{21} - k_2$$

1. Ampicillin Kinetics: Application of the Two-Compartment Model with Injection

Jusko and Lewis (1973) applied the two-compartment type of model shown in Figure 6.33 to the rapid intravenous injection of the antibiotic ampicillin, and obtained the data shown in Figure 6.34. Elimination from the body was considered to occur by renal (urinary) and extrarenal (bile secretion and metabolism) routes, as illustrated. Analysis of their data showed a good fit to this model for the parameter values

$$k_{12} = 0.38\ \text{hr}^{-1}$$

$$k_{21} = 0.73\ \text{hr}^{-1}$$

$$k_b = 0.17\ \text{hr}^{-1}$$

$$k_e = 1.55\ \text{hr}^{-1}$$

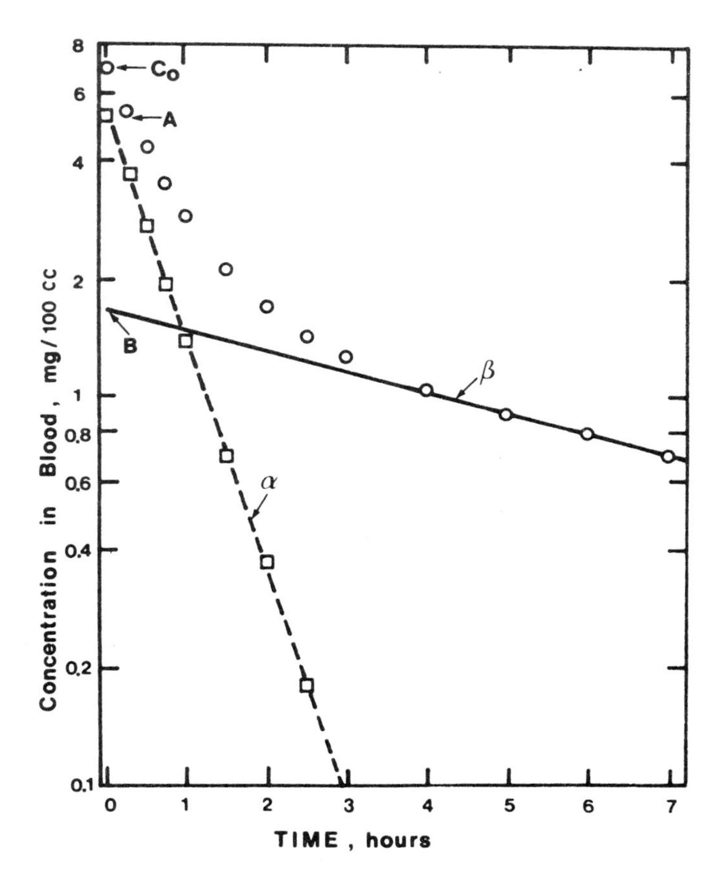

FIG. 6.32. Application of the method of feathering to blood level data. [From Notari (1971).]

central compartment volume = 12.0 liters

peripheral compartment volume = 4.9 liters

The central compartment presumably contains blood plus some other readily accessible fluid(s). However, the investigators did not attempt to specify what the contents of the two compartments actually were.

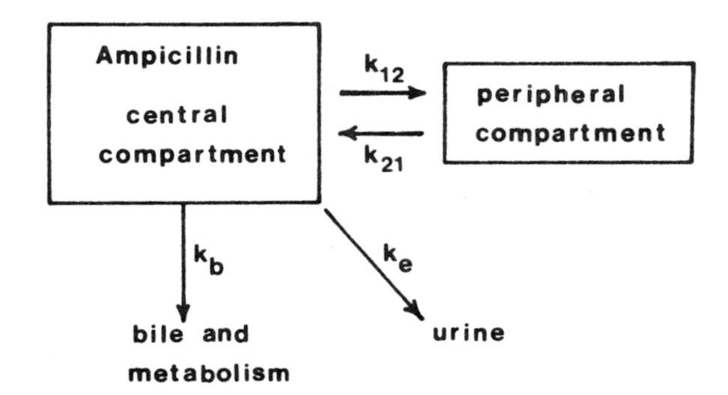

FIG. 6.33. Multicompartment pharmacokinetic model of Jusko and Lewis (1973).

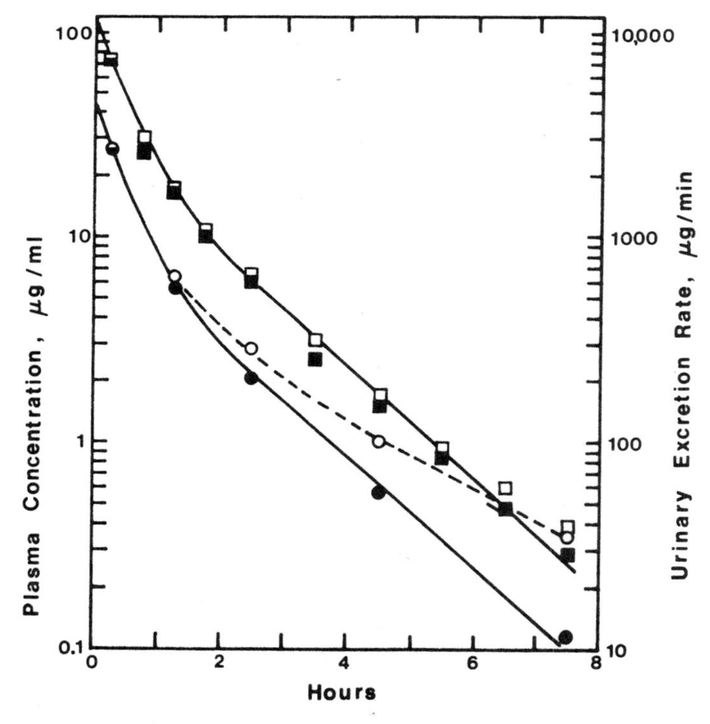

FIG. 6.34. Plasma concentrations (circles) and urinary excretion rates (squares) of ampicillin as a function of time after intravenous administration of 570 mg. Closed symbols are results of microbiological assay, and open symbols are measurements by fluorometry. [From Jusko and Lewis (1973).]

2. *Modeling Plasma Levels and Pharmacologic Effects of LSD in Humans*

Levy et al. (1969) investigated the effects of intravenously administering LSD (lysergic acid diethylamide) at a dosage level of 2 μg/kg of body weight. Plasma concentration data were fitted to the following two models, the first of which is the same type of two-compartment model with intravenous injection that we considered above:

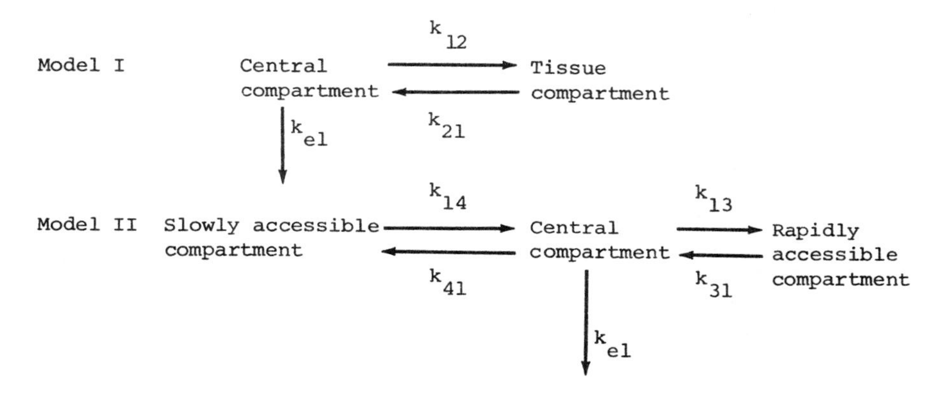

From model I, the following biexponential equation was found to describe the dependence of the central compartment plasma concentration P (in nanograms per milliliter) on time (in hours)

$$P = 5.47e^{-7.62t} + 6.92e^{-0.23t}$$

The best values for the model I rate constants were found to be $k_{el} = 0.41\ hr^{-1}$, $k_{12} = 3.08\ hr^{-1}$, and $k_{21} = 4.36\ hr^{-1}$.

For the more complex model II, the plasma concentration equation and kinetic constants were found to be

$$P = 14.64e^{-26.2t} + 2.02e^{-2.5t} + 6.53e^{-0.22t}$$

and $k_{el} = 0.74\ hr^{-1}$, $k_{13} = 14.54\ hr^{-1}$, $k_{31} = 10.21\ hr^{-1}$, $k_{14} = 1.57\ hr^{-1}$, and $k_{41} = 1.88\ hr^{-1}$.

Figures 6.35 and 6.36 show how the equations for P match the experimental data. Both models appear to fit the data quite well and one really cannot say which is better at this stage.

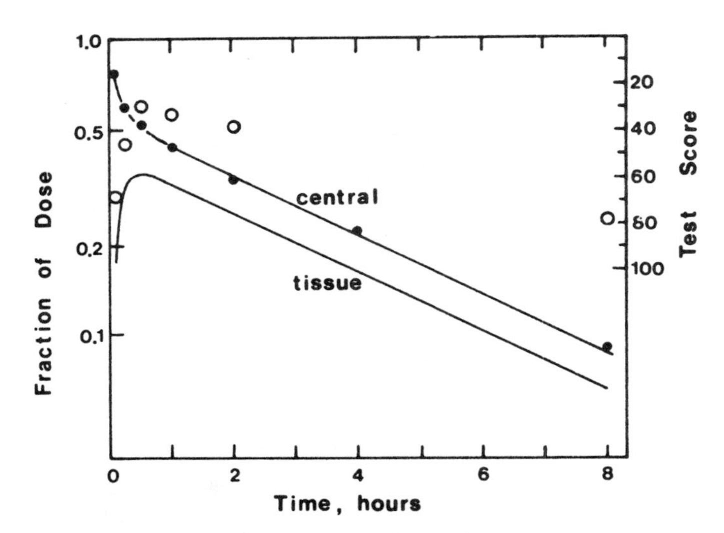

FIG. 6.35. LSD amounts versus time in the central and tissue compartments as predicted using model I. Closed circles are relative plasma concentrations (relative to the concentration at time zero). Open circles are test scores. [From Levy et al. (1969).]

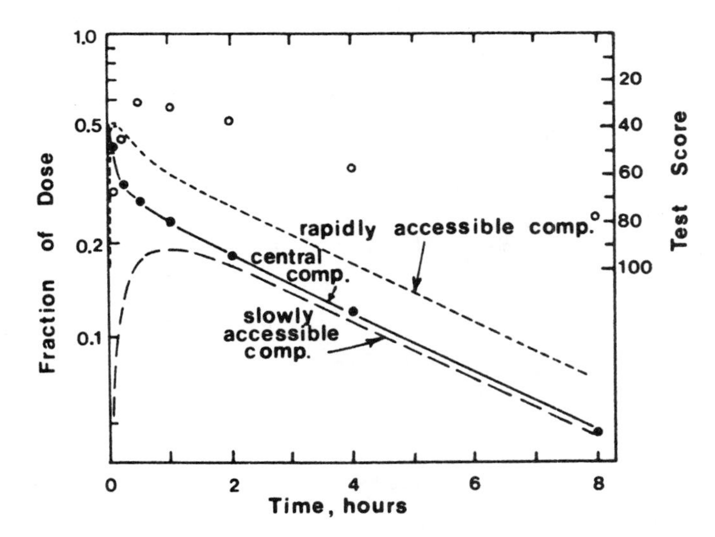

FIG. 6.36. LSD amounts in various compartments versus time, as predicted from model II. Closed circles are relative plasma concentrations; the open circles are test scores. [From Levy et al. (1969).]

Levy et al. also measured performances in solving certain mathematical problems as a function of time. These scores are also shown in Figures 6.35 and 6.36. Hypothesizing that the pharmacological effect of LSD (lowered test performance) would be related, for model I, to the concentration of LSD in the tissue compartment (Figures 6.35 and 6.36 show clearly that the effects are not related to the central compartment concentrations) Levy constructed the plot shown in Figure 6.37. Clearly, a simple time-independent relationship does not exist.

Levy then tried to correlate test performances versus various compartmental concentrations in the model II system. This led to the successful correlation shown in Figure 6.38. Now it is evident that the site of action of LSD is in some slowly accessible compartment.

Several conclusions can be drawn from this study. First, determining the validity of different models cannot always be done on the basis of concentration data alone (e.g., model I fitted the concentration data well but turned out to be invalid). Second, even

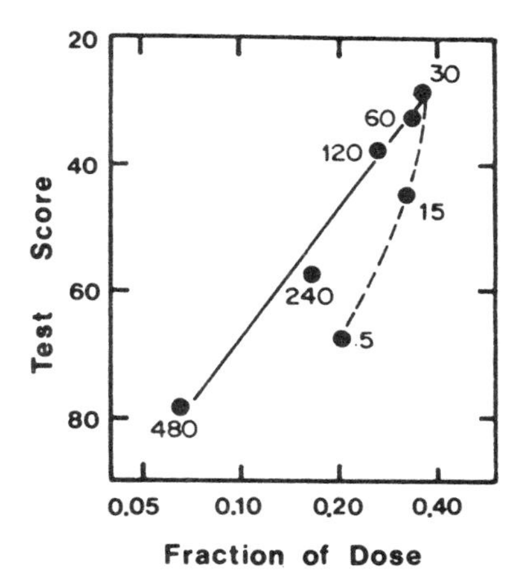

FIG. 6.37. Relation between test scores and the fraction of LSD in the tissue compartment of model I. Numbers next to the points indicate time (in minutes) at which the measurement was made. [From Levy et al. (1969).]

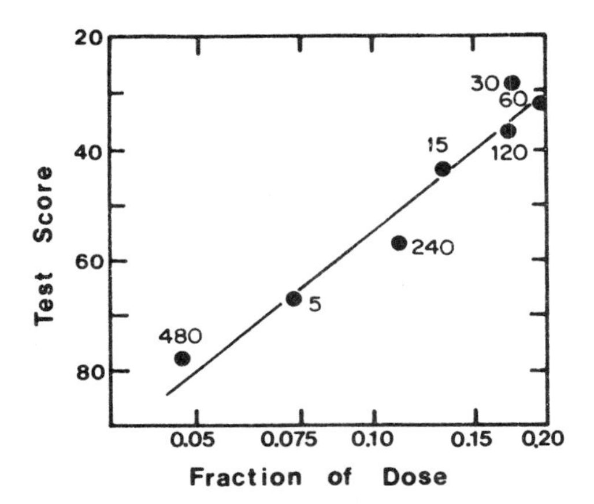

FIG. 6.38. Relation between test scores and the fraction of LSD in the slowly accessible compartment of model II. [From Levy et al. (1969).]

model II may not be strictly correct; several other three-compartment models were tested (ones involving elimination from the easily accessible compartment) and were found to fit the concentration data just as well. Third, it is possible that a four (or more)-compartment model would be even more realistic. However, there would probably be no practical way to determine this. Even with model II, although we know that the slowly accessible compartment is the important one pharmacologically, its physical nature and location is still undetermined (at least based on the data presented).

H. Comment About One-Compartment Versus Two-Compartment Models

Several writers have pointed out that when a drug is administered orally or intramuscularly, the solution to the one-compartment model involves two exponential terms and the solution to the two-compartment model involves three exponential terms. In many cases, it becomes difficult to determine which model fits the data better. Part of this is due to there being a fairly large number of adjustable parameters, and part is often due to one process (e.g., elimination) overshadowing the other processes present. When one finds that two models, each with different parameter values, fit the data equally well, it is clear that the physiological validity of the parameter values is in doubt.

This dilemma tends not to arise in cases of intravenous drug administration, since the drug absorption process is not involved and the models yield solutions having only one and two exponential terms, instead of two and three.

IX. BLOOD/TISSUE MODELS (LOCAL REGION MODELS)

The models just described generally lump the body into one compartment and therefore no fluid streams are explicitly drawn as entering or leaving the body compartment. Solute (drug) streams enter only by absorption and exit only by metabolization and elimination. These processes are all characterized in a chemical kinetic fashion, even though, as in the case of urinary elimination, an actual convective flow exists.

When one wishes to model a local region the substantial inward and outward fluid flows of blood (lymph flow is usually neglected) across the compartment boundaries must be accounted for. When modeling the body as a whole no fluid flows are considered to cross the boundaries (at least, for purposes of modeling) and convective solute transfer processes are not explicitly involved.

A. *Two-Compartment Local Model That Assumes Equilibrium*

Perhaps the simplest local model is the one depicted in Figure 6.39. Here the main compartment is considered to consist of blood and tissue subregions, each of which is assumed to be homogeneous (i.e., well stirred). Moreover, blood and tissue are assumed to be in equilibrium. A mass balance for a solute (drug) across this compartment is

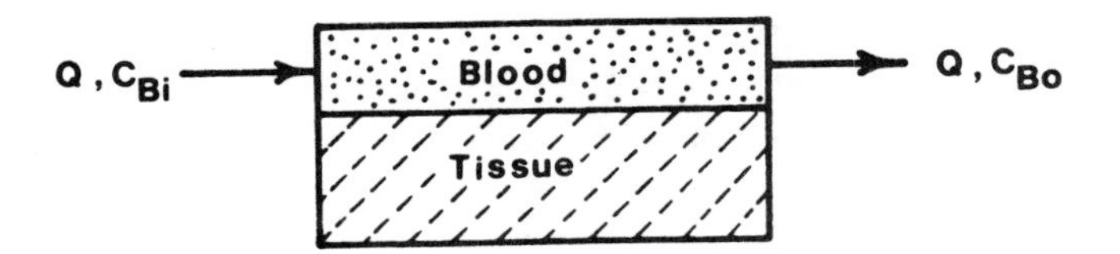

FIG. 6.39. Two-compartment local model.

$$Q(C_{Bi} - C_{Bo}) = V_T \frac{dC_T}{dt} + V_B \frac{dC_B}{dt}$$

where Q is the volumetric blood flow rate; C_{Bi}, C_{Bo} are the concentrations of solute in the inlet and outlet bloodstreams; C_B, C_T are the concentrations of solute in the blood and tissue regions; and V_B, V_T are volumes of the blood and tissue regions.

In many regions of the body, the volume of blood is much less than the volume of tissue, i.e., $V_B << V_T$, and hence the total compartment volume V is roughly equal to V_T. Hence, we can write the right-hand side of the mass balance as $V(dC_T/dt)$. Also, because equilibrium exists between blood and tissue, we can relate C_B and C_T by the expression

$$C_B = \alpha C_T$$

where we have assumed that a linear equilibrium relation exists (α is the partition coefficient). Since the outlet concentration in the blood, C_{Bo}, equals C_B, we may then write the mass balance as

$$\frac{V}{\alpha} \frac{dC_B}{dt} = Q(C_{Bi} - C_B)$$

For the case where a drug is suddenly introduced at a constant rate into the blood, i.e., C_{Bi} goes from zero to a constant value C^0_{Bi} at $t = 0$, the equation just given has the solution

$$C_B = C^0_{Bi}\left[1 - \exp(-\frac{Q\alpha t}{V})\right]$$

The response of the outlet blood to the step change is therefore exponential (note that C_T can be obtained using this solution and the fact that $C_T = C_B/\alpha$).

As suggested earlier, this one-compartment model with <u>fluid</u> streams can be related to the type of model shown in Figure 6.40, which represents all mass transport processes in chemical-kinetic fashion. This latter model is characterized by

$$\frac{dX}{dt} = V\frac{dC_X}{dt} = k_1D - k_2X$$

or

$$\frac{dC_X}{dt} = \frac{k_1D}{V} - \frac{k_2X}{V} = \frac{k_1D}{V} - k_2C_X$$

For a step change at $t = 0$ from $D = 0$ to $D = D_0$ this has the solution

$$C_X = \frac{k_1D_0}{k_2V}\left[1 - e^{-k_2t}\right]$$

The nature of the correspondence between these two models is now clear. That is,

$$C_X = C_B$$

$$C_{Bi}^0 = \frac{k_1D_0}{k_2V}$$

$$k_2 = \frac{Q\alpha}{V}$$

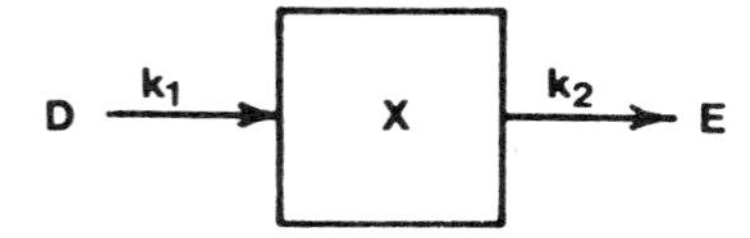

FIG. 6.40. Simple one-compartment model.

Either model may be used to represent a physical system, depending on whichever seems more appropriate.

B. *Two-Compartment Local Model That Assumes a Finite Mass Transfer Resistance*

This model is the same as the one just discussed except that mass transfer equilibrium between blood and tissue is not assumed. One must therefore characterize intercompartmental transfer, and the usual way this is done is to state that the amount transferred from blood to tissue per unit time is equal to $KS(C_B - \alpha C_T)$, where K is a mass transfer coefficient, S is the interfacial area between the blood and tissue (e.g., total area of capillary walls), and $(C_B - \alpha C_T)$ represents the difference between the prevailing blood concentration (C_B) and the value it would have if equilibrium were to exist (i.e., αC_T). Solute balances for this system are

$$\text{Tissue:} \quad V_T \frac{dC_T}{dt} = KS(C_B - \alpha C_T)$$

$$\text{Blood:} \quad V_B \frac{dC_B}{dt} = Q(C_{Bi} - C_{Bo}) - KS(C_B - \alpha C_T)$$

where it has been assumed that the subregions are both uniform in concentration.

For a step change of C_{Bi} from zero to C_{Bi}^0 at $t = 0$, these equations have the solution

$$C_B = C_{Bi}^0[Ae^{-at} + (1 - A)e^{-bt}]$$

where A, a, and b are parameters related to K, S, V_B, V_T, α, and Q. The exact relations are not important for present purposes. What is significant is the biexponential nature of the solution. This is the same form that the two-compartment open model has, as shown earlier. This is to be expected because of the great similarities of the models. One can relate the parameters of the present flow model to the earlier chemical-kinetic model, of course (as we just did for the previous local model), but we will omit doing so here.

C. *Parallel-Compartment Models That Assume Blood/Tissue Equilibrium*

As Middleman (1972) has pointed out, the biexponential type of solution obtained above (for a two-subregion compartment with finite mass transfer resistance) also arises for models consisting of two parallel one-region compartments in which equilibrium exists. Figure 6.41 illustrates such a system. Agreement of experimental data with a biexponential mathematical expression can therefore imply either type of physical system. In such a case, physiological reasoning must be employed in order to decide which system is more likely.

We shall now consider two situations in which multiexponential system responses are clearly the result of the existence of two or more distinct compartments in parallel, rather than the result of one large compartment having two or more subregions that are not in equilibrium.

1. *Blood Flow to White and Gray Matter in the Brain*

A clear demonstration of a situation involving two compartments in parallel is provided by the data of Lassen et al. (1963), who

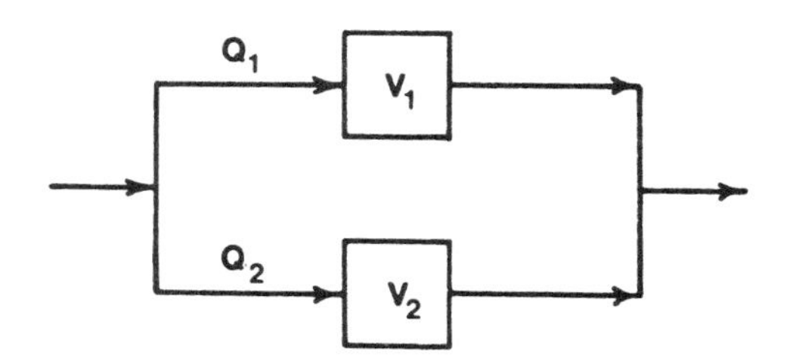

FIG. 6.41. Two-parallel-compartments model.

studied the clearance of radioactive krypton (^{85}Kr) from brain tissues. Compartment 1 was found to correspond to the white matter of the brain (mainly bundles of nerve axons) and compartment 2 was found to relate to the gray matter (clusters of nerve cells) in the brain.

Experimentally, a slug (1-3 ml) of saline solution containing dissolved ^{85}Kr was injected rapidly (in 10 sec or less) into one of the carotid arteries, which lead to the brain. The radioactive ^{85}Kr thus reached the brain quickly, and then was carried throughout the various brain tissues according to the different perfusion routes of the blood. The total ^{85}Kr in the brain cavity at any time was determined by counting gamma-ray activity with a conventional detector placed on a suitable location of the skull. Experimentally, the data on counts per second versus time show the exponential decay typical of solutes being gradually washed out of a tissue region.

If we assume that each major brain compartment (white, gray) consists of well-mixed blood and tissue subregions and if we further assume that these subregions are in equilibrium, then we may write, as shown above,

$$\frac{V}{\alpha}\frac{dC_B}{dt} = Q(C_{Bi} - C_B)$$

for each compartment. In this case, since $C_{Bi} = 0$ for $t > 0$ (after cessation of ^{85}Kr infusion) we can write

$$\frac{V}{\alpha}\frac{dC_B}{dt} = -QC_B$$

for each compartment. Integration gives

$$C_{B1} = C_{B1}^{o} \exp\left(\frac{-Q_1\alpha_1}{V_1}t\right)$$

$$C_{B2} = C_{B2}^{o} \exp\left(\frac{-Q_2\alpha_2}{V_2}t\right)$$

where C_{B1}^{o} and C_{B2}^{o} are initial concentrations.

Now if $f_1 = Q_1/Q$ and $f_2 = Q_2/Q$ are the fractions of the total flow rate Q which flow to each compartment, we may write, for the overall outlet concentration (resulting after mixing of the two outlet streams),

$$C_B = f_1 C_{B1} + f_2 C_{B2} = C^o_{B1} f_1 e^{-k_1 t} + C^o_{B2} f_2 e^{-k_2 t}$$

where $k_1 = \alpha_1 Q_1/V_1$ and $k_2 = \alpha_2 Q_2/V_2$. The overall concentration is thus a combination of two exponential terms. Therefore, if one plots concentration-time data on semilogarithmic paper, the overall curve can be resolved into two exponential contributions. The procedure involved was previously described for the general one-compartment open model and for the two-compartment model with intravenous infusion, both cases of which led (as in this case) to a biexponential equation.

Figure 6.42 shows the data of Lassen et al. and the two exponential relationships into which they may be resolved (these appear as straight lines on semilogarithmic paper, of course). The

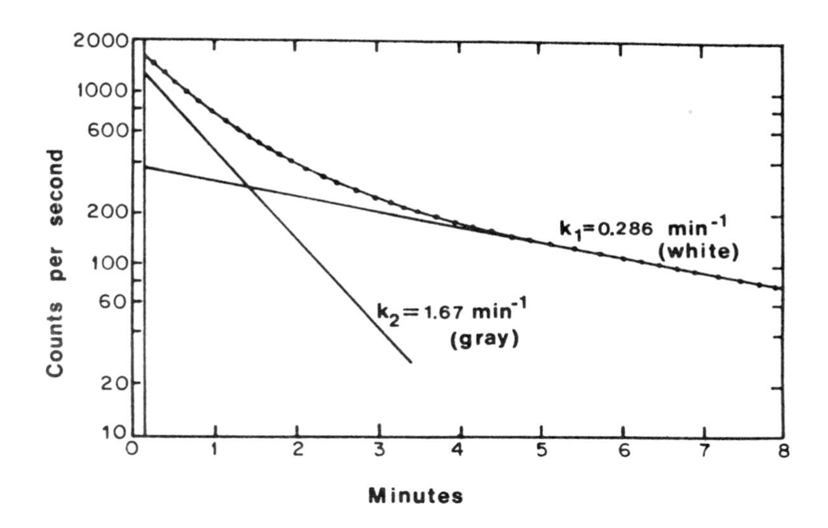

FIG. 6.42. Clearance of ^{85}Kr from the brain. [From Lassen et al. (1963).]

white matter of the brain is seen to have a rate constant of $k_1 = 0.286\ \text{min}^{-1}$ and the gray matter a rate constant of $k_2 = 1.67\ \text{min}^{-1}$. Hence the gray matter (nerve cells) is more accessible than the white matter (axon bundles). The intercepts of the straight lines are seen, from the equation above, to be equal to $f_1 C^o_{B1}$ and $f_2 C^o_{B2}$. If one assumes $C^o_{B1} = C^o_{B2} = C^o_B$, then it is clear that $f_1 = (f_1 C^o_{B1})/C^o_B$, the value of the intercept divided by the initial total concentration (and similarly for f_2). On this basis the data in Figure 6.42 suggest that $f_1 = 0.2$ and $f_2 = 0.8$; hence the white matter (axons) appears to be far less perfused with blood than the gray matter (nerve cells).

2. *Inert Gas Clearance from the Body*

The compartments-in-parallel kind of model we are considering here can be applied to the clearance of inert gases (N_2, He, H_2, A, Kr, Xe) from the human body. Clearance experiments involving these gases are usually done by (a) having the subject breathe air or oxygen containing a certain fraction of the inert gas until his body is fully saturated with the inert material, (b) then, at time zero, switching the subject to the breathing of pure air or oxygen, and (c) following the amount of inert gas cleared from the body tissues by expiration from the lungs as a function of time, by recording the volume of gas expired and by sampling the gas to determine compositions.

What one finds is that almost all inert gases are cleared from the body at similar rates, even though it is known that the relative rates of diffusion of different gases through tissues are very different. For example, independent experiments have shown the following:

Gas	Diffusion rate through representative tissue (relative to N_2 rate)
N_2	1.00
He	2.57
H_2	3.20
A	0.84
Kr	0.58
Xe	0.36

One can therefore conclude that inert gas clearance from the body is <u>blood flow limited</u> rather than <u>diffusion limited</u>. That is, the rates at which such gases diffuse from the tissues to the perfusing blood are intrinsically much faster than the rate at which the blood can carry such gases away (determined by the blood flow rate). Therefore, if one wishes to model any body region (e.g., lungs, liver) as two subregions, blood and tissue, one can justifiably assume equilibrium exists between the blood and tissue subregions. If one further assumes each subregion is well mixed, and that $V_B << V_T$, one can write

$$V_T \frac{dC_T}{dt} = Q(C_{Bi} - C_{Bo})$$

for each body region, as shown previously. If elimination of the inert gas in the lungs is efficient (it will be, in general), then the blood returning to a body region will have a concentration $C_{Bi} \cong 0$. Hence

$$V_T \frac{dC_T}{dt} = -QC_{Bo}$$

But, since $C_{Bo} = \alpha C_T$, we can rewrite this equation as

$$V_T \frac{dC_T}{dt} = -Q\alpha C_T$$

This can be integrated, with the initial condition that $C_T = C_T^o$ at $t = 0$, to give

$$\frac{C_T}{C_T^o} = \exp\left[\frac{-Q\alpha}{V_T} t\right] = e^{-kt}$$

where $k = Q\alpha/V_T$. Now $C_T/C_T^o = A/A^o$, where A stands for the amount of gas present in the body region (e.g., milliliters of gas referred to STP). Moreover, we can define the removal rate R of gas from a body region (milliliters of gas per minute, for example) as

$$R = \frac{-dA}{dt} = \frac{-d(A^o e^{-kt})}{dt} = kA^o e^{-kt}$$

For the whole body, which can be viewed as consisting of a set of many compartments in parallel (note that if any two compartments are really in series, they must be combined into one compartment in order to conform to this view), one can write

$$A = A_1^o e^{-k_1 t} + A_2^o e^{-k_2 t} + A_3^o e^{-k_3 t} + \cdots$$

$$R = R_1^o e^{-k_1 t} + R_2^o e^{-k_2 t} + R_3^o e^{-k_3 t} + \cdots$$

where $R_1 = A_1^o k_1$, $R_2^o = A_2^o k_2$, and so on.

a. Modeling N_2 Clearance. Body tissues at atmospheric pressure contain roughly 0.01 ml N_2(STP)/ml of nonfatty tissue and about 0.05 ml N_2(STP)/ml of fatty tissue. While fatty tissue has approximately the same vascularity as resting muscle (i.e., same blood perfusion rate), the relatively high solubility of N_2 in fat, as compared to blood and nonfatty tissue, causes the fractional removal rate of N_2 from fatty tissues to be slower by a factor of 5 than the fractional removal rate from muscle tissue.

Behnke et al. (1935) have resolved N_2 elimination into two components, as expressed by

$$A = 364e^{-0.098t} + 500e^{-0.0085t}$$

where

364 = ml N_2 in the nonfatty tissue
500 = ml N_2 in the fatty tissue
0.098 = k for the nonfatty tissue, in min^{-1}
0.0085 = k for the fatty tissues, in min^{-1}

Figure 6.43 shows the general form of gas exchange rate data (a plot of log R versus time) and how the overall curve can be resolved into three different compartments: the viscera, other nonfatty tissues, and fat. With very accurate data and elaborate mathematical techniques one can resolve the overall curve into even more components. For example, the following model equation has been claimed to represent N_2 elimination from a five-compartment system:

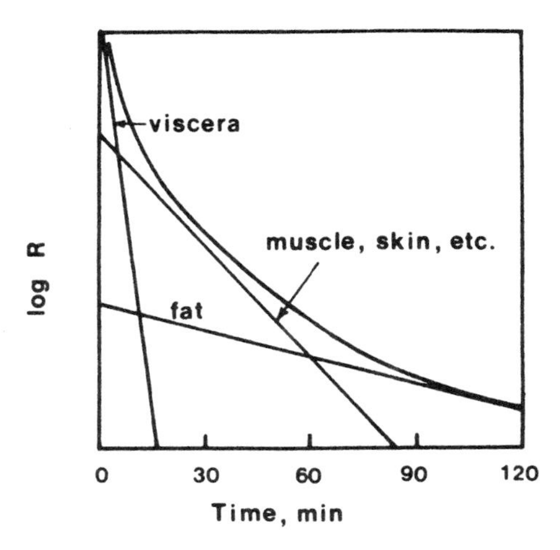

FIG. 6.43. General form of the rate-of-gas exchange curve as a function of time.

$$A = 111e^{-0.462t} + 193e^{-0.087t} + 428e^{-0.024t}$$

$$+ 95e^{-0.008t} + 600e^{-0.0025t}$$

The units of the A^{o} and k parameters are again, milliliters of N_2 and reciprocal minutes, respectively. However, one must seriously question whether resolution of data into such a large number of compartments can really be done with validity.

Table 6.2 shows regional blood perfusion rates, N_2 volumes, and removal rates determined individually for specific body regions. With such data, it is valid to construct (rather than resolve, which is the opposite process) a multicompartment model for N_2 elimination, e.g.,

$$A = \underset{\text{(lungs)}}{12.0e^{-4.8t}} + \underset{\text{(thyroid)}}{0.2e^{-5.0t}} + \underset{\text{(kidneys)}}{2.7e^{-5.0t}} + \ldots$$

Such elaborate models for gas clearance are perhaps not needed, but some sort of model (e.g., a two- or three-compartment one) is of great use in certain practical applications, e.g., in quantifying the problem of N_2 or helium elimination during decompression of deep-sea divers.

D. *A General Two-Compartment Local Model*

Several other types of blood/tissue models have been proposed in the literature. Perhaps the best way to summarize them is to develop a very general blood/tissue model and then to show how each particular model derives as a special case of the general model.

Allowing for unsteady-state behavior, axial diffusion and dispersion, and finite mass transfer resistance, one can derive the mass balances for the model given in Figure 6.44, which have the forms

$$\text{Blood:} \quad \frac{\partial C_B}{\partial t} + u\frac{\partial C_B}{\partial z} + \frac{W}{V_B} = D_B\frac{\partial^2 C_B}{\partial z^2}$$

TABLE 6.2

Regional Blood Perfusion Rates and Dissolved N_2 Exchange Rates for a 70-kg Man

Tissue	Volume of tissue (ml)	Volume of N_2 (ml)	Blood flow rate (liters/min)	Rate constant k (min^{-1})
Lungs	1200	12.0	5.8	4.8
Thyroid	30	0.2	0.2	5.0
Kidneys	270	2.7	1.33	5.0
Heart	300	3.0	0.15	0.5
Adrenals, 7 ml				
Testes, 50 ml	78	0.8	0.08	1.0
Prostate, 21 ml				
Salivary glands	35	0.4	0.02	0.5
Brain	1400	14.0	0.76	0.5
Marrow (hemopoietic)	1400	30.0	0.30	0.15
Hepatic portal				
Liver	1560	17.0	—	0.27
Spleen	150	1.5		
Pancreas	85	0.9	1.5	0.5
Intestines				
Stomach	1350			0.7
Colon				
Intestinal contents	1500	100		0.008
Muscle (40 liters)			0.8	0.025
Connective tissue (5 liters)	45,000-55,000	450-550	0.1	0.02
Skin (5 liters)			0.3	0.07
Fat (12 liters)	15,000-5000	750-250	0.2	0.004
70-kg man, 1.85 m^2		1383-983		

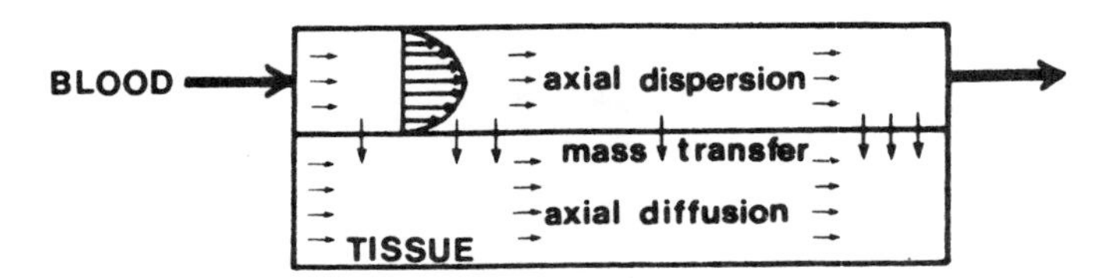

FIG. 6.44. Two-compartment local model with axial diffusion and dispersion and mass transfer resistance.

$$\text{Tissue:} \quad \frac{\partial C_T}{\partial t} = \frac{W}{V_T} - R + D_T \frac{\partial^2 C_T}{\partial z^2}$$

where u is the space-averaged blood velocity; D_B, D_T are the axial diffusion coefficients; and R is the rate of consumption of the solute by metabolism, per unit volume of tissue. W is the rate of interfacial mass transfer (mass per time), and for nonequilibrium situations can be represented by $KS(C_B - \alpha C_T)$, as previously stated. Most local models invariably assume that the metabolic consumption term can be neglected in comparison to the other terms. Although this is often a poor assumption, we shall assume likewise in all that follows.

E. Steady-State Transfer to a Large Tissue Region

This model assumes that the tissue region is so large that $C_T = 0$ for a long period of time. If one also assumes that steady-state conditions have been achieved ($\partial C_B/\partial t = 0$) and that axial diffusion in the blood is negligible in comparison to convective transport, one is left with

$$u \frac{dC_B}{dz} = -\frac{KS}{V_B} C_B$$

This has the solution $C_B = C_{Bi} \exp[-(KS/uV_B)z]$. A situation to which this model would apply would be, for example, the continuous intravenous delivery of a highly tissue-soluble drug.

F. Unsteady-State Transfer to a Finite Tissue Region

Assuming again that axial diffusion is neglectable, we have the following equations to solve for the unsteady-state case:

$$\frac{\partial C_B}{\partial t} + u\frac{\partial C_B}{\partial z} + \frac{KS}{V_B}(C_B - \alpha C_T) = 0$$

$$\frac{\partial C_T}{\partial t} = \frac{KS}{V_T}(C_B - \alpha C_T)$$

These equations are coupled, since C_B and C_T appear in both, but they may nevertheless be solved analytically. By analogy to the solutions obtained for a chromatographic problem, namely mass transfer between a fluid and a bed of adsorbent, under conditions of a linear equilibrium relationship and a linear interphase rate law [see Bird et al. (1960), pp. 702-705] we may write the following solution for the case of a step change in concentration at the compartment inlet at $t = 0$:

$$\frac{C_B}{C_{Bi}} = J(\zeta, \tau)$$

where

$$\zeta = \frac{KS}{uV_B} z$$

$$\tau = \frac{KS\alpha}{V_T}\left(t - \frac{z}{u}\right)$$

and the "J function" is given by

$$J = 1 - \int_0^{\zeta} \exp[-(\tau + \xi)] J_o[i(4\tau\xi)^{1/2}]\, d\xi$$

with J_o being a zero-order Bessel function of the first kind, and $i = \sqrt{-1}$. Values of the J function have been computed by many investigators and are graphically presented by Hiester and Vermeulen (1952). For a step change in the inlet blood drug concentration from zero to some value C_{Bi}, a typical response of the system looks like that shown in Figure 6.45. The concentration profiles in the tissue region have the same shape as those for the blood region. In general, the broadness or sharpness of these curves depends primarily on the magnitude of the mass transfer coefficient and area product, KS. And the time required for breakthrough to occur depends primarily on the values of α and u (i.e., capacity of tissue region for the drug and how fast the drug is being carried into the system).

G. *Models That Assume Equilibrium and Axial Diffusion*

If mass transfer is rapid, we know that W will be large. However, W can no longer be conveniently represented by $KS(C_B - \alpha C_T)$ since it approaches the indeterminate form of $\infty \cdot 0$ (i.e., large KS but small $C_B - \alpha C_T$, since $C_B \cong \alpha C_T$). In this case, we merely multiply the general blood and tissue balances by V_B and V_T, respectively, and add them. The terms containing W cancel and we have left

$$V_B \frac{\partial C_B}{\partial t} + uV_B \frac{\partial C_B}{\partial z} + V_T \frac{\partial C_T}{\partial t} = D_B V_B \frac{\partial^2 C_B}{\partial z^2} + D_T V_T \frac{\partial^2 C_T}{\partial z^2}$$

Since $C_B = \alpha C_T$ we can rewrite this as

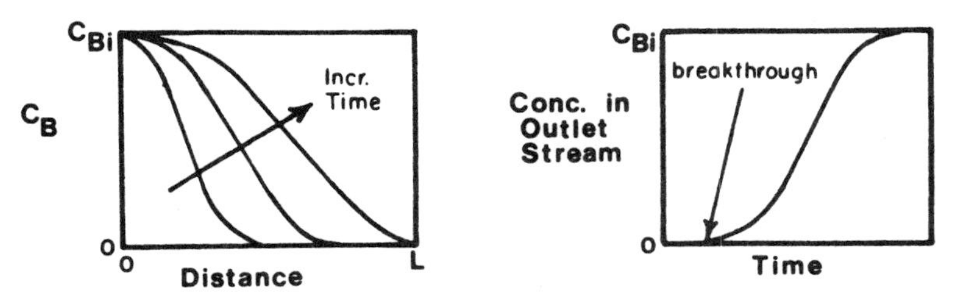

FIG. 6.45. Concentration profiles and breakthrough curve for drug uptake in a finite tissue region.

$$\left(V_B + \frac{V_T}{\alpha}\right) \frac{\partial C_B}{\partial t} + uV_B \frac{\partial C_B}{\partial z} = \left(D_B V_B + \frac{D_T V_T}{\alpha}\right) \frac{\partial^2 C_B}{\partial z^2}$$

or

$$\frac{\partial C_B}{\partial t} + u' \frac{\partial C_B}{\partial z} = D' \frac{\partial^2 C_B}{\partial z^2}$$

where

$$u' = \frac{uV_B}{V_B + V_T/\alpha}$$

$$D' = \frac{D_B V_B + D_T V_T/\alpha}{V_B + V_T/\alpha}$$

For the case of a constant-rate intravenous infusion, i.e., the inlet drug concentration is raised from zero to C_{Bi} and kept there, this equation has the following solution, again by analogy to fixed-bed adsorption theory, which calls this the dispersion model of adsorption

$$\frac{C_B}{C_{Bi}} = \frac{1}{2} + \frac{1}{2} \operatorname{erf} \left[\left(\frac{zu'}{D'}\right)^{1/2} \frac{\alpha Qt - V}{(4\alpha QtV)^{1/2}} \right]$$

where erf is the error function, Q is the blood flow rate, and $V = V_T + V_B$.

The concentration profiles and effluent curves predicted by this dispersion model are of the same shapes as those predicted by the preceding model (often called the mass transfer model). In fact, the two models can be shown to give nearly identical results if the relationship

$$\frac{KS}{V_B} = \frac{V_B u'^2}{VD'} \left(\frac{V_T}{V_B + V_T}\right)^2$$

is satisfied. The reason for this similarity is that nonequilibrium (finite mass transfer rate) and dispersion both have the same effects on a concentration profile in the blood—both cause spreading of the profile in a nearly symmetrical fashion.

The reader is urged to consult Middleman (1972) who discusses many of these same models in detail and cites examples of their use. Since our purpose is to provide a brief but broad introduction to the field, we will stop at this point.

X. USE OF INDICATORS TO DETERMINE REGIONAL BLOOD VOLUMES AND BLOOD FLOW RATES

Clinically, great use has been made of certain indicator substances (usually dyes), which have the property of not being able to enter any tissue, to provide information about the volume and flow rate of blood in a specific region (e.g., an organ such as the heart).

Considering our previously developed models for a region comprised of blood and tissue it is clear that for substances that cannot enter tissue our description reduces to

$$V_B \frac{dC_B}{dt} = Q(C_{Bi} - C_{Bo})$$

If a slug of indicator (dye) is injected upstream of a region, one observes that as the slug passes through the region there is a period during which $C_{Bi} > C_{Bo}$ and a later period when $C_{Bo} > C_{Bi}$ (no matter how spread out, or dispersed, the slug gets). If we integrate the mass balance as follows

$$\int_0^\infty V_B \left(\frac{dC_B}{dt}\right) dt = \int_0^\infty Q(C_{Bi} - C_{Bo})\ dt$$

it is clear that the left-hand side (the average rate of accumulation) must be zero, since there is no net retention of dye by the region. Therefore, looking at the right-hand side we can say

$$Q\int_0^{\infty} C_{Bi}\, dt - Q\int_0^{\infty} C_{Bo}\, dt = 0$$

But since $Q\int_0^{\infty} C_{Bi}\, dt$ is just the mass of dye introduced (M), then

$$Q = \frac{M}{\int_0^{\infty} C_{Bo}\, dt}$$

Hence, if one monitors the outlet concentration of dye in the blood as a function of time, one can determine (knowing the mass of dye injected) the blood flow rate to the region.

The volume of blood in a region may also be determined as follows. The mean residence time of a tracer in the region is defined as

$$t_R = \frac{\int_0^{\infty} tC_{Bo}\, dt}{\int_0^{\infty} C_{Bo}\, dt}$$

or

$$t_R = \frac{Q}{M}\int_0^{\infty} tC_{Bo}\, dt$$

However, t_R must also equal V/Q, where V is the volume of the region. Hence,

$$V = \frac{Q^2}{M}\int_0^{\infty} tC_{Bo}\, dt$$

One therefore needs only to evaluate the integral in the last equation from the data, and use the previously obtained Q value, in order to arrive at a value for V. It might be noted that, were the C_{Bo}

versus time curve symmetrical (it usually is not), one could obtain t_R directly as the time corresponding to the peak concentration.

Calculating the quantity $\int_0^\infty C_{Bo}\, dt$ is frequently complicated by the fact that blood is continually recirculated throughout the body. Thus, some of the dye that first comes out of the region may return back and pass through a second time before the dye concentration would have normally gone to zero (this complication depends greatly on the region studied; obviously for the coronary circulation this effect could be rather large). Much analysis has shown that the best way to remove the recirculation effect is to extrapolate the $C_{Bo}(t)$ data on a semilogarithmic plot, as shown in Figure 6.46.

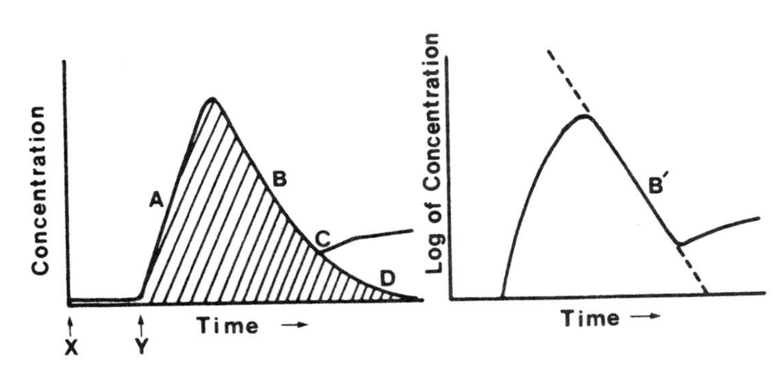

FIG. 6.46. The concentration curve at the sampling site in the rapid injection, indicator dilution technique. X, time of injection at the injection site. Y, time of first arrival at sampling site. A, rising part of concentration curve as more indicator arrives. B, exponential decay part of curve. C, beginning of recirculation. D, continuation of curve if there had been no recirculation. The shaded area gives $\int_0^\infty C_{Bo}\, dt$, from which the flow rate can be calculated. On the right, the semilogarithmic plot gives a straight line (B') for the exponential part of the curve, B. Extrapolation of this line allows part D of the curve to be calculated, and thus the total area, free from the recirculation error. The calculation is strictly valid only for steady flow. [From A. C. Burton, *Physiology and Biophysics of the Circulation*, 2nd ed., copyright· 1972 by Yearbook Med. Pub., Chicago, Illinois. Used by permission.]

PROBLEMS

1. Derive Equation 6.5, starting with Equations 6.3 and 6.4. Then obtain an expression for the asymptotic value of B as $t \to \infty$. Discuss the physical significance of the numerator and denominator of this expression, and why it is logical that the asymptotic value of B should be equal to their ratio.

2. Write unsteady-state differential equations (solute mass balances) for each compartment shown in Figure 6.5. Define intercompartment mass transfer coefficients and contact areas as needed (e.g., K_{12}, A_{12}, etc.).

3. *Characterizing alcohol uptake and dissipation in man.* Levett (1973) has reported experimental data on blood alcohol concentrations versus time following the ingestion of different amounts of alcohol by a 170-lb man, under both fasting and nonfasting conditions (see Figure 6.47).

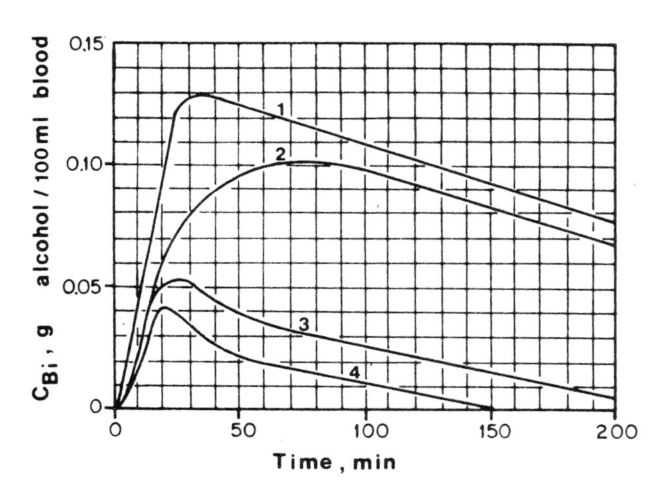

FIG. 6.47. Blood alcohol concentrations for several test conditions.

The curves shown are for the following test conditions:

Curve 1 3 oz alcohol taken in 3 sec, fasting

Curve 2 3 oz alcohol taken over 6 min, fasting

Curve 3 1 1/2 oz alcohol taken in 3 sec, nonfasting

Curve 4 1 oz alcohol taken in 3 sec, nonfasting

One may conveniently apply the one-compartment open model to the data of curves 1, 3, or 4 (3-sec ingestion time) shown in the figure. Since modeling cases involving prolonged ingestion time [e.g., 6 min (curve 2)] requires use of a more complex model, we will omit consideration of such cases here.

Our one-compartment open model equation, developed earlier, indicates that the concentration of alcohol <u>in the body</u> at any time is given by

$$C_B = \frac{B}{V_d} = \frac{A_0 k_1}{(k_2 - k_1)V_d}\left(e^{-k_1 t} - e^{-k_2 t}\right)$$

For the concentration of alcohol <u>in the blood</u>, Levett proposes the equation (no derivation is presented)

$$C_{Bl} = \frac{0.95K}{T_1 - T_2}\left(e^{-t/T_1} - e^{-t/T_2}\right)$$

where T_1 and T_2 are time constants for the absorption and elimination processes. These time constants are identical to the reciprocals of the rate constants we have been using, i.e., $T_1 = 1/k_1$ and $T_2 = 1/k_2$. Hence, Levett's equation can be written

$$C_{Bl} = \frac{0.95Kk_1k_2}{k_2 - k_1}\left(e^{-k_1 t} - e^{-k_2 t}\right)$$

If one assumes that the concentration <u>in the blood</u> is directly proportional to that <u>in the body</u> as a whole (e.g., $C_{Bl} = mC_B$), then we can write <u>our</u> equation as

$$C_{B1} = \frac{mA_0k_1}{(k_2 - k_1)V_d}\left(e^{-k_1t} - e^{-k_2t}\right)$$

Comparing this with Levett's equation indicates that

$$\frac{0.95Kk_1k_2}{(k_2 - k_1)} = \frac{mA_0k_1}{(k_2 - k_1)V_d} = \alpha$$

i.e., Levett's quantity K is equal to $mA_0/(0.95k_2V_d)$. Therefore K is seen to be proportional to the size of the dose of alcohol ingested (the other quantities are fixed).

Because $k_1 > k_2$ for this situation (the absorption is rapid relative to the elimination) the methods outlined in the text for determining k_1, k_2, and α from the experimental data can be used.

The current problem is to find values for these three parameters using the data of Levett's curve 1.

4. *N_2 depletion from the body during surgery.* During a surgical procedure, a patient usually is being administered a high-O_2-content gas, and therefore depletion of the N_2 that is normally dissolved in the body tissues gradually occurs. No harmful physiological effects seem to result from this. However, it would be interesting to determine how much N_2 would be depleted in, say, a half-hour operation. Using the five-compartment equation given in the text ($A = 111e^{-0.462t} + \cdots$), plot (a) the fraction of N_2 left in the body and (b) the rate of N_2 removed in milliliters per minute, for times ranging from 0 to 30 min.

5. *Dye dilution.* A dye is injected at a uniform rate into the blood upstream of some region of interest for a period T sec and then is stopped. If the region of interest is well mixed (as in the left ventricle of the heart), then

$$V\frac{dC_{Bo}}{dt} = Q(C_{Bi} - C_{Bo})$$

describes the behavior of C_{Bo} versus time. Integrate this (a) for $t \leq T$, when $C_{Bi} = C_{Bi}^{o}$, and (b) for $t > T$, when $C_{Bi} = 0$. Sketch the shapes of the $C_{Bo}(t)$ curves for $t \leq T$ and $t > T$, as predicted by your theoretical integrated equations. What would the $t > T$ solution look like on semilogarithmic paper?

REFERENCES

Behnke, A. R., Thomson, R. M., and Shaw, L. A., Rate of elimination of dissolved nitrogen in man in relation to fat and water content of the body, *Am. J. Physiol.*, 114, 137 (1935).

Bird, R. B., Stewart, W. E., and Lightfoot, E. N., *Transport Phenomena*, Wiley, New York, 1960.

Bischoff, K. B., and Brown, R. G., Drug distribution in mammals, *Chem. Eng. Prog. Symp. Ser.*, 62, No. 66, 33 (1966).

Bischoff, K. B., Dedrick, R. L., and Slater, S. M., A model to represent bile transport of drugs, *Proc. Ann. Conf. Eng. Med. Biol.*, 23, 89 (1970a).

Bischoff, K. B., Dedrick, R. L., and Zaharko, D. S., Preliminary model for methotrexate pharmacokinetics, *J. Pharm. Sci.*, 59, 149 (1970b).

Dedrick, R. L., Gabelnick, H. L., and Bischoff, K. B., Kinetics of urea distribution, *Proc. Ann. Conf. Eng. Med. Biol.*, 21, 36-1 (1968).

Edelman, I. S., and Liebman, J., Anatomy of body water and electrolytes, *Am. J. Med.*, 27, 256 (1959).

Hiester, N. K., and Vermeulen, T., Saturation performance of ion exchange and adsorption columns, *Chem. Eng. Prog.*, 48, 505 (1952).

Hills, B. A., Chemical engineering principles in medicine and biology, *Br. Chem. Eng.*, 16, 700 (1971).

Huckaba, C. E., Biomedical engineering, *Chem. Eng.*, 78 (1), 126 (1971).

Jusko, W. J., and Lewis, G. P., Comparison of ampicillin and hetacillin pharmacokinetics in man, *J. Pharm. Sci.*, 62, 69 (1973).

Lassen, N. A., Hoedt-Rasmussen, K., Sorensen, S. C., Skinhoj, E., Cronquist, S., Bodforss, B., and Ingvar, D. H., Regional blood flow in man determined by krypton, *Neurology*, 13, 719 (1963).

Levett, J., Uptake and dissipation of alcohol in man, *Proc. Ann. Conf. Eng. Med. Biol.*, 15, 106 (1973).

Levy, G., Gibaldi, M., and Jusko, W. J., Multicompartment pharmacokinetic models and pharmacologic effects, *J. Pharm. Sci.*, 58, 422 (1969).

Middleman, S., *Transport Phenomena in the Cardiovascular System*, Wiley-Interscience, New York, 1972.

Notari, R. E., *Biopharmaceutics and Pharmacokinetics*, Marcel Dekker, New York, 1971.

Rowland, M., and Beckett, A. H., Mathematical treatment of oral sustained release drug formulations, *J. Pharm. Pharmacol.*, 16, 156T (1964).

Schanker, L. S., and Morrison, A. S., Physiological disposition of guanethidine in the rat and its uptake by heart slices, *Int. J. Neuropharmacol.*, 4, 23 (1965).

Scholer, J. F., and Code, C. F., Rate of adsorption of water from stomach and small bowel of human beings, *Gastroenterology*, 27, 565 (1954).

Wagner, J. G., *Biopharmaceutics and Relevant Pharmacokinetics*, Drug Intelligence Publ., Hamilton, Illinois, 1971.

Wiegand, R. G., and Taylor, J. D., Kinetics of plasma drug levels after sustained release dosage, *Biochem. Pharmacol.*, 3, 256 (1960).

BIBLIOGRAPHY

Rescigno, A., and Segre, G., *Drug and Tracer Kinetics*, Blaisdell, Waltham, Massachusetts, 1966.

Atkins, G. L., *Multicompartment Models for Biological Systems*, Methuen, London, 1969.

Chapter 7

TRANSPORT THROUGH CELL MEMBRANES

The means by which the blood conveys materials (nutrients, wastes) to and from the billions of capillaries in the body were discussed in some detail in Chapter 4. Filtration of plasma through the porous walls of the capillaries produces an interstitial, or extracellular, fluid which surrounds the individual tissue cells. Although this extracellular fluid does move slowly in preferred directions, ultimately being collected by the lymphatic system (which discharges it back into the blood), it can be considered to be fairly stagnant for present purposes.

The fundamental processes of transport of nutrients <u>to</u> the cell membrane and transport of wastes <u>from</u> the cell membrane (and back into the plasma in the capillaries) are driven primarily by ordinary diffusion. Although diffusional transfer is not efficient over large distances, the fact that each cell in the body is usually within 20-

30 μm, or two or three cell diameters, of a capillary does lead to very good extracellular transport of species in the body.

As shown in Table 2.3, the extracellular fluid and plasma are essentially identical in composition. The extracellular fluid generally lacks only the larger molecular species that are unable to penetrate the capillary walls freely. This same table shows, howeever, that the intracellular fluid is vastly different in composition than the extracellular fluid, especially with respect to Na^+, K^+, Mg^{2+}, Cl^-, phosphates, and glucose. Figure 7.1 makes the comparison a bit more clearly. Obviously, a highly nonequilibrium situation exists here in which tremendous gradients for mass transport across the cell membrane exist. Since all species listed in Figure 7.1 are found on both sides of the membrane barrier, they

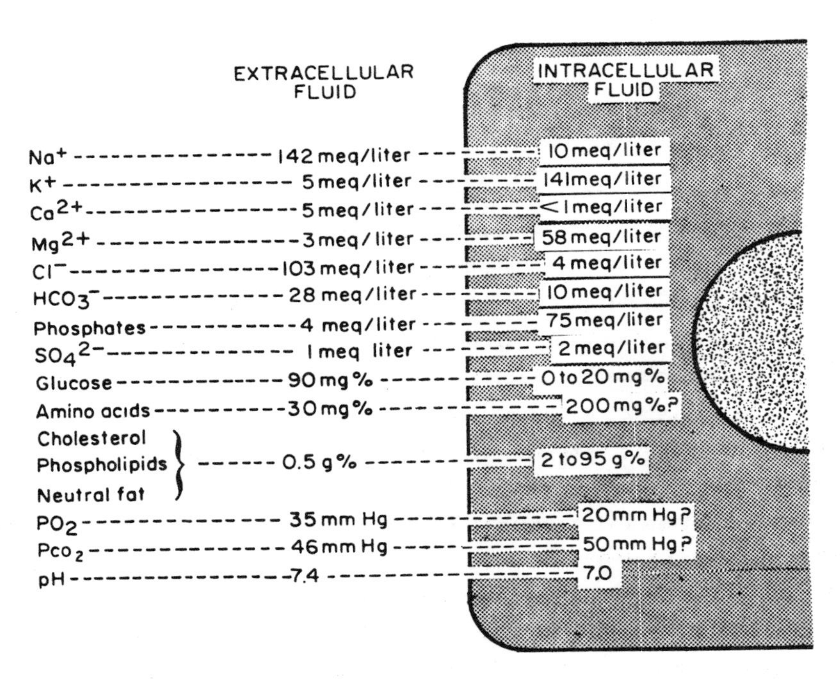

FIG. 7.1. Chemical compositions of extracellular and intracellular fluids. [From Guyton (1971), p. 39.]

must be able to transfer through the membrane. One might wonder how these steady-state differences in concentrations are maintained. It is certain that considerable energy must be required to maintain a system in such a state.

The subject of the present chapter is to investigate the mechanisms of transport of species through cell membranes. We will see that ordinary "passive" diffusion, "facilitated" diffusion (species aided by a "carrier"), and "active" transport (carrier-aided transfer against a concentration gradient, requiring biochemical energy) are all operative. Quantitative descriptions and examples are offered for some of these mechanisms. We begin, however, by discussing the structure and properties of the membranes themselves.

The basic function of the cell membrane is quite clear and may be summarized in brief fashion: to selectively control the transport of all species (charged/uncharged, large/small, etc.) into and out of the cell, so as to maintain the optimum internal and external environments for the functioning of the cell.

I. MEMBRANE STRUCTURE, COMPOSITION, AND PERMEABILITY

The cell membrane is thin (roughly 80-100 Å thick) and elastic. Chemically, membranes typically consist of 50-60% protein, 30-35% lipids, and 5-10% polysaccharides (some RNA and other species are also often present). The protein portion consists mainly of long, fibrous, elastic kinds of proteins. Table 7.1 gives some available data on membrane compositions for some microorganisms and mammals. For humans alone, membrane composition does not vary too widely, e.g., RBC, skin, liver, and muscle cell membranes are quite similar in makeup.

The lipid portion is comprised of several major classes, but the predominant types and typical percentages are phospholipids 65%, cholesterol 25%, and other lipids (e.g., glycolipids) 10%. Table 7.2 presents a breakdown of the lipids in human RBC membranes. Chemical

TABLE 7.1

Chemical Composition of Isolated Cell Membranes[a]

Species or tissue	Protein (%)	Lipid (%)	Other constituents or comments
Microorganisms			
Mycoplasmas sp.	47-60	35-37	Only 10% lipid is cholesterol; also present, 4-7% carbohydrate
Micrococcus lysodeiktius	63-65	15-26	About 2% RNA
Sarcina lutea	53-61	20-27	About 5% RNA
Bacillus lichenformis	75	28	About 0.8% RNA
Staphylococcus aureus	41	22.5	
Bacillus megaterium	70	25	Lipid largely cephalin
Amoeba proteus	25	32	15% polysaccharide
Pseudomonas aeruginosa	60	35	
Saccharomyces cerevisiae ETH 1022	37	35	
Saccharomyces cerevisiae NCYC 366	49	45	
Avian erythrocyte	89	4	
Mammalian cells			
Muscle, rat	65	15	Lipid largely phospholipid
Liver, rat	85	10	Half phospholipid is lecithin; cholesterol is one-third total lipid
Nerve myelin, ox brain	18-23	73-78	As liver. Over 90% protein is proteolipid, chloroform-methanol soluble
Human erythocyte	53	47	

[a]Adapted from Stein (1967).

TABLE 7.2

Chemical Composition of Human Erythrocyte Membranes[a,b]

Total protein	Total lipid	Total cholesterol	Total phospholipid	% Total phospholipid as		
				Lecithin	"Cephalin"	Sphingomyelin + lysophosphatide
17.7	3.99	1.20	2.27		60	
—	3.94	—	—			
—	4.95	1.13	2.88	30	40	22
—	—	—	—	38	25	37
6.0	5.24	1.42	3.15	27	27(PE)[c]	22
5.61	4.95	1.08	3.15	20	36	25
—	4.76	1.17	—	30	41	24
—	4.80	1.13	2.73			

[a]From Stein (1967).

[b]All values recorded as $10^{13} \times$ g substance per red cell.

[c]Here PE stands for phosphatidylethanolamine.

formulas for a typical phospholipid and for cholesterol are shown in Figure 7.2.

The exact structure of the cell membrane remains strongly debated even today, but the most accepted model is the "bimolecular lipid leaflet" structure shown in Figure 7.3. This consists of two rows of phospholipid molecules arranged with their hydrophobic (fatty acid) chains oriented inward and their hydrophilic (polar phosphate radical) groups oriented outward. An interrupted layer of proteins lies on each side, and a mucopolysaccharide coating is thought to exist on top of the outside protein layer. Many experimentally observed facts are explained by this model: (a) the fact that lipid-soluble species penetrate easily and other species do not (the protein layer is broken at intervals, allowing entrance of all species, yet the central continuous lipid portion controls transport of only lipid-soluble ones), (b) the membrane is hydrophilic (pro-

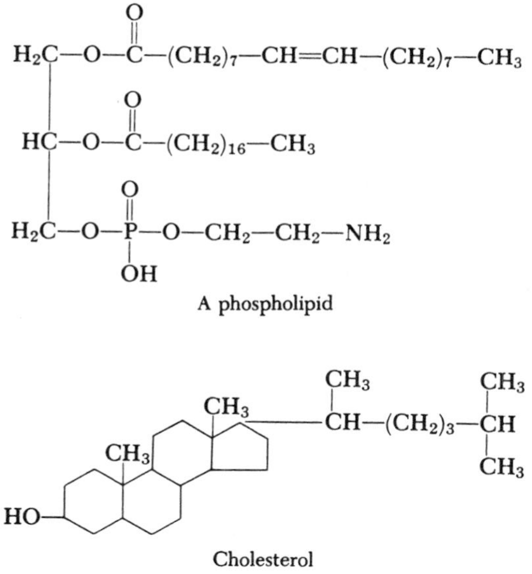

$$H_2C{-}O{-}C({=}O){-}(CH_2)_7{-}CH{=}CH{-}(CH_2)_7{-}CH_3$$
$$HC{-}O{-}C({=}O){-}(CH_2)_{16}{-}CH_3$$
$$H_2C{-}O{-}P({=}O)(OH){-}O{-}CH_2{-}CH_2{-}NH_2$$

A phospholipid

HO, CH_3, CH_3, CH_3, $CH{-}(CH_2)_3{-}CH$, CH_3, CH_3

Cholesterol

FIG. 7.2. Chemical structures of a phospholipid and cholesterol.

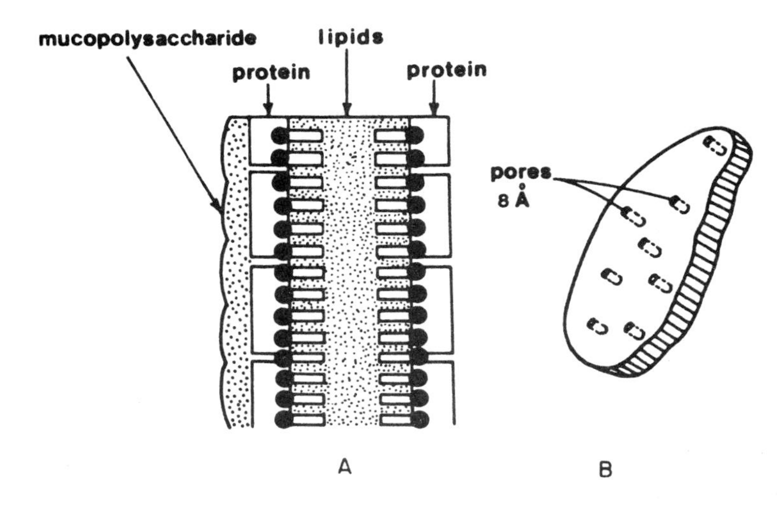

FIG. 7.3. (A) Postulated molecular organization of the cell membrane. (B) Pores in the cell membrane. [From Guyton (1971), p. 15.]

tein and mucopolysaccharide layers account for this), and (c) the mucopolysaccharide on one side might account for observed differences in the chemical aspects of the two sides.

This model as shown fails, however, to account for the fact that, while most species which have low lipid solubility do not transfer by ordinary diffusion through the membrane, some species like water, urea, and dissolved ions penetrate very freely. Therefore, the existence of membrane "pores" of an equivalent diameter (they are not necessarily cylindrical) of about 8 Å has been postulated. These pores, extending right through the membrane, would account for the species diffusion rates given in Table 7.3. Based on water flux rates it has been estimated that roughly 1/1600 of the membrane area consists of pores. In spite of this small fraction, the water flux out of a typical cell is large enough to shrink it to essentially nothing in a few hundredths of a second, were it not for the equal flux of water inward. Table 7.3 shows a vast difference between the diffusion rates of hydrated Cl^- and K^+ ions, even

TABLE 7.3

Relationship of Effective Diameters of Different Substances to Pore Diameter[a]

Substance	Diameter (Å)	Ratio to pore diameter	Approximate relative diffusion rate
Water molecule	3	0.38	50,000,000
Urea molecule	3.6	0.45	40,000,000
Hydrated chloride ion			
(red cell)	3.86	0.48	36,000,000
(nerve membrane)	—	—	200
Hydrated potassium ion	3.96	0.49	100
Hydrated sodium ion	5.12	0.64	1
Lactate ion	5.2	0.65	?
Glycerol molecule	6.2	0.77	?
Ribose molecule	7.4	0.93	?
Pore size	8 (Av.)	1.00	—
Galactose	8.4	1.03	?
Glucose	8.6	1.04	0.4
Mannitol	8.6	1.04	?
Sucrose	10.4	1.30	?
Lactose	10.8	1.35	?

[a]These data have been gathered from different sources but relate primarily to the red cell membrane. Other cell membranes have different characteristics. [From Guyton (1971), p. 42.]

though they are nearly the same size. From such information, it has been postulated that positively charged groups, probably adsorbed Ca^{2+} ions or parts of protein molecules, line the pores, as illustrated by Figure 7.4.

Table 7.3 shows clearly the very critical influence of the molecule/pore diameter ratio on diffusion rates. Note that what counts here is the hydrated molecular diameter. It is also indicated that the simple sugars are too large to fit through the pores. We know also that simple sugars have poor lipid solubility, yet they do transfer quite well into cells. As we shall see later, the explanation for this surprising behavior is that the sugars are probably carried inside by certain larger lipid-soluble molecules.

Data concerning the permeabilities of cell membranes to a variety of chemical species are available. If we exclude from consideration the relatively few species that are small enough to transport through the membrane pores, and those that transport by carrier mechanisms (i.e., not by ordinary passive diffusion), we find the correlation shown in Figure 7.5 between permeability and oil/water partition coefficient (this is presumably indicative of the lipid/water solubility ratio). Permeability P is defined by the equation

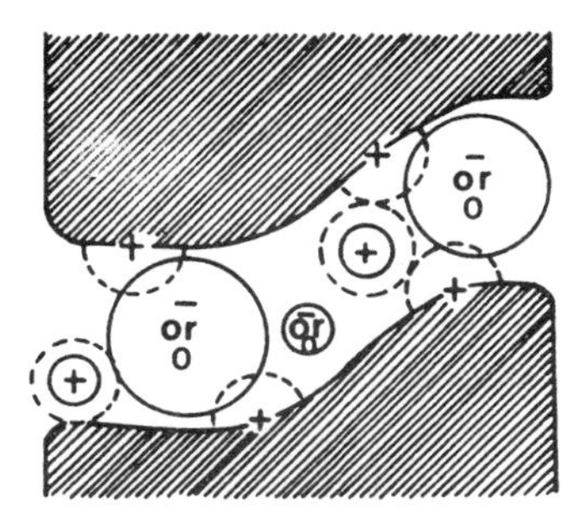

FIG. 7.4. Postulated structure of the cellular pore, showing the sphere of influence exerted by charges along the surface of the pore. [Modified from Solomon, A. K., *Sci. Am.*, 203 (6), 146 (1960).]

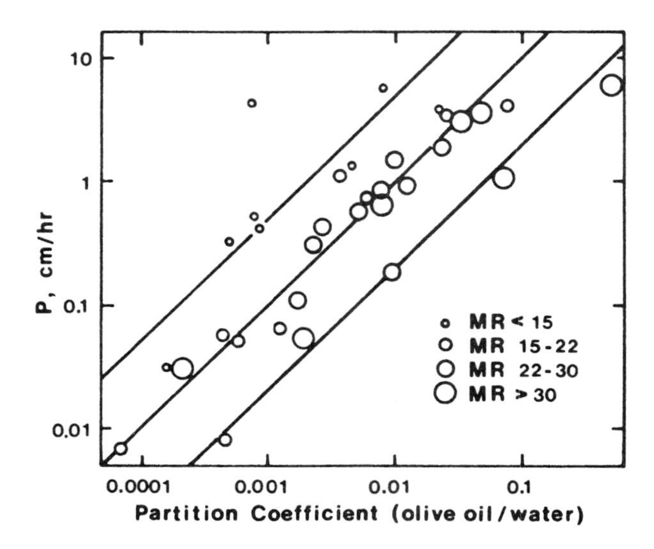

FIG. 7.5. The permeability of cells of *C. ceratophylla* to organic nonelectrolytes of different oil solubility and different molecular size. MR is the molar refraction of the molecules depicted, a parameter proportional to the molecular volume. [From Stein (1967), p. 74.]

$$P = \frac{-N_i}{\Delta C_i}$$

where N_i is the flux of species i g-mol/cm^2-sec, and ΔC_i is the concentration difference in the fluid from one side of the membrane to the other (g-mol/cc). The minus sign is needed because, if the flux (a vector) occurs in the +Z direction, then the change in C_i in the +Z direction must be negative. P is then always positive, by definition. Figure 7.5 also shows that permeability decreases with increasing molecular volume (the solid lines, by the way, connect series of compounds that are "homologous," i.e., of the same basic chemical constitution). The dependence of permeability on molecular size is shown more explicity in Figure 7.6. Since kinetic theory tells us that heavier molecules move at slower speeds, and therefore

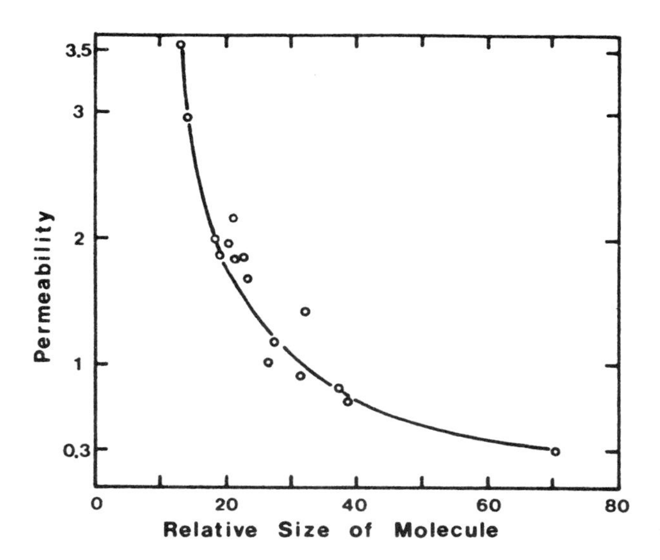

FIG. 7.6. Relation between molecular size and permeability in *Beggiatioa*. Scales are essentially arbitrary.

diffuse slower than lighter molecules, these results are not surprising.

Stein (1967) shows quite clearly the effects on permeability of adding extra -OH or extra -CH- groups to various molecules. His diagrams, presented here as Figures 7.7 and 7.8, demonstrate that decreased hydrophilic nature (less -OH) and increased hydrophobic nature (more -CH-) raise lipid solubilities (and, therefore, permeabilities).

II. SOLVENT MOVEMENT ACROSS MEMBRANES: OSMOSIS

The substance that moves in greatest amounts through cell membranes (about 100 "cell volumes" worth per second, in and out) is the solvent itself, namely water. Natural membranes are all <u>semi-</u>

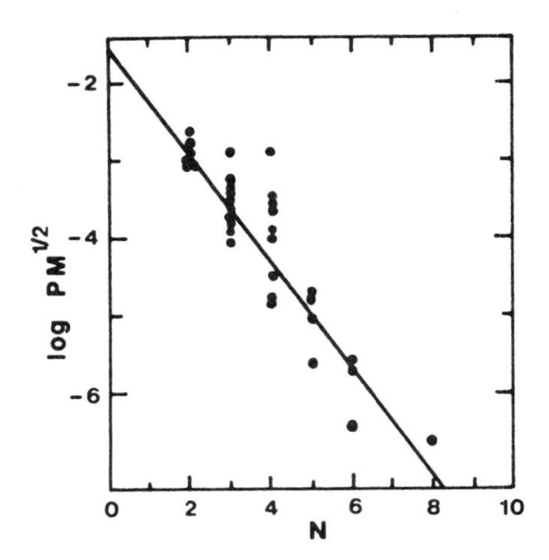

FIG. 7.7. The permeability data of Figure 7.5 replotted to show the variation of log $PM^{1/2}$ (P in centimeters per second) on the ordinate with the number N of hydrogen-bond-forming groups in the permeant on the abscissa. [From Stein (1967), p. 77.]

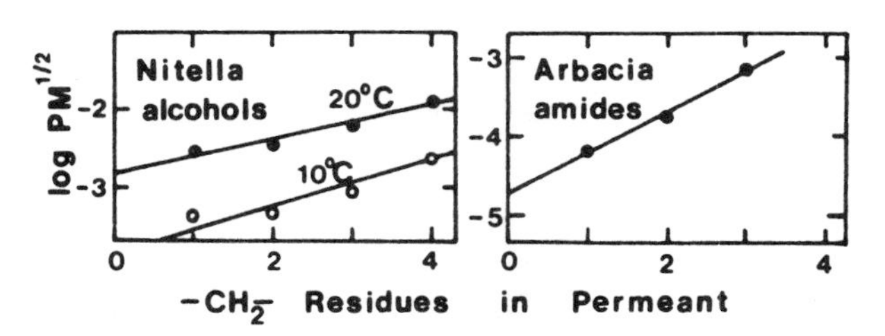

FIG. 7.8. Influence of length of hydrocarbon chain on the rate of penetration of some amides and alcohols. [From Stein (1967), p. 82.]

permeable to some extent, i.e., some substances (usually the larger ones, or those with negligible lipid solubility) do not transport through. This property gives rise to osmotic water flow.

To illustrate the phenomenon of osmotic water transport, let us assume that we have the conditions shown in Figure 7.9, with pure water on one side of a membrane and a NaCl solution on the other side. Let us assume NaCl cannot move through the membrane (this is

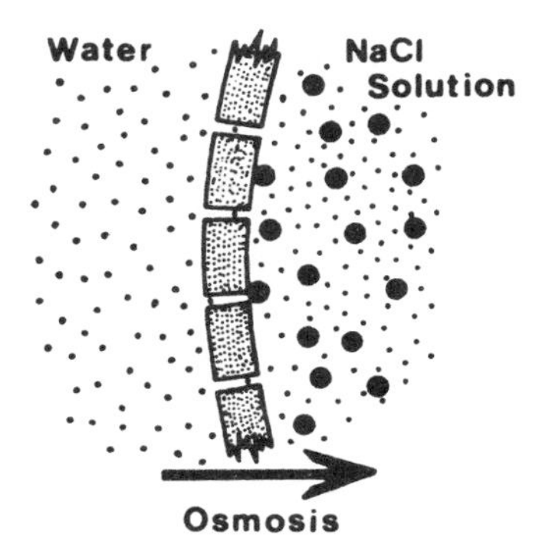

FIG. 7.9. Osmosis at a cell membrane when a sodium chloride solution is placed on one side of the membrane and water on the other side. [From Guyton (1971), p. 45.]

true for many membranes whose active transport mechanisms have been "poisoned").

Because of the presence of NaCl on one side, the concentration of water itself will be lower than on the pure water side. Thus, more water molecules will strike the membrane per unit time on the pure side than on the solution side, and this imbalance will cause a net diffusional flow of water into the solution. This is called osmosis, and the process will tend to occur until the concentration of water on both sides is equalized—in this case, this can occur only at infinite dilution of the solution.

This osmotic solvent flow can be stopped, however, if the solution side is pressurized to the proper degree, causing the solution volume to decrease to the point where the number of water molecules per unit volume in the solution equals the number per unit volume in the pure solvent. The pressure difference ΔP required to do this is called the osmotic pressure π. A more formal way to express this is to write the expression for the "chemical potential" μ of water

$$\mu = -RT \ln X_w$$

Here X_w is the mole fraction of water in the solution, T is the absolute temperature, and R is the universal gas constant (82.05 cm^3-atm/g-mol-°K). For $X_w = 1$ (pure water) we get a reference value of $\mu = 0$. One can also write the equation given above as

$$\mu = -RT \ln (1 - \Sigma X_j)$$

where ΣX_j is the sum of the mole fractions of <u>all</u> of the <u>solute</u> species. One can show from thermodynamics that the quantity μ is equal to $\tilde{V}\,\Delta P$, where $\tilde{V}$ is the molar volume of water (18.136 cc/g-mol at 37°C), and ΔP is the pressure difference required to halt osmotic flow (i.e., π). Thus, the osmotic pressure of any solution relative to <u>pure</u> water is just

$$\pi = -\frac{RT}{\tilde{V}} \ln(1 - \Sigma X_j)$$

For <u>low</u> solute concentrations, we can perform the expansion

$$\ln(1 - X) \cong -X - \frac{X^2}{2} - \frac{X^3}{3} - \cdots$$

and justify dropping all but the leading term. We then end up with the familiar Van't Hoff equation

$$\pi \cong \frac{RT}{\tilde{V}} \Sigma X_j = RT\Sigma C_j$$

where ΣC_j is the sum of the concentrations of all solutes, in moles per unit volume.

The osmotic pressure of a solution is not really so much a pressure as it is a measure of the concentration (or activity to be more exact) of the solvent. Note that osmotic pressure rises as water concentration decreases (solute concentration increases). In another sense, then, the osmotic pressure of a solution is a measure of the <u>deficit</u> of water concentration created by the presence of solute.

The last equation contains concentration in units of moles per volume. It should be stressed that what counts in osmosis is the number (i.e., moles) of solute molecules present, not the mass present. The reason for this is that each particle in solution, regardless of its mass, exerts essentially the same pressure on the membrane, since the kinetic energies of the particles are nearly the same. Molecules with greater mass move more slowly than lighter molecules, of course, but the product mv^2 is nevertheless about the same for all. Therefore, large solutes (like proteins) generally add surprisingly little to the total solution osmotic pressure, even though their mass concentrations may be quite substantial (as in plasma).

A. *Osmolarities and Tonicities*

Because osmotic water transport is so important physiologically it is common practice to speak of the total solute content of a solution in terms of "osmoles." One osmole is equal to one gram-mole of a solute which does not dissociate in solution. For a solute like NaCl, which dissociates into two ions in solution, a gram-mole equals two osmoles. Hence, a 1M (1 g-mol/liter) glucose solution is also a 1 osmolar solution, and a 1M NaCl solution is 2 osmolar (osmoles are thus the same as "equivalents"). Osmolarity is related to the term tonicity, often used by physiologists. "Isotonic saline" is an NaCl solution that has the same osmotic pressure as blood plasma, and it is commonly employed in medical treatments. Hypertonic and hypotonic solutions are those that have higher and lower osmolarities, respectively, than blood plasma.

To give one an idea of the magnitude of the osmotic pressure values of various fluids, we cite the fact that 1 Osm/liter is equivalent to an osmotic pressure of 19,300 mm Hg (equal to the pressure of a column of water about 860 ft high). In the limit of complete reduction of water concentration to zero (pure solute) we would have an osmotic pressure of 1,073,000 mm Hg relative to pure water. Clearly, the driving force for net solvent transport by osmosis is high, when an osmotic differential exists.

Another term commonly used by physiologists is colloid osmotic pressure. This simply refers to the contribution to the total solution osmotic pressure which is due to the colloids (macromolecules, such as proteins). The reason this parameter is important is that many membranes, such as capillary vessel walls, are permeable to all solutes except the colloids. One rule regarding osmotic pressures is that if the two solutions on either side of the membrane have the same amounts of a particular solute, then that solute can be disregarded—its osmotic contributions on both sides are the same and they counterbalance. Hence, when two solutions are virtually identical, except that one contains colloids, then the overall osmotic pressure difference equals the excess on one side due to the colloids.

B. *Quantitative Representation of Osmotic Flux*

Clearly, when neither of the two solutions is pure solvent, the osmotic driving forces must be written as $\Delta\pi$, the difference in the solutions' osmotic pressures. If both are dilute, then

$$\Delta\pi = RT\ \Delta(\Sigma C_j)$$

The total volumetric flow of solvent across a membrane is usually characterized by the equation

$$Q = kA(\Delta\pi - \Delta P)$$

where k is osmotic permeability. Note that $\Delta\pi$ must be reduced by the hydrostatic pressure difference across the membrane, <u>if</u> any exists. The parameter k must be experimentally measured for each membrane, as no adequate theory exists for its prediction.

Although osmosis is driven by a water "concentration difference," it must be pointed out that it cannot be regarded as simple diffusion of water through a membrane. As Ruch and Patton (1965) mention, measurements with isotopic tracers indicate that osmotic fluxes are far higher than diffusion theories would predict. Even though random molecular movements drive both osmosis and ordinary diffusion, somehow they are quite different. As yet no satisfactory explanation for this exists.

C. *Corrections for Solute Activity*

Although in the equations presented above we wrote $\pi \cong -(RT/\tilde{V}) \times \ln(1 - \Sigma X_j)$, we should mention that solute activities rather than concentrations should be used. That is, more correctly,

$$\pi = \frac{-RT}{\tilde{V}} \ln(1 - \Sigma \gamma_j X_j)$$

where γ is the activity coefficient (which is one for infinitely dilute solutions). For dilute solutions, γ is still needed, i.e.,

$$\pi \cong RT\ \Sigma \gamma_j C_j$$

Figure 7.10 shows how γ varies with concentration for NaCl solutions. For isotonic saline, the activity coefficient is only about 0.75; i.e., its "effective" concentration is only 75% of its actual concentration. This effect is much larger for charged solutes than for neutral ones, since charged particles in solution tend to be surrounded by others of opposite charge. Thus, when an ion moves it must either drag along these particles, or break away from them; in either event its rate of movement is hindered. The value of γ for NaCl will depend also on the concentrations of other ions present, as well as its own concentration, since all ions affect the electrical environment. It turns out that, in blood plasma, the activity coefficients of all univalent ions are roughly the same, about 0.7. Polyvalent ions have even lower activity coefficients. As an approximation it is common practice, when looking at the balance of

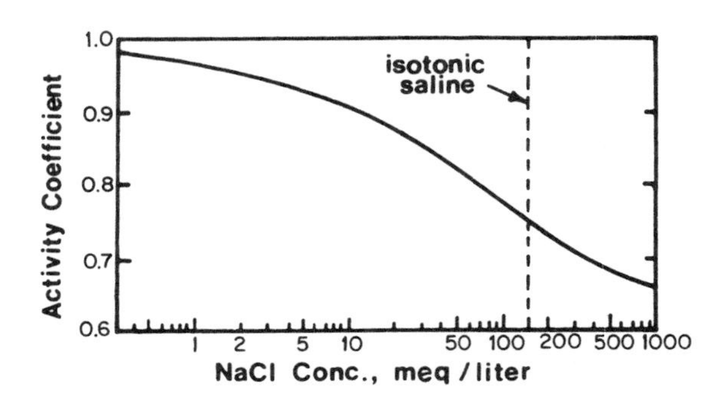

FIG. 7.10. The activity coefficient at increasing sodium chloride concentrations. [From Ruch and Patton (1965), p. 826.]

osmotic pressures in physiological situations, to disregard the concept of activity coefficients and work only in terms of concentrations. This is justified by the fact that nearly all body fluids have the same overall activity correction factors. Table 2.3, which gives the compositions and corrected osmolar activities for plasma, interstitial, and intracellular fluids, shows this clearly, and also indicates that overall activity coefficients are about 0.93 (the nonelectrolytes strongly counterbalance the low ionic activities).

Denbigh (1968) mentions that the activity coefficient may be estimated from the Debye-Hückel theory as

$$-\log \gamma = \alpha \nu_{+} |\nu_{-}| I^{1/2}$$

where $\nu_{+}|\nu_{-}|$ is the product of the ionic charges for the particular electrolyte (e.g., NaCl) and I is the ionic strength of the solution defined as

$$I = \frac{1}{2} \Sigma \nu_i^2 c_i$$

the summation being made over all ions in the solution. The value of α has been determined as 0.509 at 25°C and 0.488 at 0°C, for water as solvent. However, this formula is limited to quite dilute solutions. A better empirical formula to use is

$$-\log \gamma = \alpha \nu_+ |\nu_-| \frac{I^{1/2}}{1 + I^{1/2}}$$

with α having the same value as before.

D. *Osmotic Shrinking and Bursting of Red Blood Cells*

The effects of osmotic water shifts on cells in general and on red blood cells in particular can be observed easily experimentally by exposing red blood cells, whose inner fluid is isotonic with 0.15M NaCl solution, to hypertonic and hypotonic saline. When exposed to hypertonic saline, water leaves the cells, causing them to shrink (crenate) into distorted shapes of various kinds (easily observed microscopically). Exposure to hypotonic solutions causes rapid swelling, which may actually result in the bursting of some cells (lysis). Figure 7.11 shows a so-called fragility curve for red blood cells, a plot of percent hemolyzed versus hypotonic concentration (isotonic level 0.9 g/100 ml). These data are conven-

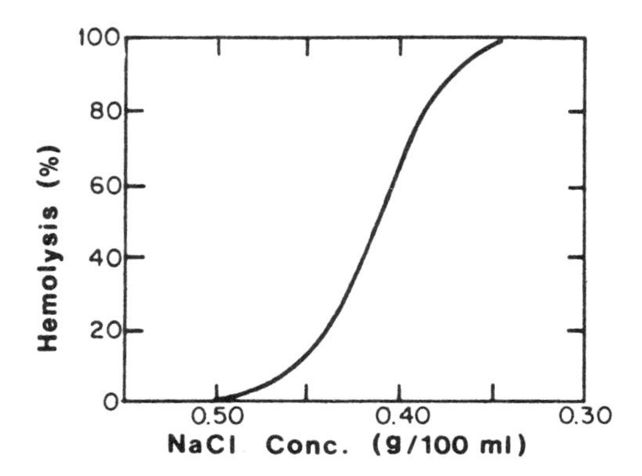

FIG. 7.11. Fragility curve for human erythrocytes.

iently obtained by measuring the amount of free hemoglobin in the plasma (which results from lysis).

As a final point with respect to osmosis, it should be pointed out that for nearly all cells in the body there is normally a balance between inner and outer osmolarities, and hence little net water flux occurs. In certain areas, such as in capillary walls, there does occur a steady and significant net water flux by osmosis (this is how lymph is formed). However, in this case the flow is not really flow into or out of cells, but rather flow through actual pores in the capillary wall.

III. PASSIVE DIFFUSION OF NONELECTROLYTES

We begin our treatment of true cell membrane diffusion, as opposed to osmosis, with the simple case of nonelectrolyte transport. As shown by several writers [refer, for example, to Bird et al. (1960)], Fick's law for diffusion has the form

$$N_i - X_i \Sigma N_j = -D_i C \nabla X_i$$

where N_i is the molar flux of solute i (e.g., moles/cm^2-sec) relative to stationary coordinates, ΣN_j is the sum of all species molar fluxes (including the solvent and i) relative to stationary coordinates, C is the total molar concentration of the fluid, and ∇X_i is the gradient of the mole fractional concentration of solute i.

The term ΣN_j represents the bulk flow of the whole solution and manifests itself in an increase or decrease of the total moles of species in the cell with time. The amount of species i that is carried in with (or out with) this bulk flow is clearly the mole fraction of i times the molar bulk flow rate. Since substantial bulk flow would normally result in a volume change of a cell we can assume that ΣN_j is usually neglectable (one exception is where osmotic flow of solvent is large, as in red blood cell crenation or lysis). Another way of stating this is to say that equimolal counter-diffusion exists. The term on the right is the diffusive flux relative to bulk flow. D_i, the diffusion coefficient, is roughly constant for any particular situation, but can vary with concentration somewhat.

When diffusion is unidirectional, as in a membrane, we may assume that

$$\nabla X_i = \frac{\partial X_i}{\partial x} + \frac{\partial X_i}{\partial y} + \frac{\partial X_i}{\partial z} = \frac{dX_i}{dz}$$

where z is the transport direction. For normal cases, then,

$$N_i \cong -D_i C \frac{dX_i}{dz} = -D_i \frac{dC_i}{dz}$$

Most membranes are quite thin, and it is common practice to assume that the concentration gradient is linear, i.e., $dC_i/dz = (C_{i2} - C_{i1})/\Delta z$ where C_{i2} is the concentration of i in the membrane at the outer boundary, C_{i1} is the concentration of i in the membrane at the inner boundary, and $\Delta z = z_2 - z_1$ is the membrane thickness.

Since one normally knows, not the bounding concentrations in the membrane, but the concentrations in the fluids, one usually writes

$$N_i = \frac{-D_i K_{Di} (C_{si2} - C_{si1})}{\Delta z}$$

where C_{si} is the concentration of i in the solutions and K_{Di} is the partition coefficient for solute i (like a solubility in the membrane). K_{Di} is the ratio of the concentration in the membrane to the concentration in solution (see Figure 7.12). This approach assumes K_{Di} is constant, i.e., independent of concentration. If one uses bulk C_{si} values, this implicitly assumes that no concentration gradients exist in the solutions, i.e., diffusion is much slower in the membrane than in the solutions. This may not always be true.

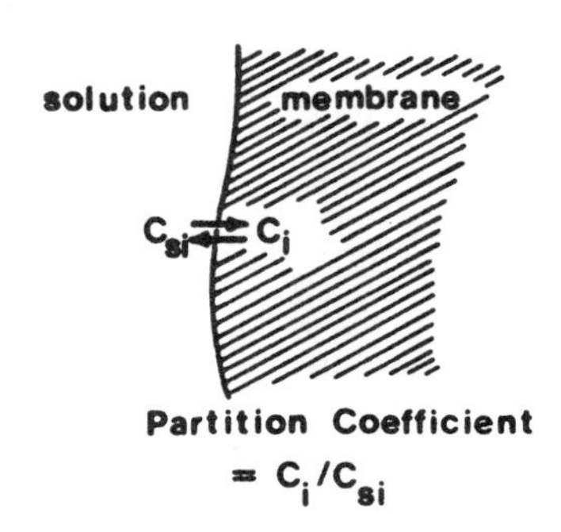

FIG. 7.12. The partition coefficient. [From Ruch and Patton (1965), p. 822.]

Comparing the above with an earlier equation we see that the so-called solute permeability P is equal to $D_i K_{Di}/\Delta z$. It is now clear why observed solute permeabilities correlate directly with lipid solubility (see Figures 7.5-7.8): Diffusion theory predicts it! The dependence of P on molecular weight is also now explained. The kinetic theory of gases predicts quite explicitly that $D_i \propto MW_i^{-1/2}$. For liquids as well (which is more like our case), this same relationship is generally true [as is discussed by Davson (1964) in detail]. Thus, permeabilities should decrease with molecular size, and data presented earlier indicate they do.

IV. PASSIVE DIFFUSION OF ELECTROLYTES

When the diffusing species is a charged ion, an additional force besides the ion's concentration gradient can cause diffusion. This other force is the prevailing electrical potential gradient. Assuming that the fluxes produced by both forces are linearly additive, we have, for unilateral transport and zero bulk flow

$$N_i = -D_i\left(\frac{dC_i}{dz} + \nu_i \beta C_i \frac{d\phi}{dz}\right)$$

where $\beta = F/RT$, F is Faraday's constant (the net charge per mole of univalent ions, 96,496 coulombs), ϕ is the electrical potential, and ν_i is the valence.

This result may be rewritten as (dropping the subscript i)

$$N = -De^{-\nu\beta\phi} \frac{d}{dz} (Ce^{\nu\beta\phi})$$

The quantity in parentheses, $Ce^{\nu\beta\phi}$, is often called the electrochemical activity and represents the effective concentration of the species under the influence of the electrical potential. It is related to the electrochemical potential μ by the equation

$$\mu - \mu_0 = RT \ln (Ce^{\nu\beta\phi}) = RT \ln C + \nu F\phi$$

where μ_0 is a standard state potential.

A. *The Zero Net Flux Case*

Let us assume that a particular species is in equilibrium and no net flux of the species occurs across the membrane. Therefore,

$$-De^{-\nu\beta\phi} \frac{d}{dz}(Ce^{\nu\beta\phi}) = 0$$

Since D is finite and $e^{-\nu\beta\phi}$ is finite (only for $\phi = \infty$ would this not be so), then it <u>must</u> be true that

$$\frac{d}{dz}(Ce^{\nu\beta\phi}) = 0$$

that is, $Ce^{\nu\beta\phi}$ must be a constant. If "1" and "2" are the inner and outer boundaries of the membrane, then

$$C_1e^{\nu\beta\phi_1} = C_2e^{\nu\beta\phi_2}$$

or

$$\phi_2 - \phi_1 = \frac{1}{\nu\beta} \ln \frac{C_1}{C_2}$$

This is one form of the general Nernst equation. For 37°C, one can show that $1/(\nu\beta) = 26.5/\nu$ mV.

Ruch and Patton (1965) mention several major applications of the Nernst equation. First, by testing whether data for a particular solute agree with the equation one can deduce whether or not passive transport is the sole means by which the solute moves (nonagreement indicates that some facilitated or active transport mechanism must also be operative). Second, one can use the Nernst equation to predict the overall membrane potential, $\phi_2 - \phi_1$. However, to do this one usually must employ a more general equation which accounts for more than just one solute. The more general Nernst equation is developed below.

B. Derivation of the General Nernst Equation

Since the flux of any single ion is given by the equation

$$N_i = -D_i\left(\frac{dC_i}{dz} + \frac{\nu_i F}{RT} C_i \frac{d\phi}{dz}\right)$$

the current carried by this type of ion is equal to $N_i \nu_i F$ coulombs/cm^2-sec. If one now assumes that the electrical potential gradient across the membrane is linear (the Goldman assumption), i.e.,

$$\frac{d\phi}{dz} = \frac{E}{\delta}$$

(where $E = \phi_2 - \phi_1$ and $\delta = z_2 - z_1$), we can write that the current I is

$$I = -\nu FD \frac{dC}{dz} - \frac{(\nu F)^2 DCE}{RT\ \delta}$$

Integrating, it can be shown that

$$I = -\frac{(\nu F)^2 DE}{RT\delta}\left(\frac{C_2 - C_1 e^{-EF\nu/RT}}{1 - e^{-EF\nu/RT}}\right)$$

When one considers the current carried by all ions, it must be true that at equilibrium electroneutrality prevails, i.e.,

$$\Sigma I_i = 0$$

where the summation is made over all negative ions and all positive ions. This requirement, combined with the preceding equation, permits derivation of the general Nernst equation:

$$-E = \frac{RT}{F} \ln \frac{D_{Cl}Cl_1 + D_K K_2 + D_{Na}Na_2 + \cdots}{D_{Cl}Cl_2 + D_K K_1 + D_{Na}Na_1 + \cdots}$$

If one or two ions dominate by having large products of their diffusion coefficients times their concentrations, then the terms for the other species may be neglected. This can be illustrated as follows.

C. *Resting Membrane Potentials in Nerve Cells*

Electrical potentials exist across the membranes of essentially all cells in the body but especially in muscle and nerve cells. A nerve cell has, in its unexcited state, a transmembrane potential of about -75 mV (inside negative with respect to the outside). This potential is local, i.e., confined to the immediate neighborhood of the membrane; the bulk fluids are, of course, electrically neutral.

Active transport creates and maintains the large differences in the ionic compositions of intracellular and extracellular fluids which were presented earlier (Table 2.3). It turns out that the permeability of the resting nerve cell membrane to K^+ is much larger (∿75 times) than its permeability to Na^+. Thus K^+ tends to move outward from the cell, causing a local excess of positive charges on the outer side and the presence of negative charges along the inner side. Chloride, which only diffuses about 1/60 as fast as K^+, tends to enter the cell. This also promotes the generation of a negatively charged inner wall and a positive outer wall. Other positive and negative ions behave like K^+ and Cl^- but are either present in much lower amounts or have lower diffusive permeabilities. Therefore, K^+ really dominates the transport picture.

If we accept the permeability ratios for Na^+, Cl^-, and K^+ which were mentioned above, and use the Na^+, Cl^-, and K^+ concentrations given in Figure 7.1, we can estimate the transmembrane potential as

$$\Delta\phi = -26.5 \ln \frac{(1)(141) + (1/60)(103) + (1/75)(10)}{(1)(5) + (1/60)(4) + (1/75)(142)} = -74 \text{ mV}$$

This agrees well with actual measured values of about 75 mV. If this computation were done accounting only for K^+ (no Na^+ or Cl^-), a result of 88 mV would be obtained, which is much the same.

D. Gibbs-Donnan Equilibrium

A third major application of the Nernst equation is in the analysis of the so-called Gibbs-Donnan equilibrium phenomena.

As long as all charged ions can permeate the membrane, no membrane potential can exist at equilibrium <u>if</u> passive diffusion is the sole transport mechanism. However, if some ions are too large to permeate the membrane, then an equilibrium membrane potential can exist. In biological systems the presence of nonpermeating proteins in anionic form on one side of a membrane, but not on the other side, does occur (e.g., across capillary walls).

Consider the system shown in Figure 7.13, where NaCl exists on both sides of a membrane and a large nonpermeating anion P^- exists on only one side. From the Nernst equation it is apparent that at equilibrium

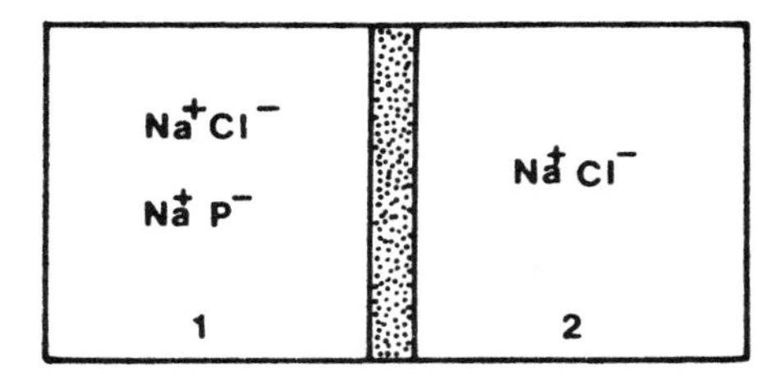

FIG. 7.13. A mixture of a protein salt, NaP, and NaCl separated from NaCl by a membrane permeable to salt and water.

$$\frac{(Na)_1}{(Na)_2} = \frac{(Cl)_2}{(Cl)_1}$$

or

$$(Na)_1(Cl)_1 = (Na)_2(Cl)_2$$

Since there are equal concentrations of positive and negative ions in each compartment (electroneutrality must be satisfied), then we may replace $(Na)_2$ by $(Cl)_2$ to obtain

$$(Na)_1(Cl)_1 = (Cl)_2^2$$

Now, $(Na)_1$ is clearly greater than $(Cl)_1$ since part of the Na^+ ions in compartment 1 are associated with Cl^- ions and part with P^- ions [it is also obvious that $(Na)_1 > (Na)_2$ and $(Cl)_1 < (Cl)_2$]. Hence, the left-hand side of the equation given above, being the product of two unequal quantities, may be represented by a rectangle, and the right-hand side by a square. One can easily prove that the sum of the sides of a rectangle is greater than the sum of the sides of a square of equal area; therefore,

$$(Na)_1 + (Cl)_1 > 2(Cl)_2$$

or

$$(\mathrm{Na})_1 + (\mathrm{Cl})_1 > (\mathrm{Na})_2 + (\mathrm{Cl})_2$$

The sum of the diffusible ion concentrations in compartment 1 is greater than that in compartment 2. In addition, because of the nondiffusible P^- ions, the total concentrations of solutes are in even greater imbalance, i.e.,

$$(\mathrm{Na})_1 + (\mathrm{Cl})_1 + (\mathrm{P}) > (\mathrm{Na})_2 + (\mathrm{Cl})_2$$

Osmotically there exists, then, a driving force for water transport into compartment 1. However, as long as Na^+ and Cl^- can freely redistribute, one can show that as long as nondiffusible ions exist in compartment 1, there will always be an osmotic imbalance favoring water flow into compartment 1. Unless opposing pressure is applied to compartment 1, no limit to the process exists and ultimately all water and solute from side 2 will pass to side 1.

In the capillaries a hydrostatic pressure greater than that in the interstitial fluid on the other side of the wall does in fact exist. This counteracts the osmotic tendency for interstitial fluid to enter the protein-rich plasma. Actually, the hydrostatic pressure difference is sufficient to cause net water transport out of the plasma.

V. PRESSURE DIFFUSION

The passive diffusion of solutes can also be driven by gradients in hydrostatic pressure. To characterize this one uses the same diffusion equation presented earlier with an added term:

$$N_i = -D_i \left(\frac{dC_i}{dz} + \frac{C_i \nu_i F}{RT} \frac{d\phi}{dz} + \frac{C_i \overline{V}_i}{RT} \frac{dP}{dz} \right)$$

where $\overline{V}_i = (\partial \tilde{V}/\partial n_i)_{T,P,n_j}$, the partial molar volume of solute i. Pressure diffusion is not normally as important as other passive diffusion mechanisms but still is often significant. Even for red blood cells where the transmembrane hydrostatic pressure is only about 1 mm Hg, the contribution of pressure diffusion is far from negligible. This mechanism should not be confused with osmotic pressure-driven solvent flow, which is really different.

VI. FACILITATED TRANSPORT

Some substances are quite insoluble in lipids, are larger than the membrane pores, and yet still transfer through cell membranes quite well. Sugars (e.g., glucose) are typical solutes of this kind. Figure 7.14 shows how transport is accomplished—at the higher concentration side of the membrane the solute combines with a carrier of some sort. The combined form, which is lipid-soluble, then transports by ordinary passive diffusion to the lower concentration side where the solute splits away from the carrier.

The rate of this facilitated carrier transport depends on (a) the concentration difference of the solute across the membrane, (b) the amount of carrier present, (c) the rate of the combination and splitting reactions, and (d) the diffusion coefficient of the carrier-solute combination. The nature of the carriers is not yet

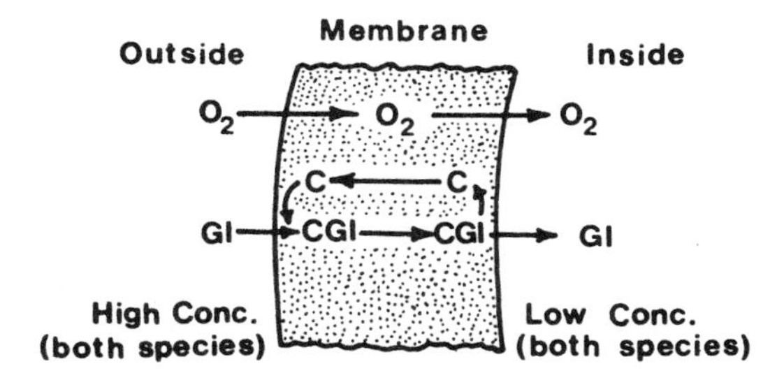

FIG. 7.14. Diffusion of substances through the lipid matrix of the membrane. The upper part of the figure shows free diffusion of oxygen through the membrane and the lower part shows facilitated diffusion of glucose. [From Guyton (1971), p. 41.]

known but it is thought that for glucose the carrier is a protein of about 50,000 molecular weight. The effects of hormones (e.g., insulin increases glucose transport rates by almost 10 times) are also not understood.

It should be pointed out that the reactions at both sides are not 100% combination or 100% splitting. Rather, reversible reactions exist, as shown in Figure 7.15. It is only the high solute concentration at one side that causes the reaction equilibrium to shift in favor of "product" (carrier-solute complex), and the low solute concentration at the other end that causes the equilibrium to shift back in favor of dissociation. The reactions may not necessarily be rapid enough so that equilibrium exists, but they are thought to be so.

Facilitated diffusion can also be significant in enhancing the transport of substances which already transport anyway (see the example below on oxygen transport through hemoglobin solutions), in contrast to sugar transport through membranes, which will not occur at all unless a carrier is operative.

The carrier transport of one substance down its concentration gradient can often be coupled with transport of another substance

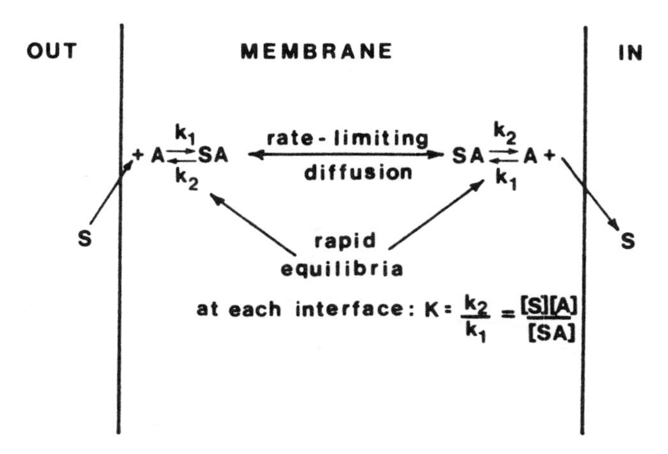

FIG. 7.15. Scheme for carrier-mediated transport.

in the opposite direction by the same carrier. Although this latter substance may proceed against its own concentration gradient, this is not to be considered a true case of active transport, i.e., countergradient transport driven by cellular biochemical energy. Rather, in this case the energy is being supplied by the established concentration gradient of the first substance. Glucose-arabinose transport in red blood cells is an example of such coupling (arabinose goes "uphill").

VII. FACILITATED DIFFUSION OF OXYGEN IN HEMOGLOBIN SOLUTIONS

Around 1960, experimental studies concerned with measuring oxygen diffusion rates through hemoglobin solutions (soaked into a Millipore filter separating two gas chambers) uncovered the fact that oxygen transported very much faster than nitrogen at low solute partial pressures. Typical results are shown in Figure 7.16. In the high partial pressure ranges the data are adequately explained by simple diffusion models, and differences between O_2 and N_2 are consistent with known O_2 and N_2 diffusivity and solubility values for aqueous solutions.

It was ultimately concluded that combination between oxygen and hemoglobin, and the subsequent diffusion of oxyhemoglobin, was augmenting the oxygen transport at low partial pressures. One can analyze the situation as follows. Let us represent the reaction as

$$O_2 + Hb \rightleftarrows HbO_2$$

Four components exist in the system: O_2, Hb, HbO_2, and water. It is clear that no net flux of water occurs ($N_w = 0$) and that the molar fluxes of Hb and HbO_2 will be equal and opposite at steady state ($N_{Hb} + N_{HbO_2} = 0$) since the carrier continually recycles. Thus, the bulk flow in the system (ΣN_j) is simply equal to the transport of O_2. Therefore,

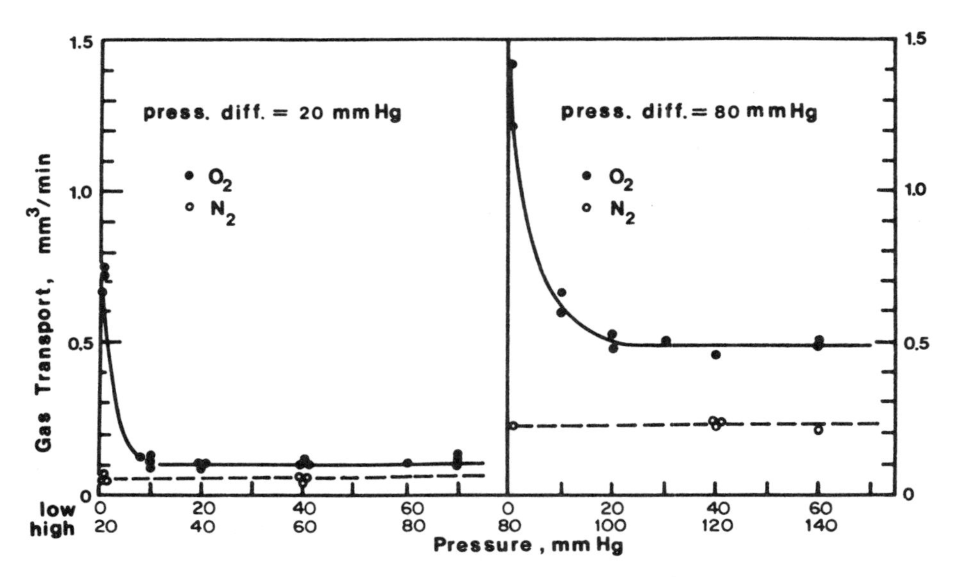

FIG. 7.16. Steady-state flux of oxygen and nitrogen through hemoglobin solutions with constant pressure differences. [From Keller and Friedlander (1966).]

$$N_{O_2}(1 - X_{O_2}) = -CD_{O_2} \frac{dX_{O_2}}{dz}$$

Pressure diffusion is neglected since pressure is kept the same on both sides, although <u>partial</u> pressures are varied. For HbO_2 we can write also

$$N_{HbO_2} - X_{HbO_2} N_{O_2} = -CD_{HbO_2} \frac{dX_{HbO_2}}{dz}$$

If the oxygen partial pressure is low, X_{O_2} will be small (the solubility of O_2 in aqueous solutions is not very great) and X_{HbO_2} will also be small (the Hb will be only partially reacted, and also the high molecular weight of Hb means the <u>mole</u> fraction of HbO_2 will not be very large), and we can therefore take them to be zero in the equations above. The total transport rate of oxygen equals that transported as dissolved O_2 and that carried in the form of HbO_2, and therefore

$$N_{O_2,tot} = N_{O_2} + N_{HbO_2} = -C\left(D_{O_2} \frac{dX_{O_2}}{dz} + D_{HbO_2} \frac{dX_{HbO_2}}{dz}\right)$$

If we assume reaction equilibrium exists everywhere (fast forward and reverse reactions), then we can write

$$\frac{dX_{HbO_2}}{dz} = \frac{dX_{O_2}}{dz} \frac{dX_{HbO_2}}{dX_{O_2}} = \frac{dX_{O_2}}{dz} \frac{dC_{HbO_2}}{dC_{O_2}}$$

where dC_{HbO_2}/dC_{O_2} is equal to the slope of the oxyhemoglobin dissociation curve, Figure 7.17 (when replotted as moles per liter HbO_2 versus moles per liter O_2, in solution). One can then express the transport of O_2 as

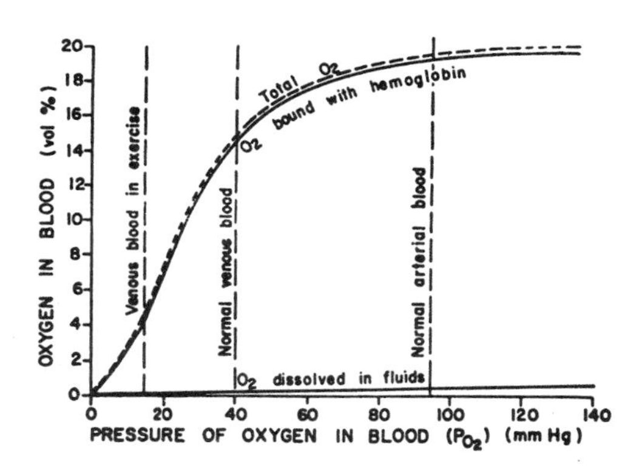

FIG. 7.17. Quantity of oxygen in each 100 ml of normal blood (a) bound with hemoglobin and (b) dissolved in the water of the blood; (c) total oxygen in both forms.

$$N_{O_2} = -CD_{eff} \frac{dX_{O_2}}{dz}$$

where the effective diffusion coefficient D_{eff} is given by

$$D_{eff} = D_{O_2} + D_{HbO_2} \frac{dC_{HbO_2}}{dC_{O_2}}$$

Note that the slope of the HbO_2 dissociation curve is very steep at lower O_2 partial pressures (0-40 mm Hg) and levels off toward zero at higher partial pressures. Thus, the effective diffusion coefficient for O_2 transport will be much higher than D_{O_2} alone at low partial pressures, and will tend toward D_{O_2} at higher partial pressures. This explains the observed behavior quite nicely.

In the concentrated solutions inside red blood cells (the data above were taken in more dilute solutions of free Hb), the value of D_{HbO_2} is quite low. Thus, the augmentation of O_2 transport is not of great physiological importance. The example above does, however, illustrate the principles of facilitated transport clearly.

VIII. ACTIVE TRANSPORT

We have seen earlier that intracellular fluid tends to have much more K^+ and much less Na^+ and Cl^- than extracellular fluids. Since these ions can indeed permeate cell membranes, the question arises as to how the large concentration differences of these ions are maintained across the cell membrane. The answer is that active transport occurs from the lower concentration zones to the higher concentration zones, which overrides the passive diffusion processes (e.g., leakage of Na^+ into the cell). Figure 7.18 shows that a

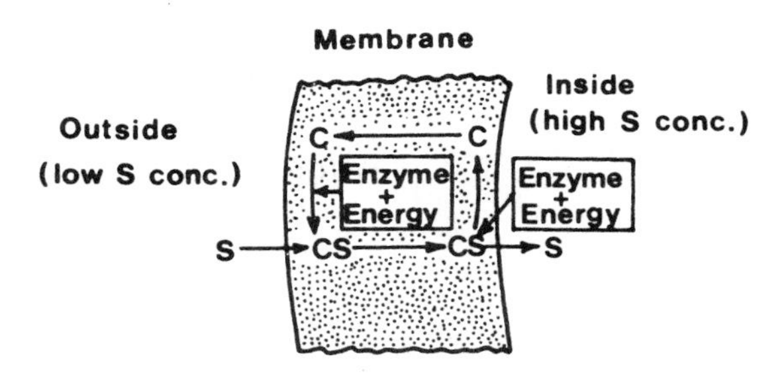

FIG. 7.18. Basic mechanism of active transport. [From Guyton (1971), p. 47.]

carrier is again involved. In this case, however, transport is truely against often large concentration gradients, and therefore biochemical cellular energy is required to fuel the process.

Very little is known about active transport. Enzymes are believed to catalyze the chemical reactions between solute and carrier. The carriers, probably proteins or lipoproteins, may work in three possible ways, as depicted in Figure 7.19. Besides the usual diffusive motion type of mechanism, the carrier might (if long enough) simply pick up the solute, rotate 180 degrees, and release it at the other side. Or, the carrier (again, if long enough) may shuttle the solute along a series of active sites of some sort. These mechanisms are speculative. What is known is that the following ions actively transport: Na^+, Cl^-, K^+, Ca^{2+}, HCO_3^-, Fe ions, Mg^{2+}, H^+, I^-, ureate ions, and others. Also, amino acids and certain sugars move by this process. It is known additionally that the carriers are quite specific for each species. In some case cotransport occurs, i.e., glucose will not transport unless Na^+ does also (same carrier for both?). The transport of Na^+ and K^+ seems to be linked also, as if the carrier brings Na^+ in one direction and always carries a K^+ back on the return trip.

Active transport is often limited to certain areas or organs of the body, such as the kidneys, intestines, and liver. However, facilitated transport, when it occurs, appears to be general for nearly all cells in the body. Hormones have a particularly great

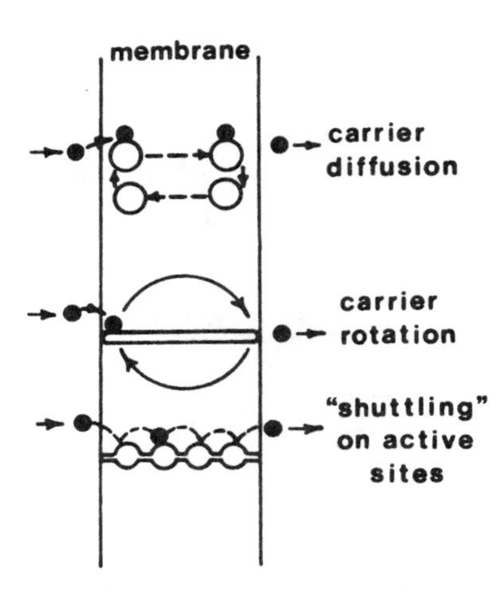

FIG. 7.19. Possible mechanisms of active transport (schematic).

influence on active transport processes, especially amino acid transport.

Figure 7.20 shows details of the postulated mechanism for Na^+-K^+ transport. The carrier Y is believed to combine with Na^+ under the action of an enzyme called adenosine triphosphatase (ATPase), with energy supplied from the reaction MgATP $\rightarrow$ MgADP + a phosphate radical. Upon delivery of Na^+ to the opposite side, splitting occurs which slightly alters the carrier's configuration (it is now therefore called X). A similar combination, this time with K^+, then occurs under the action of another (the same?) enzyme, and the process continues as indicated. This Na^+-K^+ "pump" is extremely important as the basis for nerve impulse conduction, and for the control of osmolarity in the cells. Note that a continuous leakage of Na^+ and K^+ by passive diffusion through pores occurs (easily verified experimentally by poisoning the carrier mechanism).

IX. PINOCYTOSIS

A final transport mechanism which we shall mention only briefly is pinocytosis, a mechanism by which the membrane invaginates

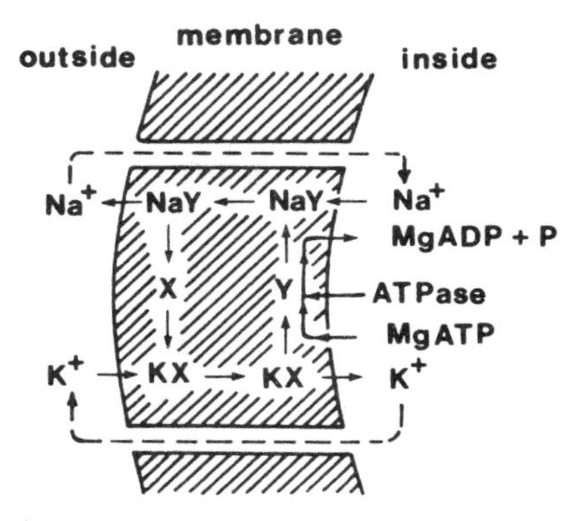

FIG. 7.20. Postulated mechanism for active transport of sodium and potassium through the cell membrane, showing coupling of the two transport mechanisms and delivery of energy to the system at the inner surface of the membrane. [From Guyton (1971), p. 49.]

(creates a cavity) and actually engulfs a large molecule or particle. This process is depicted schematically in Figure 7.21. After the membrane surrounds the entity the invaginated portion breaks off, forming a vesicle which then transports through the membrane by some means. The molecule may be delivered to the other side and released, or, in the case of particles like bacteria, digested.

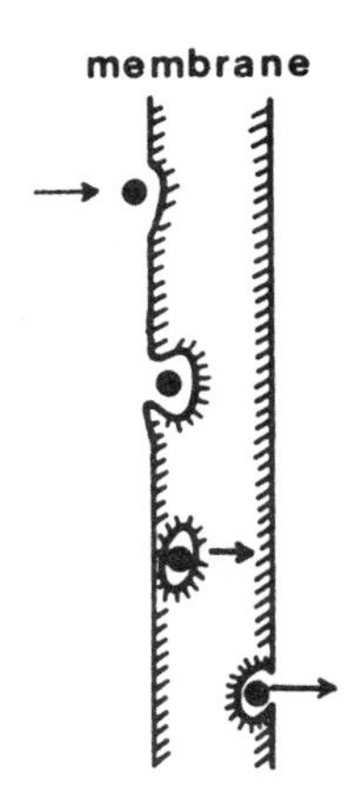

FIG. 7.21. Successive stages in pinocytotic transport through a membrane. [From Ruch and Patton (1965), p. 824.]

Pinocytosis is important in that it is the only known way that proteins can pass through the cell membrane (which they do).

PROBLEMS

1. *Osmosis.* Compute the osmotic pressure of a 0.14N NaCl solution at 37°C using (a) the exact equation for π and (b) the Van't Hoff equation for "dilute" solutions. Assume ideal behavior ($\gamma = 1$).

2. *Estimation of activity coefficients.* Estimate the activity coefficient at 37°C for a 0.14N NaCl solution using the Debye-Hückel equation for "dilute" solutions and the more accurate formula for nondilute solutions. Assume $\alpha = 0.519$ at 37°C. Compare your values to the value suggested by Figure 7.10.

3. *Diffusion of a nonelectrolyte.* In artificial kidney devices (see Chapter 9) blood containing waste materials is passed on one side of a membrane and a waste-free saline solution is passed on the other side. Wastes diffuse from the blood, through the membrane, and into the saline solution, and the blood is thereby cleansed.

   An important waste is urea, $(NH_2)_2CO$. Estimate the flux (in g/m^2-hr) of urea through a cellulosic membrane 1 mil (i.e., 0.001 in.) thick, if the blood at the membrane surface contains urea at a concentration of 100 mg% (i.e., 100 mg/100 ml) and the saline solution at the membrane surface is urea free. The diffusion coefficient for urea in a cellulose membrane is about 2.9×10^{-6} cm^2/sec, based on assuming the partition coefficient to be 1.0 [value from Colton et al. (1971)]. The flux calculated in this way will be the flux in the inlet region of a parallel-flow artificial kidney. At other locations the flux will be somewhat less. Why?

4. *Magnitude of the reversal potential created by nerve cell discharge.* A nerve cell (resting potential 75 mV; inside negative) fires when some stimulus affects the nerve cell membrane and causes it to suddenly become highly permeable to Na^+ ions. Depolarization occurs as Na^+ ions rush inside the cell. At the height of this

process, enough Na^+ ions are inside the cell to actually make the interior positively charged relative to the exterior; that is, the potential becomes the reverse of normal.

Assuming that the cell membrane Na^+ permeability during depolarization is 1000 times greater than during the resting state, and that the K^+ and Cl^- permeabilities are the same as in the resting state, estimate the magnitude of the reversal potential.

5. *Gibbs-Donnan equilibrium.* Let us assume that blood, flowing inside a capillary, has a total cation content equivalent to Na^+ = 157 meq/liter, a total small anion content equivalent to Cl^- = 156 meq/liter, and a total large anion (protein) content equivalent to P^- = 1 meq/liter. On the other side of the capillary wall, which is impermeable to proteins since they are too large to pass, is an interstitial fluid. What are the concentrations of the cations and anions in the interstitial fluid, expressed as equivalents per liter of Na^+ and Cl^-? How do the total ionic contents of the blood and interstitial fluids compare? Does a driving force for osmosis exist? If so, what hydrostatic pressure in millimeters of mercury would be needed to counteract the osmotic flux?

6. *Facilitated diffusion of oxygen.* Oxygen is diffusing through a thin membrane soaked with a hemoglobin solution, with the oxygen partial pressures set at 20 and 40 mm Hg on the two sides of the membrane. Estimate the ratio of the oxygen flux to that which would exist if no facilitation effect occurred for this situation. Take $D_{O_2} = 1.2 \times 10^{-5}$ cm^2/sec and $D_{HbO_2} = 1 \times 10^{-7}$ cm^2/sec. The average value of dC_{HbO_2}/dC_{O_2} between 20 and 40 mm Hg P_{O_2} is about 145.

REFERENCES

Bird, R. B., Stewart, W. E., and Lightfoot, E. N., *Transport Phenomena*, Wiley, New York, 1960.

Clarke, H. T., ed., *Ion Transport Across Membranes*, Academic, New York, 1954.

Colton, C. K., Smith, K. A., Merrill, E. R., and Friedman, S., Diffusion of urea in flowing blood, *A.I.Ch.E.J.*, 17, 800 (1971).

Davson, H., *Textbook of General Physiology*, 3rd ed., Williams & Wilkins, Baltimore, Maryland, 1964.

Denbigh, K. B., *The Principles of Chemical Equilibrium*, 2nd ed., Cambridge Univ. Press, London and New York, 1968, p. 312.

Guyton, A. C., *Textbook of Medical Physiology*, 4th ed., Saunders, Philadelphia, Pennsylvania, 1971.

Keller, K. H., and Friedlander, S. K., Investigation of steady-state oxygen transport in hemoglobin solution, *Chem. Eng. Prog. Symp. Ser.*, 62, No. 66, 88 (1966).

Ruch, T. C., and Patton, H. D., eds., *Physiology and Biophysics*, 19th ed., Saunders, Philadelphia, Pennsylvania, 1965.

Stein, W. D., *The Movement of Molecules Across Cell Membranes*, Academic, New York, 1967.

Chapter 8

THE HUMAN KIDNEYS

The human kidneys are the most complex and fascinating mass transfer separation devices in the body. Besides excreting the major end products of protein metabolism (urea, creatinine, uric acid) and other wastes (sulfates, phenols), the kidneys remove excess amounts of many ions (Na^+, Cl^-, K^+), control body fluid volume via water excretion, and regulate the acid-base balance of the body by appropriate elimination of H^+ or HCO_3^-. Other important functions of the kidneys could be noted, but are secondary to the present discussion.

I. STRUCTURE AND GENERAL FEATURES OF OPERATION

Figure 8.1 shows the overall gross anatomy of the kidneys, the important portions being the outer cortex region, the inner medulla

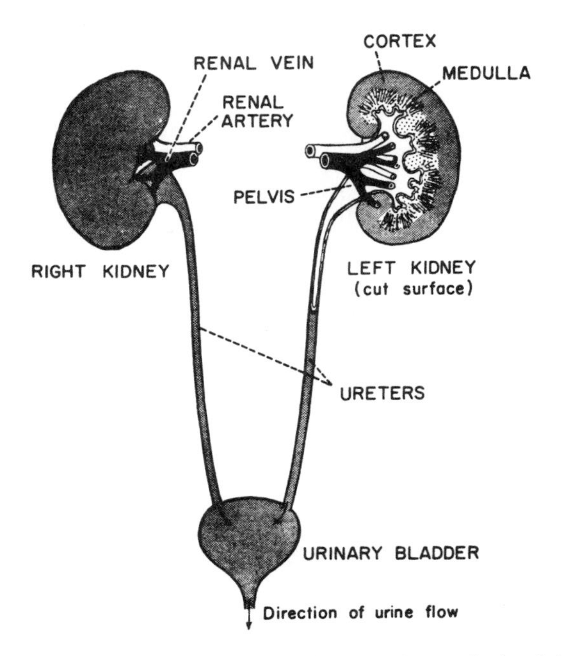

FIG. 8.1. The general organizational plan of the kidney. [From Guyton (1971), p. 393.]

area, and the converging tissue section called the renal pelvis, which feeds into the ureters. Note also the renal arteries and veins. The microscopic anatomical features center on the nephron, the functional unit of the kidneys (there are about 500,000 in each kidney). Figure 8.2 details the nephron structure. Blood from the arterial side enters the tuft of about 50 capillaries known as the glomerulus, which sits in Bowman's capsule. Here plasma filters, under a pressure difference, through the glomerular capillary walls, which are 25 times more permeable than ordinary capillary walls. About 1200 ml/min of blood flows to the two kidneys (20-25% of the cardiac output), resulting in roughly 125 ml/min of filtrate. The filtrate is essentially the same as blood plasma except that it lacks plasma proteins, which are strained out during filtration (actually about 30 g/day of protein does get through, but this is equivalent

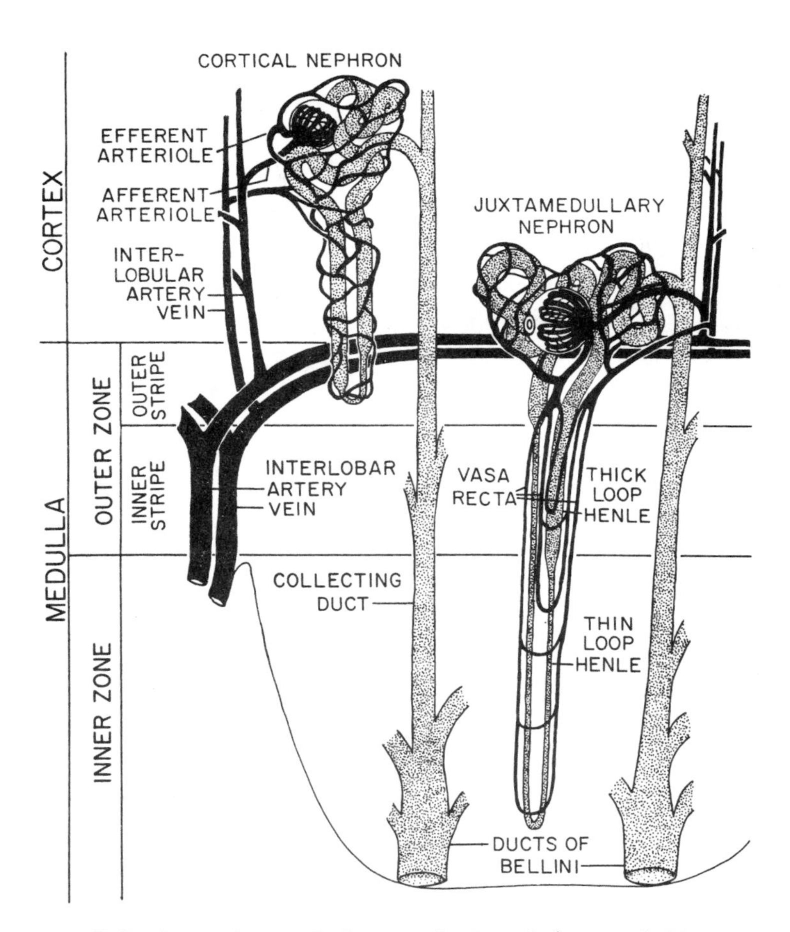

FIG. 8.2. Comparison of the cortical and juxtamedullary nephrons. [From *Physiology of the Kidney and Body Fluids*, 3rd ed., R. F. Pitts, copyright 1974 by Yearbook Med. Publ., Chicago, Illinois. Used by permission.]

to a concentration of only 0.03% in the filtrate). From Bowman's capsule, the filtrate (∿180 liters/day) flows through various ducts—the proximal tubule, Henle's loop, the distal tubule, the collecting tubule, and the collecting duct (from which it proceeds as urine to the ureters and bladder). During the passage of the filtrate through these regions, the solutes that the body wishes to retain (e.g., nutrients like glucose and amino acids) are reabsorbed almost completely, wastes (urea, creatinine, etc.) are essentially not reabsorbed at all, and ions such as Na^+ and Cl^- are reabsorbed only to the degree desired by the body. Other solutes may actually be secreted by the tubule epithelium into the fluid. Water is reabsorbed in the proper amounts required to regulate body fluid volume, but normally 99.4% is reabsorbed to yield 1 liter of urine per day from 180 liters/day of original filtrate.

Using the figures for a glomerular filtration rate (GFR) of 125 ml/min and a renal blood flow rate of 1200 ml/min, it is clear that roughly 10% of the blood is filtered and processed per pass, equivalent to the processing of about 20% of the plasma per pass.

Figure 8.3 gives a more schematic diagram of the nephron and makes clearer what takes place on the "blood side." On either side of the glomerular capillaries are the afferent and efferent arterioles which, by constricting or dilating, can control the blood pressure level in the capsule, and thus the amount of filtration. Figures 8.4 and 8.5 give the pressure distribution in the nephron and indicate how the net filtration pressure in the capsule (the GFR is of course proportional to this) is affected by afferent/efferent arteriolar constriction and by colloid osmotic pressure. After passing the efferent arteriole, blood enters the peritubular capillaries, which surround the tubules (containing the flowing filtrate). This provides good mass transfer contact with the tubules. Off of the peritubular capillary bed there are long straight capillary loops called the vasa recta which extend alongside the lower part of Henle's loop. Only about 1 or 2% of the total blood flow goes through the vasa recta, but good mass transfer contact with the lower Henle's loop is nevertheless achieved. Figure 8.6 shows the variation of filtrate flow rate with location in the tubular passage, and it is

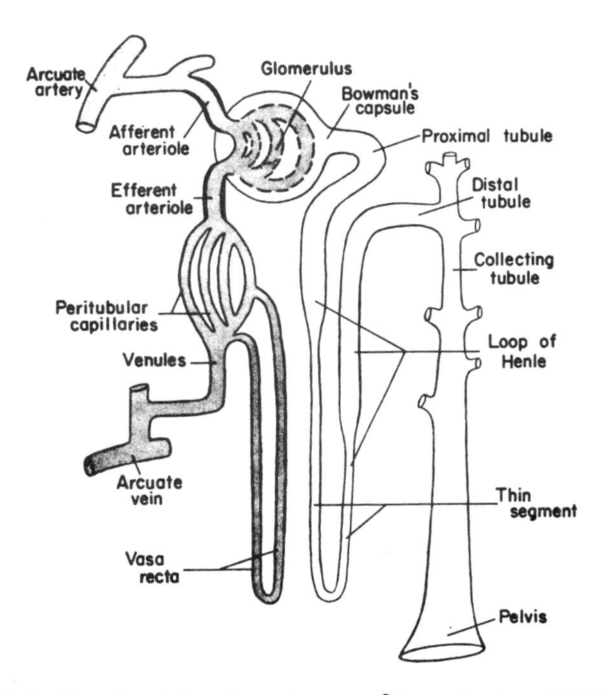

FIG. 8.3. The functional nephron. [From Guyton (1971), p. 394.]

clear that because of tremendous water reabsorption in the proximal tubule, the filtrate flow in Henle's loop is only about one-sixth of the GFR. Hence, the ratio of total vasa recta blood flow to Henle's loop filtrate flow is roughly 12-24 to 20 ml/min. The 1 or 2% of the blood in the vasa recta is therefore fully capable of accepting significant solute from the glomerular filtrate. Figure 8.2 points out that two basic kinds of nephrons exist: cortical and juxtamedullary (numbers of each are in the ratio of $\sim$85/15). The basic functioning of both types is the same, but some anatomical differences are evident, e.g., the much longer Henle's loop (and associated vasa recta) of the juxtamedullary kind.

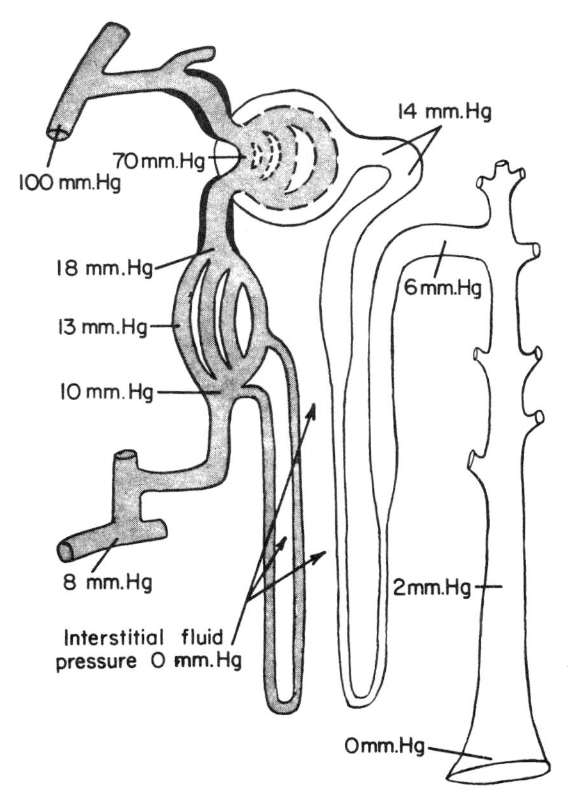

FIG. 8.4. Pressures at different points in the vessels and tubules of the functional nephron and in the interstitial fluid. [From Guyton (1971), p. 395.]

II. TRANSPORT MECHANISMS IN THE TUBULES

Osmotic, active, and passive transport mechanisms are all operative in the tubules. Figure 8.7 illustrates the active transport of Na^+ from the inside (lumen) of the proximal tubule into the peritubular fluid, the interstitial fluid surrounding the peritubular capillaries, where it is picked up by the capillary blood. Note that Na^+ is actively transported only on one side of the tubular epithelial cell membrane. This active transport (a) creates an electrical potential of -70 mV in the membrane interior, and (b) lowers the Na^+

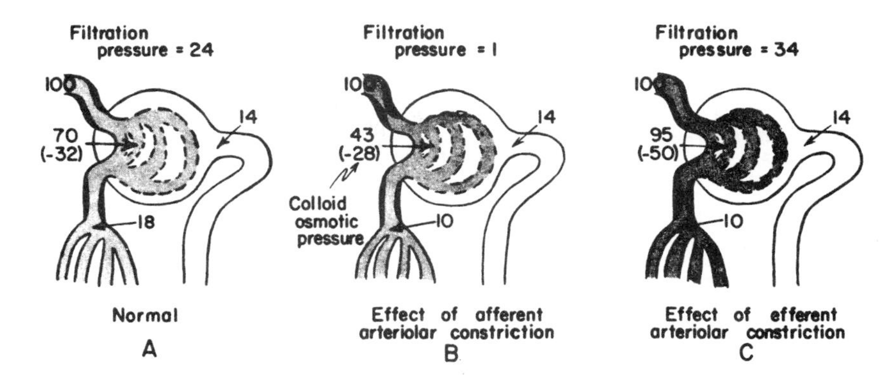

FIG. 8.5. (A) Normal pressures at different points in the nephron, and the normal filtration pressure. (B) Effect of afferent arteriolar constriction on pressures in the nephron and on filtration pressure. (C) Effect of efferent arteriolar constriction on pressures in the nephron and on filtration pressure. [From Guyton (1971), p. 398.]

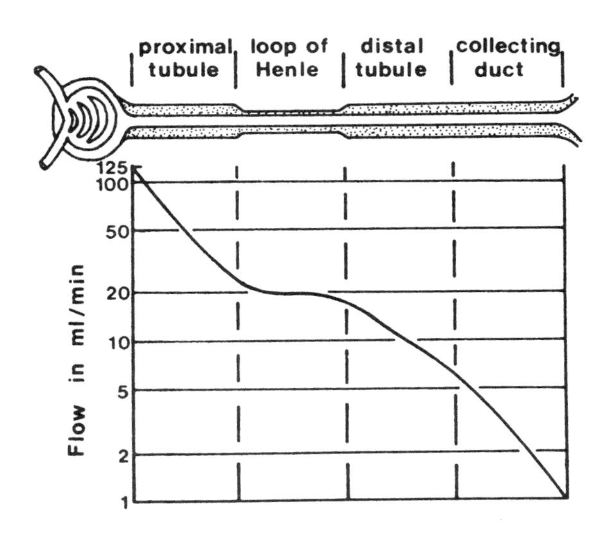

FIG. 8.6. Volume flow of fluid in each segment of the tubular system per minute. [From Guyton (1971), p. 401.]

concentration in the membrane. The latter effect induces Na^+ transport by passive diffusion (aided here by both favorable electrical potential and concentration gradients) into the membrane from the inside of the tubule. The former effect causes passive transport of

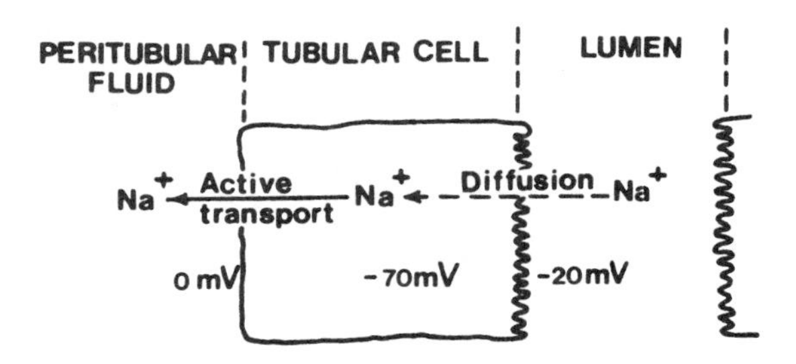

FIG. 8.7. Mechanism for transport of sodium from the tubular lumen into the peritubular fluid. [From Guyton (1971), p. 399.]

negative ions from the tubule to the peritubular fluid (e.g., Cl^-, PO_4^{2-}, HCO_3^- "follow" the Na^+ because of the electrical potential gradient created by Na^+ transport). Besides Na^+ other species such as glucose, amino acids, Ca^{2+}, K^+, PO_4^{2-}, and urate ions are actively transported in the same manner. Active secretion of some substances (e.g., H^+, K^+) occurs in other regions (the distal tubules and collecting ducts) by the reverse process. It should be mentioned that the passive secretion of K^+ can also occur in the distal and collecting tubules, when active Na^+ transport from the tubules is so large that a highly negative potential is generated inside the lumen, which "pulls" K^+ into the lumen.

Water always transports osmotically. For example, in the case described above, Na^+ transport out of the tubules and into the peritubular fluid makes the peritubular fluid hyperosmotic relative to the filtrate in the tubules. Hence, water will transport out of the tubules by osmotic means. This water shift, in turn, concentrates urea and other nonactively transported substances, in the tubules. Urea and similar solutes will therefore diffuse passively into the peritubular fluid. The diffusion rate will depend strongly on the amount of water that shifts and the permeability of the tubule membrane to the particular solute.

Figures 8.8 and 8.9 show typical amounts (milligrams per minute, milliequivalents per minute) of nonionic and ionic solutes in the tubules as a function of location (water rates at various points are

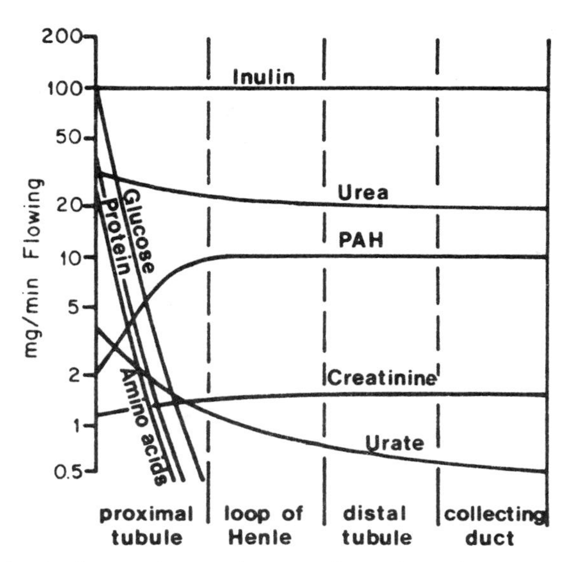

FIG. 8.8. Reabsorption and secretion of various substances in the tubules. [From Guyton (1971), p. 402.]

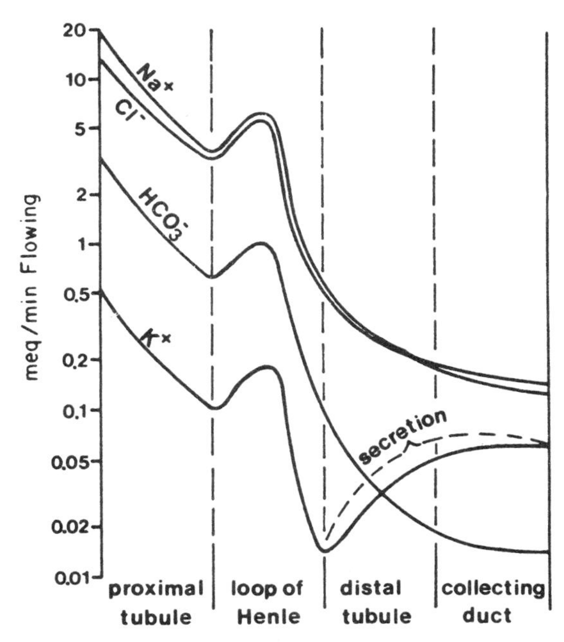

FIG. 8.9. Reabsorption of different ions in the tubules. [From Guyton (1971), p. 403.]

very nearly the same as the total solution flow rates given in Figure 8.6). Note the very quick and complete reabsorption of nutritionally important substances such as glucose and amino acids (via active transport) and proteins (via pinocytosis, digestion into amino acids, and subsequent active transport of the amino acids). Wastes like urea are poorly reabsorbed (because of low solubility in the tubular membrane). Creatinine and para-aminohippuric acid (PAH) are secreted weakly and strongly, respectively. Inulin (a fructose polymer, molecular weight 5200) is neither reabsorbed nor secreted. The positive ions, as described above, are generally strongly reabsorbed by active means (except for K^+ secretion in the latter part of the tubules, as also mentioned) and most negative ions passively follow because of electrical potential effects. H^+ ions (not shown) are actively secreted in all regions except Henle's loop. It should be mentioned in this connection that the reabsorption of bicarbonate ions actually occurs as the result of the reaction of secreted H^+ with HCO_3^- to give CO_2, which is then passively reabsorbed (CO_2 is highly soluble in the tubule membranes). The actual permeability of the tubule membranes to HCO_3^-, per se, is small. When the body fluids are alkaline (fewer than usual H^+), then HCO_3^- is not as strongly reabsorbed, and vice versa. This is a prime means by which the acid-base balance of the body is regulated. It should also be remarked here that the reason for the <u>rise</u> in the amount of ions in Henle's loop is the passive diffusion of these ions <u>into</u> the tubules in the medullar regions of the kidneys where the lower reaches of Henle's loops are located (no active transport here).

Figure 8.10 shows the data of the preceding two figures plotted as <u>concentrations</u> versus distance. Inulin, for example, which does not undergo any change in the amount per time at different locations, nevertheless rises in concentration, since water removal is continually occurring. Table 8.1 shows similar data in a more easily compared form. Note how some species (e.g., creatinine) are much more concentrated in the urine than in the original glomerular

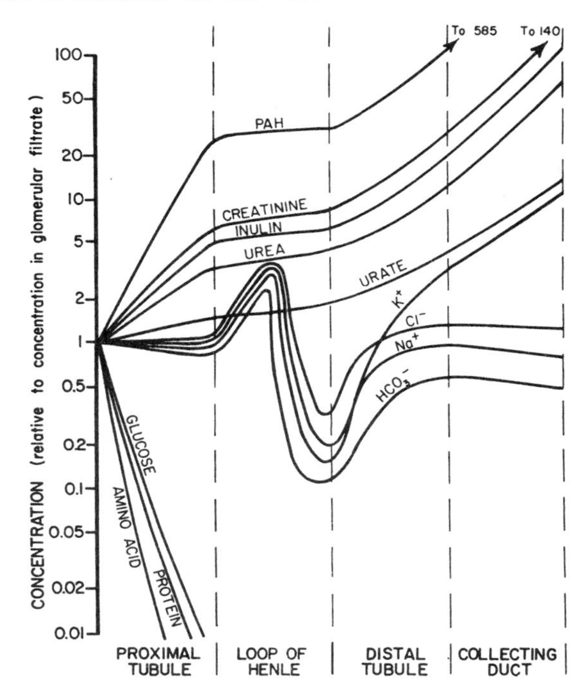

FIG. 8.10. Average changes in concentrations of different substances at different points in the tubular system. [From Guyton (1971), p. 403.]

filtrate (or plasma). Others, like glucose, are completely recovered by the body.

Figure 8.11 shows the change in the total solute concentration in the tubular fluid in a typical nephron, expressed as osmolarity versus location. The cross-hatched area indicates the range of possible osmolarities that can be produced, depending on whether the kidney wishes to create a dilute or concentrated urine.

An important aspect of the kidneys' reabsorption processes is the fact that there exist, for the actively transported solutes, upper limits to the rates of transport. Figure 8.12 shows this with regard to glucose. When the tubular load (milligrams per minute of solute in the filtrate) becomes larger than about 250 mg glucose/min, the active transport mechanism for glucose reabsorp-

TABLE 8.1

Relative Concentrations of Substances in the Glomerular Filtrate and in the Urine[a]

	Glomerular filtrate (125 ml/min)		Urine (1 ml/min)		Conc. urine/conc. plasma (plasma clearance per minute)
	Quantity/min	Concentration	Quantity/min	Concentration	
Na^+	17.7 meq	142 meq/liter	0.128 meq	128 meq/liter	0.9
K^+	0.63	5	0.06	60	12
Ca^{2+}	0.5	4	0.0048	4.8	1.2
Mg^{2+}	0.38	3	0.015	15	5.0
Cl^-	12.9	103	0.134	134	1.3
HCO_3^-	3.5	28	0.014	14	0.5
$H_2PO_4^-$ / HPO_4^{2-}	0.25	2	0.05	50	25
SO_4^{2-}	0.09	0.7	0.033	33	47
Glucose	125 mg	100 mg%	0 mg	0 mg%	0.0
Urea	33	26	18.2	1820	70
Uric acid	3.8	3	0.42	42	14
Creatinine	1.4	1.1	1.96	196	140
Inulin	—	—	—	—	125
Diodrast	—	—	—	—	560
PAH	—	—	—	—	585

[a]From Guyton (1971), p. 404.

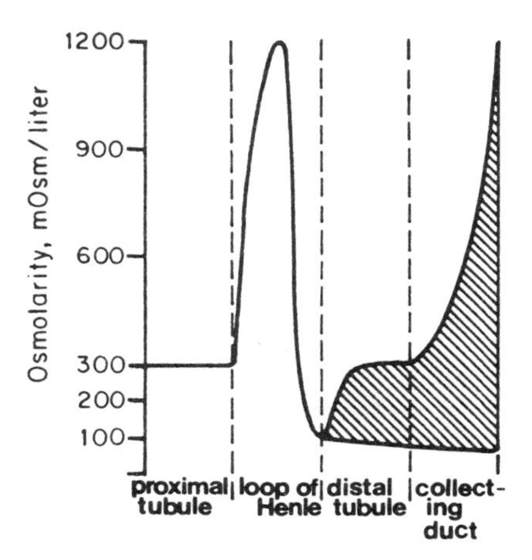

FIG. 8.11. Changes in osmolarity of the tubular fluid as it passes through the tubular system. [Redrawn from Guyton (1971), p. 409.]

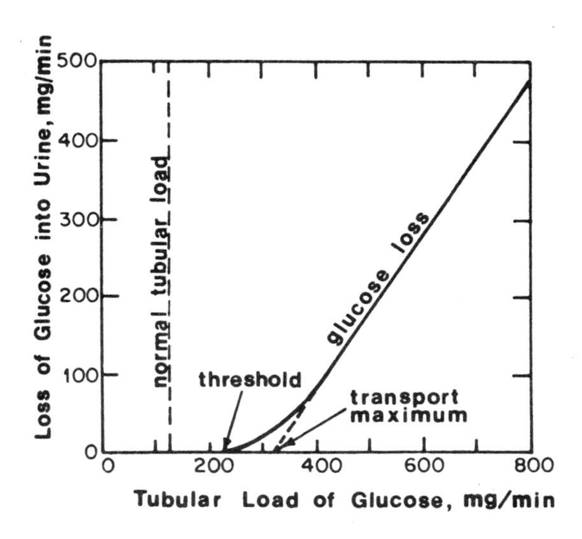

FIG. 8.12. Relationship of tubular load of glucose to loss of glucose into the urine. [Redrawn from Guyton (1971), p. 413.]

tion reaches a saturation level—i.e., all of the carrier and/or specific enzymes available for glucose transport are being fully utilized. As suggested by Figure 8.12, the point at which saturation is reached is not sharply defined; therefore, it is common practice to obtain values for the "transport maximum" of a solute by the extrapolation procedure illustrated. The transport maximum is an ideal index of the maximum rate of transport of a solute, and it is implied that when the tubular load is less than or equal to the transport maximum, then all of the solute is reabsorbed. Actually, as indicated, less than complete reabsorption begins to occur above some threshold tubular load which is somewhat less than the tubular load corresponding to the transport maximum. The tubular load is, of course, equal to the plasma concentration of the solute times the GFR. Hence, for a GFR of 125 ml/min and a glucose "threshold load" of 220 mg/min, the "threshold concentration" of glucose in the plasma would be 220 mg/125 ml, or 180 mg%. Transport maxima for various substances are given in Table 8.2. Na^+, which is not listed, does not appear to have a transport maximum, which is very significant. Transport maxima for solutes that are actively secreted are also listed in Table 8.2.

III. PORE MODELS OF THE GLOMERULAR TUFT

It remains strongly debated even today as to whether the glomerular capillary walls contain actual stable pores or whether the walls are gel-like in structure. Independent measurements of the wall membrane thickness (by electron microscopy), of fluid pressures on each side of the membrane (by micropuncture) of glomerular filtration rate (by measuring plasma and urine inulin contents), and of colloid osmotic pressures have established that the wall membrane is 400-600 Å thick, that the net filtration pressure is usually around 20-30 mm Hg, and the filtration rate is 1.9-4.5 ml/mm Hg-min-100 g of kidney. Diffusion measurements using tritiated water

TABLE 8.2

Transport Maxima of Important Substances Absorbed from the Tubules[a]

Glucose	320	mg/min
Phosphate	0.1	mmol/min
Sulfate	0.06	mmol/min
Amino acids	1.5	mmol/min
Vitamin C	1.77	mg/min
Urate	15	mg/min
Plasma protein	30	mg/min
Hemoglobin	1	mg/min
Lactate	75	mg/min
Acetoacetate	Variable	(about 30 mg/min)

Transport maxima for secretion

	mg/min
Creatinine	16
PAH	80
Diodrast	57 (of iodine)
Phenol red	56

[a]From Guyton (1971), p. 413.

(whose diffusion coefficient is known accurately) indicate a total "open" area for diffusion of 500-1000 cm^2/100 g of kidney, or about 5-10% of the total glomerular membrane area.

These numbers are summarized in Table 8.3. On the basis that straight cylindrical pores exist and that Poiseuille's law can describe the flow through these pores (both of these assumptions are quite tenuous), the glomerular filtration rate would be given by

$$GFR = \frac{n\pi r^4 \, \Delta P}{8\mu L}$$

One can then deduce that the pores must have an average diameter of

TABLE 8.3

Operational Characteristics of Glomerular Capillaries[a]

Total glomerular capillary area	5,000-15,000 cm^2/100 g kidney
Total capillary pore area	500-1000 cm^2/100 g kidney
Fractional pore area	1/10-1/20
Pore diameter	70-100 Å
Pore length	400-600 Å
Filtration coefficient	1.9-4.5 ml/min-mm Hg-100 g
Pressure drop across capillary wall	45-65 mm Hg
Colloid osmotic pressure	25-35 mm Hg
Pressure to overcome viscous resistance to flow	20-30 mm Hg

[a]From Pappenheimer, J. R., Über die Permeabilität der Glomerulummembranen in der Niere, *Klin. Wechnschr.*, 33, 362 (1955).

about 70-100 Å. This model of the glomerular membrane is supported by data showing that solutes of molecular weight of approximately 70,000 or less pass through the membrane. From diffusion measurements it is known that the effective diameter of serum albumin molecules (molecular weight 69,000) is about 71 Å (the word "effective" is used because albumin is not spherical in shape).

IV. A MODEL FOR GLOMERULAR FILTRATION IN THE RAT

Deen et al. (1972) have developed a mathematical model for glomerular filtration in the rat, and have used this model to interpret experimental data. Their model idealizes the glomerular capillary bed as a single capillary of length L. Since glomerular capillaries are freely permeable to small solutes, equal concentrations of these will exist on both sides of the capillary wall. Thus, their osmotic pressure contributions on both sides will cancel. One can therefore consider the system to have only two components, protein and water.

A differential balance along the capillary (x direction) yields

$$\frac{dQ}{dx} = -\frac{kS}{L} P_{UF}$$

where Q is the volumetric plasma flow rate, k is an "hydraulic permeability," S is the total surface area of the capillary, and P_{UF} is the net pressure causing ultrafiltration. P_{UF} can, in turn, be related to the hydrostatic pressure in the capillary P_c, to the hydrostatic pressure in Bowman's capsule P_B, to the colloid osmotic pressure in the capillary π_c, and to the colloid osmotic pressure in the filtrate π_B as follows:

$$P_{UF} = (P_c - P_B) - (\pi_c - \pi_B)$$

Assuming π_B is negligible because very little protein passes through into the filtrate, this can be written as

$$P_{UF} = \Delta P - \pi_c, \text{ where } \Delta P = P_c - P_B$$

Deen et al. have also shown how π_c can be related to the protein concentration C according to

$$\pi_c = a_1 C + a_2 C^2$$

by fitting available experimental data on π_c versus C to a quadratic functional form. Hence, one can write

$$\frac{dQ}{dx} = -\frac{kS}{L}[\Delta P - a_1 C - a_2 C^2]$$

Noting that C = m/Q, where m is the mass flow rate of protein (a constant), and that therefore

$$\frac{dQ}{dx} = -\frac{m}{C^2}\frac{dC}{dx}$$

one can recast the preceding mass balance into the form

$$\frac{dC}{dx} = \frac{kS}{mL}[\Delta P - a_1C - a_2C^2]C^2$$

This equation was integrated numerically by Deen and his coworkers for a variety of assumed parameter values (inlet concentration C_0, k, S, L, m). To do this, a further assumption regarding how ΔP varies with x was needed. Experimental data on P_c values obtained by random micropuncture of glomerular capillaries in the rat suggested that P_c is essentially constant (the axial pressure drop from inlet to outlet being probably no greater than 2 or 3 mm Hg). Hence, P_c was taken to be constant at a measured value of about 45 mm Hg.

From the numerically determined C(x) profiles, it was then possible to determine $\pi_c(x)$ profiles, and therefore $P_{UF}(x)$ profiles. It should be mentioned that P_B was assumed to be constant at 10 mm Hg, a measured value. From $P_{UF}(x)$ profiles, one can then obtain capillary average P_{UF} values, denoted by $\overline{P}_{UF}$.

Deen et al. used their model to determine, for rats, experimental values for K_f, an "ultrafiltration coefficient" that is equal to the product kS. Inlet and outlet P_c values and π_c values were measured, as well as the glomerular filtration rates for single capillaries, using micropuncture techniques. Since GFR = $K_f\overline{P}_{UF}$, one can determine K_f if the GFR and $\overline{P}_{UF}$ are known.

In order that $\overline{P}_{UF}$ be determinable it is necessary that P_{UF} not go to zero prior to the end of the capillary. Under normal conditions, P_{UF} does reach zero before the outlet is attained (a condition labeled "filtration pressure equilibrium" in which π_c has risen far enough to equal the magnitude of $P_c - P_B$). Hence, to force P_{UF} to be nonzero at the capillary outlet, the flow rate of plasma to the kidneys of the subject rats had to be artificially increased by infusing extra plasma (equal to 5% of the rats' body weights) into the rats prior to the experiments.

The experiments of Deen et al. suggest that K_f = 0.08 nl/sec-mm Hg for rats over a wide range of plasma flow rates. Low plasma flow rates were achieved by constricting the abdominal aorta, and high plasma flows were obtained by occluding the carotid arteries. The measured GFR values were always proportional to the plasma flow rates (surprisingly, P_C and $\bar{P}_{UF}$ values remained relatively normal during the aortic constriction and carotid occlusion procedures, presumably because of simultaneous constriction of the efferent arteriole and dilation of the afferent arteriole, respectively). K_f values did not change significantly during these tests. Because the GFR is proportional to the plasma flow rate to the kidneys, the filtration fraction (fraction of entering plasma which ends up as filtrate) is independent of the plasma flow rate to the kidneys.

Based on anatomical data for the subject rats, S was estimated to be about 0.0019 cm^2 per capillary. Hence, $k = K_f/S = 0.08/0.0019 =$ 41 nl/sec-cm^2-mm Hg. This hydraulic permeability value can be compared to the following known values for capillaries in various other tissues: frog mesentery k = 0.65 - 1.0; rat cremaster muscle k = 0.88; rat peritubular k = 1.0; rabbit omentum k = 0.3-9. Clearly, the glomerular permeability is one or two orders of magnitude higher than these values. This explains why glomerular filtration can proceed at a rapid rate despite the fact that the average $\bar{P}_{UF}$ under normal conditions may be as low as 5 mm Hg (under normal conditions, P_B = 10 mm Hg, P_C = 45 mm Hg, π_C = 20 mm Hg at the inlet and 35 mm Hg at the outlet; hence, P_{UF} = 15 mm Hg at the inlet, 0 mm Hg at the outlet, and $\bar{P}_{UF}$ = 5 mm Hg on a capillary-average basis).

Deen and coworkers have also performed experiments on rats with aortic constriction and without prior plasma infusion. In this case, autoregulation fails to maintain $P_C - P_B$ at near normal values (it becomes 25 mm Hg instead of 35 mm Hg). Moreover, the GFR falls by two-thirds, from 27 to 9 nl/min, even though the plasma flow rate to the kidneys is only about 40% less than normal. These observations are taken to imply that the magnitude of the transcapillary pressure difference, $P_C - P_B$, affects K_f. In particular, K_f is lower when $P_C - P_B$ is lower.

V. THE COUNTERCURRENT MECHANISM OF URINE FORMATION

The human body sometimes needs to reject substantial amounts of water (e.g., when much fluid is imbibed) and at other times must conserve as much water as possible. Therefore, the kidneys must be capable of producing urine that ranges from very dilute to rather concentrated. Creating a urine less concentrated than the glomerular filtrate (which is about 300 milliosmolar) is achieved, in essence, by allowing active and passive transport of solutes out of the glomerular filtrate without permitting a large amount of water to follow. Generating urine more concentrated than about 300 mOsm/liter is accomplished basically by having the filtrate come into contact with a hyperosmotic interstitial fluid (up to 1200 mOsm/liter) across a water-permeable membrane. This occurs in the collecting duct region, where water removal from the tubular fluid can create a urine that may be as concentrated as 1200 mOsm/liter (this is about the upper limit: a certain minimum amount of water is needed just to carry away the normal production of metabolic wastes, and generation of urine of osmolarity > 1200 simply requires too much energy). When concentrated urines are desired, ADH (antidiuretic hormone) is secreted into the blood by the body. This hormone causes the distal tubule and collecting duct walls to become highly permeable to water. When a dilute urine is desired, ADH is not secreted and therefore these regions become areas of negligible water transfer. Water stays in the tubular fluid while solute transfer processes continue; hence, dilute urine results.

How is the large hyperosmotic level of the interstitial fluid (in the region where the collecting ducts pass, i.e., the medulla) developed, since it is the key to making concentrated urine? The answer can be given in terms of the countercurrent mechanism illustrated in Figure 8.13. Active transport of Na^+ out of the ascending limb of Henle's loop (Cl^- follows) causes a concentration gradient favoring the passive diffusion of NaCl into the descending limb of Henle's loop. The countercurrent flow of fluid in Henle's

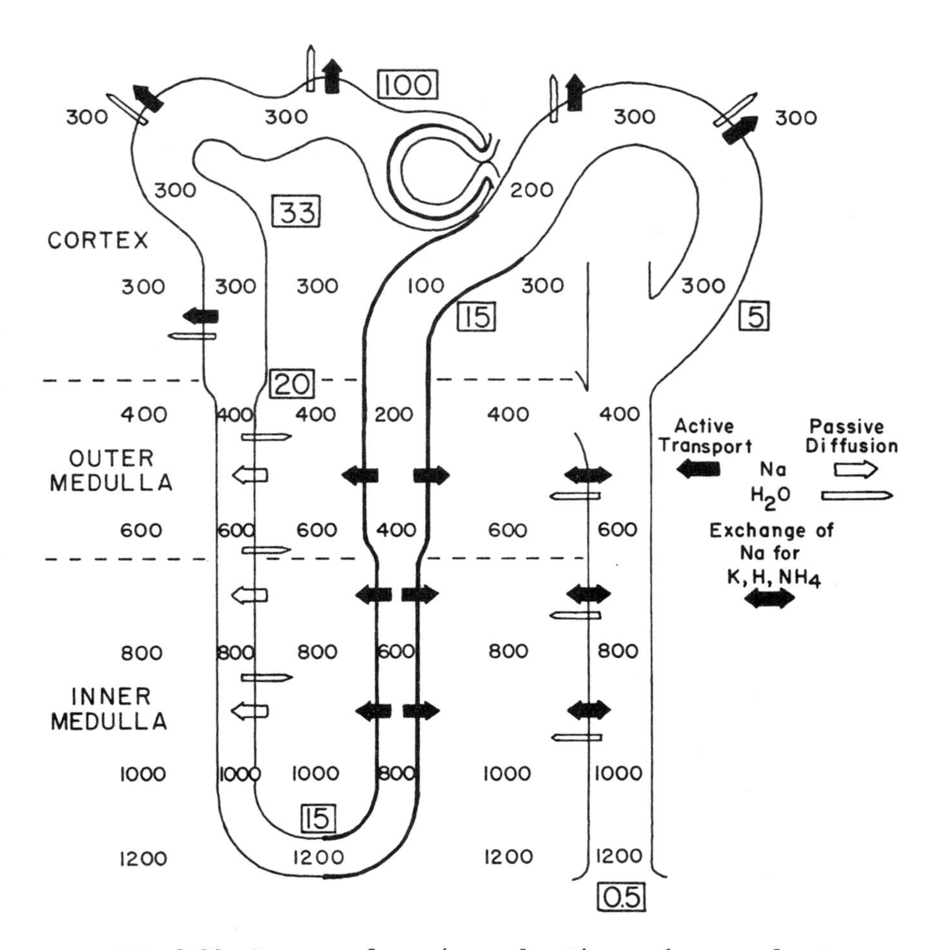

FIG. 8.13. Summary of passive and active exchanges of water and ions in the nephron in the course of elaboration of hypertonic urine. Concentrations of tubular urine and peritubular fluid in milliosmoles per liter; large, boxed numerals, estimated percentage of glomerular filtrate remaining within the tubule at each level. [From R. F. Pitts, *Physiology of the Kidney and Body Fluids*, 3rd ed., copyright 1974 by Yearbook Med. Publ., Chicago, Illinois. Used by permission.]

loop causes a concentration "multiplier" effect, such that the fluid at the bottom of the loop is highly concentrated. There is generated, then, a large concentration gradient in both limbs of the loop, and in the interstitium of the medulla.

To further clarify the urine formation process let us list some of the properties and transport mechanisms of the various portions of the tubular passage:

1. *Proximal tubule*. Strong active Na^+ (and other solute) transport into the cortical interstitium (and thence into the peritubular capillaries), Cl^- follows passively to maintain electroneutrality, and H_2O follows readily by osmosis. Osmolarity does not change from one end to the other, but total water and solute amounts decline substantially.

2. *Descending limb*. Na^+ is passively transported into the tubular duct (Cl^- follows). H_2O transports out by osmosis because the medullar region is hyperosmotic. NaCl is nearly doubled, water is reduced by about 25% from inlet end to tip of Henle's loop. Fluid inside becomes hypertonic (∿1200 mOsm/liter maximum).

3. *Ascending limb*. Na^+ actively transports out (Cl^- follows), water does not move (walls impermeable to it). NaCl leaving at the upper end of limb is about one-third that at the tip of loop; water leaving at the upper end of limb is the same as at tip of loop. Tubular fluid leaves somewhat hypotonic (∿230 mOsm/liter).

4. *Distal tubule*. Some Na^+ is actively transported out or exchanged for H^+, K^+, NH_4^+. Water flows out osmotically only if ADH is present. NaCl leaving is about one-third of entering amount—water leaving is about one-third of entering amount (if ADH is present). Fluid that leaves is isotonic (∿300 mOsm/liter if ADH is present) since some other ions have been gained (if no ADH, it leaves diluted).

5. *Collecting duct*. There is some net loss of Na^+ by active transport, but mainly exchange for H^+, K^+, NH_4^+. Water flows out osmotic-

ally _if_ _ADH_ _is_ _present_. Urine becomes very concentrated if ADH is present, somewhat more dilute than plasma if ADH is absent.

Since Figure 8.13 indicates that the cortical interstitial fluid is isotonic whereas the medullary interstitial fluid exhibits a large steady gradient with great hypertonicity in the lower portions, one might wonder how and why such a difference exists. The relatively large blood flow through the cortical region carries away excess solute and water (via the peritubular capillaries) and thus keeps the region isotonic with respect to plasma. In the medulla, the vasa recta blood flow is so low that not much solute can be carried away. More importantly, however, the looped configuration of the vasa recta (which have fairly permeable walls) means that countercurrent exchange occurs, so that nearly all of the solute picked up by the downflowing blood is lost again during upflow. The failure of the vasa recta blood to remove any significant solute serves to maintain the high hypertonicity of the lower medullary interstitium. The whole countercurrent urine concentration mechanism relies, in fact, on the parallel, looped side-by-side arrangements of the vasa recta and Henle's loops.

Figure 8.2 shows that the cortical nephrons do not have deeply penetrating Henle's loops. The juxtamedullary nephrons (15% of the total) therefore carry the whole burden of creating the top-to-bottom concentration gradient in the medulla, which is exploited by the cortical nephrons when concentrated urine is needed (since the collecting ducts of the cortical nephrons _do_ pass through the medulla).

VI. MODELS OF NEPHRON FUNCTION

Several investigators have developed mathematical models of nephron function of various degrees of complexity. One reasonably realistic model is the one of Tarica et al. (1971). This model assumes the geometrical dimensions and numbers given in Table 8.4, and, for all segments of the nephron, characterizes species transport by the following differential material balance equation:

$$\frac{d(Q_{wj}C_{ij})}{dx_j} = -2\pi R_j n J_{ij}$$

where Q_{wj} is the volume filtrate flow rate in segment j (milliliters per minute), C_{ij} is the concentration of species i in segment j (millimoles per milliliter), x_j is the position along segment j (millimeters), R_j is the segment radius (millimeters), n is the total number of nephrons in both kidneys, and J_{ij} is the molar flux of species i through walls of segment j (mmol/mm^2-min). The fluxes

TABLE 8.4

Estimates for Nephron Dimensions in Man[a]

Nephron segment	Length (mm)	Radius (μm)
Proximal tubule	14	15
Henle's loop	20	
Descending limb	10	6
Ascending thin limb	4	6
Ascending thick limb	6	10
Distal tubule	12	10
Collecting tubule	22	50
Cortical segment	10	
Medullary segment	10	
Papillary segment	2	
n(total number of nephrons)	2,500,000	
Number with long loops	350,000	
Number with short loops	2,150,000	

[a]From Tarica et al. (1971).

of the various species (water, Na^+, and urea were considered) were characterized by the rate equations

water: $J_w = k_w Q_w x$ in proximal tubule, $k_w Q_w$ elsewhere

Na^+: $J_{Na} = k_{Na}(C_{Na_i} - C_{Na_o})$ for passive transport (descending limb)

$J_{Na} = k_{Na} C_{Na_i}$ for active transport (all other places)

urea: $J_u = k_u(C_{u_i} - C_{u_o})$

Here the subscripts i and o stand for inside and outside the tubule, in the interstitium, respectively. The k's are transport coefficients estimated from available experimental data (see Table 8.5). The flux expressions for water are such that an exponential decrease with distance is predicted for the proximal tubule and a linear decrease is predicted for the other segments (however, if k_w is set equal to zero, a constant flow rate will result).

With assumed initial and boundary conditions the differential mass balances for the three species were integrated numerically to give results of the sort shown in Figure 8.14. These results are qualitatively correct. One problem encountered was that of estimating transport coefficients; frequently, these were determined by matching data for specific tubular locations to the model, a procedure that is undesirable but often unavoidable.

VII. AN ANALYTICAL MODEL FOR HENLE'S LOOP

Middleman (1972) presents a simple model for only the Henle's loop portion of the nephron based on the schematic diagram shown in Figure 8.15. Assumptions made for the model are that (a) water transfers osmotically out of the descending limb, (b) no

TABLE 8.5

Transport Coefficients for Water, Sodium, and Urea in Nephron Segments of Human Kidneys[a]

Nephron segments	Water ($10^{-6}/mm^2$)	Sodium (10^{-5} ml/min-mm^2)	Urea (10^{-5} ml/min-mm^2)
Proximal tubules	4.88	—	2.10
Henle's loop			
Descending thin limb	2.44	10.0	14.0
Ascending thin limb	0.0	1.91	10.0
Ascending thick limb	0.0	1.91	10.0
Distal tubules	3.72	0.643	0.52
Collecting tubules	0.48	0.0313	0.026

[a]From Tarica et al. (1971).

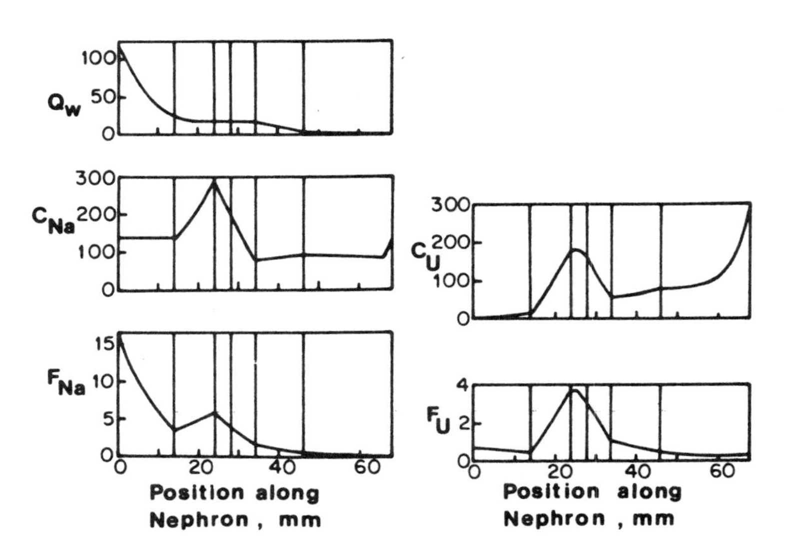

FIG. 8.14. Simulation curves for human nephron under normal conditions. Q is in milliliters per minute, C millimoles per liter, and F millimoles per minute. [From Tarica et al. (1971).]

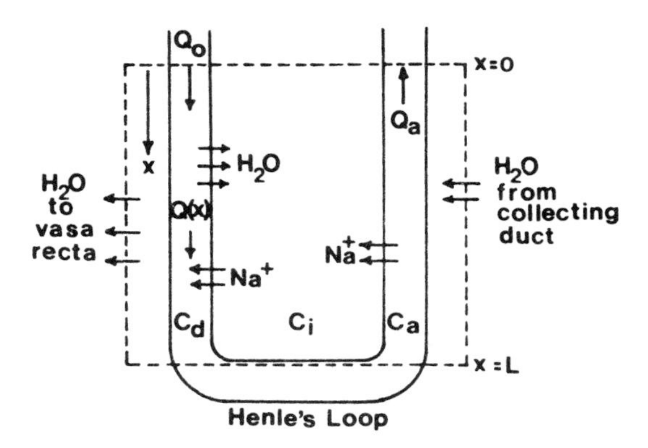

FIG. 8.15. Definition sketch for a model of Henle's loop.

water can enter the ascending limb, (c) Na^+ transfers passively into the descending limb, and (d) Na^+ transfers actively out of the ascending limb.

The basic differential equations of this model are

Na^+, descending limb: $$-\frac{d}{dx}(QC_d) = k(C_d - C_i)$$

Na^+, ascending limb: $$Q_a \frac{dC_a}{dx} = k_a C_a$$

Water, descending limb: $$-\frac{dQ}{dx} = k_o(C_i - C_d)$$

Here Q is the volumetric flow rate and the k's are transport coefficients. Q is taken as constant in the ascending limb, the active transport of Na^+ is assumed to be proportional to the Na^+ concentration (this seems reasonable), and the osmotic water transport rate is regarded as being proportional to the osmotic pressure difference or, equivalently, the Na^+ ion concentration difference (approximately correct since Na^+ is the dominant ion).

If one assumes that $k_a C_a = -k(C_d - C_i)$, i.e., all the Na^+ that is "pumped" out of the ascending limb goes into the descending limb (not really correct - some of the NaCl diffuses away toward the cortex), one can obtain the analytical solutions:

$$\frac{Q}{Q_o} = 1 - \frac{k_o Q_a C_{ao}}{Q_o k} \left[\exp\left(\frac{k_a x}{Q_a}\right) - 1 \right]$$

$$\frac{C_a}{C_{do}} = \frac{C_{ao}}{C_{do}} \exp\left(\frac{k_a x}{Q_a}\right)$$

$$\frac{C_d}{C_{do}} = \frac{Q_o}{Q} + \frac{k}{C_{do} k_o} \left(\frac{Q_o}{Q} - 1\right)$$

C_{ao} is determined from evaluation of the quadratic

$$\frac{k_o Q_a C_{do}}{Q_o k} \left[\exp\left(\frac{k_a L}{Q_a}\right) - 1 \right] \exp\left(\frac{k_a L}{Q_a}\right) \left(\frac{C_{ao}}{C_{do}}\right)^2$$

$$+ \left\{ \frac{Q_a}{Q_o} \left[\exp\left(\frac{k_a L}{Q_a}\right) - 1 \right] - \exp\left(\frac{k_a L}{Q_a}\right) \right\} \frac{C_{ao}}{C_{do}} + 1 = 0$$

Figure 8.16 shows predictions of this model and the parameter values employed. Obviously, the model and/or parameter values are too crude, since a concentration seven times the inlet concentration is predicted for the bottom of the loop (rather than about three times as high). However, all of the proper qualitative features seem to be reflected (small drop in water flow rate along descending limb, somewhat hypotonic filtrate at top of ascending limb, etc.). Better choices of the transport coefficients probably would have given more realistic concentration profiles. In any case this model, even though restricted to only part of the nephron, illustrates well the problems involved in attempting to describe accurately the function of an organ like the kidney.

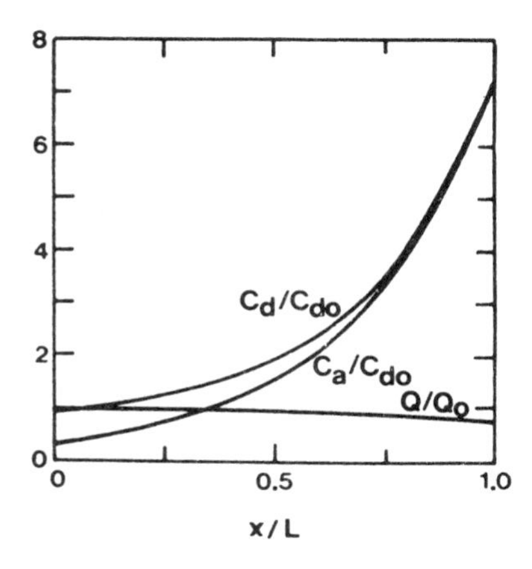

FIG. 8.16. Results of simple model of loop function. Lk/Q_o = 100, $C_{do}Lk_o/Q_o = 5$, $k_aL/Q_a = 3$, $k_a/k = 0.02$.

PROBLEMS

1. *Rate of formation of glomerular filtrate.* Given that two human kidneys weigh 250 g, and that the number of pores (of 70 Å diameter and 500 Å length) is such that the pore area in the glomerular capillary walls is 500 cm^2 per 100 g of kidney, estimate the GFR. Assume a net ΔP of 25 mm Hg (Table 8.3). If your answer seems high, can you explain why? Hint: What is the effect of protein accumulation near the pore entrances?

2. *Use of inulin to determine the glomerular filtration rate.* Inulin is a polysaccharide that happens to be neither secreted nor reabsorbed by the tubules of the kidney, and its molecular weight (5200) is low enough to permit it to pass through the glomerulus freely. It is infused at a steady rate into the blood of a person whose GFR is to be determined. After a while a steady-state plasma concentration is established.

Assume that blood samples taken after steady state has been reached show an inulin concentration of 0.1 g/100 ml of plasma. If a total of 180 ml of urine is then collected over the following 2-hr period, and analysis shows there is 0.08 g/ml in the urine, what is the GFR of the person being tested (it should be mentioned that inulin is not metabolized by the body and is excreted only in the urine)?

3. *Use of PAH to determine the rate of blood flow to the kidneys.* PAH (para-aminohippuric acid) has the property of being actively secreted from the capillaries surrounding the kidney tubules into these tubules (thus into the urine). At low plasma PAH concentrations (up to 8 mg/100 ml), the fraction of the PAH carried by the blood to the kidneys which is lost to the urine via both glomerular filtration and secretion totals 91%, as determined by sampling the blood before and after the kidneys. At higher concentrations the fraction extracted is less.

If the same procedure described in the preceding problem is carried out using PAH, the plasma concentration is 1 mg/100 ml, and the urine collected over a 1-hr period contains 0.35 g of PAH, what is the rate of plasma flow to the kidneys? If the person's hematocrit is 45%, what is the blood flow rate?

4. *Determination of transport maxima.* Transport maxima for various solutes can be determined by overloading the tubular cells with more of the solute than can be absorbed or secreted. Let us consider the case where glucose is being infused into the blood at such a rate that the plasma concentration reaches a steady value of 3.20 mg/ml. If urine sampling analysis shows that, under these conditions, 80 mg/min of glucose passes into the urine, what is the transport maximum for glucose reabsorption? In this computation, one must know the GFR, which, as determined by the procedure given in Problem 2, we shall take to be 125 ml/min.

5. *Removal of a solute from the body by the kidneys.* Assume that a drug overdose is taken, is rapidly absorbed into the body, and

distributes into the extracellular fluids (13 liters) only. If the drug is neither secreted nor reabsorbed by the kidneys, how long will it take for 90% of the drug to be eliminated in the urine? Model the extracellular fluid pool as a single perfectly stirred tank, neglect drug metabolism (not a good assumption for some drugs), use a GFR of 125 ml/min, and assume a blood flow of 1200 ml/min to the kidneys.

This example will suggest why "forced diuresis" (stimulation of high rates of urine formation by the use of certain agents) is a common technique for treating drug overdoses.

REFERENCES

Deen, W. M., Robertson, C. R., and Brenner, B. M., A model of glomerular filtration in the rat, *Am. J. Physiol.* 223, 1178 (1972).

Guyton, A. C., *Textbook of Medical Physiology*, 4th ed., Saunders, Philadelphia, Pennsylvania, 1971.

Middleman, S., *Transport Phenomena in the Cardiovascular System*, Wiley-Interscience, New York, 1972.

Pitts, R. F., *Physiology of the Kidney and Body Fluids*, Yearbook Med. Publ., Chicago, Illinois, 1963.

Tarica, R. R., Koushanpour, E., and Stevens, W. F., Mathematical simulation of renal function, *Chem. Eng. Prog. Symp. Ser.*, 67, No. 114, 28 (1971).

BIBLIOGRAPHY

Friedlander, S. K., and Walser, M., Some aspects of flow and diffusion in the proximal tubule of the kidney, *J. Theor. Biol.*, 8, 87 (1964).

Jacquez, J. A., Carnahan, B., and Abbrecht, P., A model of the renal cortex and medulla, *Math. Biosci.*, 1, 227 (1967).

Kelman, R. B., A theoretical note on exponential flow in the proximal part of the mammalian nephron, *Bull. Math. Biophys.*, 24, 303 (1962).

Koushanpour, E., Tarica, R. R., and Stevens, W. F., Mathematical simulation of normal nephron function in rat and man, *J. Theor. Biol.*, 31, 177 (1971).

Palatt, P. J., Saidel, G. M., and Macklin, M., Transport processes in the renal cortex, *J. Theor. Biol.*, 29, 251 (1970).

Pinter, G. G., and Shohet, J. L., Origin of sodium concentration profile in the renal medulla, *Nature*, 200, 1 (1963).

Wesson, L. G., Jr., A theoretical analysis of urea excretion by the mammalian kidney, *Am. J. Physiol.*, 179, 365 (1954).

Chapter 9

ARTIFICIAL KIDNEY DEVICES

Although various diseases of the kidney may initially attack a specific area of the organ (e.g., the glomeruli, the tubules) progression of the diseases often leads ultimately to severe general impairment of kidney function. A total lack of urine excretion frequently occurs. When substantial or total inability of the kidneys to remove water, metabolic wastes, and excess electrolytes from the body exists, death is normally only a matter of days away. It has been estimated that 30,000-50,000 Americans die each year from kidney disease, of which about 10,000-15,000 would be suitable candidates for artificial kidney treatment. Currently, about 8000 people are receiving such treatment in America.

I. BASIC METHODS OF ARTIFICIAL WASTE REMOVAL

A large number of techniques have been developed in an attempt to artificially remove the appropriate species from the body when natural kidney function fails. Table 9.1 summarizes the daily production of all wastes by the body; these wastes must be removed regularly to maintain life (although not necessarily each day, e.g., three days' worth of wastes can be removed every third day).

Virtually all of the procedures for waste removal operate on the basis of contacting a body fluid (usually blood) with a "dialysate" solution across a semipermeable membrane. The membrane is normally of a porosity such that all species except proteins and blood cells can potentially transfer. The dialysate, a typical

TABLE 9.1

Daily Waste Production in Normal and Uremic Persons

Component	Normal man (g/day)	Uremic patient (g/day)[a]
Water	1500	300[b]
Urea	30	12
Creatinine	0.6	0.2
Uric acid	0.9	0.4
Na^+	5	0.4
Cl^-	10	1.2
K^+	2.2	0.5
Ca^{2+}	0.2	0.1
PO_4^{3-}	3.7	1.8
HSO_4^-	8.2	—
Phenols	Trace	—

[a]Based on strict dietary control of protein, sodium, water, etc.
[b]May vary considerably.

composition of which is given in Table 9.2, is an aqueous solution that is similar in composition to the normal fluids of the body except that it contains no wastes such as urea, creatinine, uric acid, sulfates, phenols, and the like. Therefore, the body fluid contacted with the dialysate will lose urea, creatinine, uric acid, sulfates, phenols, etc., to the dialysate by diffusion across the membrane. If enough fresh dialysate is supplied to keep the concentrations of these wastes from building up in the dialysate and thereby suppressing this diffusion, the body fluid will ultimately be cleansed of these wastes. This type of membrane transport process is known as dialysis. Solutes such as NaCl, which should remain in the body in certain proper amounts, normally occur in excess in patients having kidney disease. To bring these solutes down to the correct levels but no further, the dialysate is prepared with their concentrations set at the desired ultimate values. Water must also be removed from the body since, even if no water is taken orally, oxidation of foodstuffs creates water. This removal

TABLE 9.2

Typical Dialysate Composition

Component	g/liter	Component	meq/liter
NaCl	5.8	Na^+	132
$NaHCO_3$	4.5	K^+	2.0
KCl	0.15	Cl^-	105
$CaCl_2$	0.18	HCO_3^-	33
$MgCl_2$	0.15	Ca^{2+}	2.5
Glucose	2.0	Mg^{2+}	1.5

Note that the dialysate is physiologic with respect to only a few electrolytes. Thus, depletion of any other transferable substances (e.g., amino acids) will occur during each dialysis. There is some evidence that, over a long term, such depletions may become physiologically significant.

is usually achieved by either (a) applying a net hydrostatic pressure difference between the body fluid and dialysate (this causes ultrafiltration of water) or (b) adding extra glucose (or another sugar) to the dialysate, thereby making it hyperosmotic. The latter method will cause some net diffusion of sugar into the body fluid, but this creates no problem since it simply provides food to the patient. A certain excess of sugar is always added to the dialysate even if only an isotonic solution is desired, in order to match the osmotic pressure of the body fluid proteins.

Many methods for waste removal from the body involve flowing dialysate either periodically or continuously into natural body cavities which are enclosed by natural membranes. Some examples are as follows:

1. *Peritoneal dialysis*. Dialysate is admitted to the abdominal cavity, which is completely enclosed by the peritoneal membrane, allowed to approach equilibrium with the surrounding body fluids, and then drained. The process is then repeated as many times as necessary.
2. *Gastrodialysis*. A cellophane bag is placed into the stomach and periodically filled and drained of dialysate. The access tube reaches the bag via the mouth and esophagus of the anesthetized patient.
3. *Intestinal dialysis*. Dialysate is run continuously for about 8 hr through a 6- or 7-ft length of intestine which has been connected to external tubing.
4. *Pleural dialysis*. The lung cavity, which is surrounded by the pleural membrane, is employed in the same fashion as in peritoneal dialysis.

These methods have the advantages of the avoidance of handling blood (no hemolysis, no blood leakage problems) and simplicity of equipment, but have several disadvantages: (a) poor efficiency in most cases, (b) uncomfortableness, (c) loss of proteins in some methods (e.g., in peritoneal dialysis), (d) a disturbing incidence of membrane infection, and (e) the necessity that the dialysate be extremely sterile.

Before turning our attention in detail to the method normally used, the dialysis of blood outside the body (hemodialysis), we might also mention here some other extracorporeal blood treatment approaches that have been tried:

1. *Fixed bed adsorption columns*, containing activated charcoal, ion exchange resins, etc., or a combination of these materials, either directly exposed to the blood or encapsulated in bead form in semipermeable membranes. These devices suffer from (a) lack of good total adsorption capacity per unit volume, (b) poor selectivity (e.g., they capture uric acid well, urea poorly), (c) lack of ability to remove water, and (d) their tendency to filter blood cells out of the bloodstream.

2. *Ultrafiltration methods*, where blood is fed to a chamber having a supported-membrane bottom and pressurized, driving out plasma (no proteins though) with its entrained waste materials. A makeup solution which is essentially like the dialysate solution previously described is added back to the blood to reconstitute it. Variations include adding the makeup solution prior to filtration, and continuous rather than batch operation. This approach has been a promising one, but the tendency of the membranes to "foul" with gummy protein has been a serious problem. The equipment is often complex also.

II. HEMODIALYSIS

The procedure most often used to clear the body of metabolic wastes and excess species is to connect tubing to a major blood vessel, feed blood to a device containing a membrane (where the blood flows on one side of the membrane and dialysate flows on the other side), and to route the partially cleansed blood back to the body via tubing connected to another large vessel. Artificial kidneys of this type in common use vary somewhat in operation: Some use blood pumps, others use the natural arterial to venous pressure difference to provide blood flow; some use countercurrent or cocurrent flow of blood and dialysate, others use cross flow; some use membranes aligned in parallel flat sheets, others use flattened membrane tubing rolled into coils, and still others use large numbers of parallel cylindrical semipermeable "hollow fibers"; some use dialysate on a once-through basis, others use dialysate recycle (with or without makeup and "bleed" streams); and so forth.

To establish a frame of reference for evaluating such differences it would be useful to enumerate at this point those features or aspects which would be generally considered to characterize the ideal artificial kidney:

1. The device should be efficient in removing nitrogenous and toxic products of metabolism and excess ionic species.

2. The device should be capable of efficiently removing water either by the use of hyperosmotic dialysate or by ultrafiltration (hydrostatic pressure difference).

3. It should have a fairly small (∿500 ml or less) internal blood-side volume so that the patient's own blood can be used to "prime" (fill) the unit, thereby avoiding the need to use bank blood.

4. The blood-side flow resistance of the device should be low enough so that adequate blood flow rates can be achieved without a blood pump, utilizing the natural arterial-venous pressure difference of the patient as the motive force. Having a blood pump in the circuit requires added, often complicated safety features, and is apt to cause undue hemolysis.

5. The part of the device which contains the dialysis membrane should be preassembled, prepackaged, presterilized, and disposable (i.e., cheap enough to be discarded after one use).

6. The unit should be constructed from nontoxic, blood-compatible materials which produce insignificant hemolysis and which do not adsorb or filter out vital blood components.

7. Reliability, safety, repeatability of performance, and ease of operation are necessary.

8. Low costs for the disposable dialyzer portion of the system and for maintenance of the overall system are very important.

No hemodialyzer in current use meets all or most of these criteria. However, we shall briefly describe those devices that are most often used in clinical practice. These devices may generally be classified as flat plate membrane types or coiled membrane types.

A. *Flat Plate Type of Hemodialyzers*

These dialyzers are exemplified by the two-layer Kiil dialyzer shown in Figure 9.1, which is the most popular one of this type. The assembled unit is roughly 40 in. long by 14 in. wide and is 3 in. high (excluding the clamps) and consists of parallel epoxy boards having lengthwise grooves and carved-out lengthwise channels (as shown in the figure). Two sheets of cellophane or "Cuprophane" membrane are inserted between each board-to-board joint. Appropriate headers at each end of the unit direct blood to the channels between the cellophane sheets and dialysate to the spaces between the cellophane and the boards (down the grooved channels). Flow is normally countercurrent. A four-layer Kiil unit is also popular.

B. *Coil Type of Hemodialyzers*

The most popular type of this kind of device, called the Kolff Twin Coil, is shown in Figure 9.2. The membrane consists of two cellophane tubes, each 9 cm in circumference and 10.8 m long, which

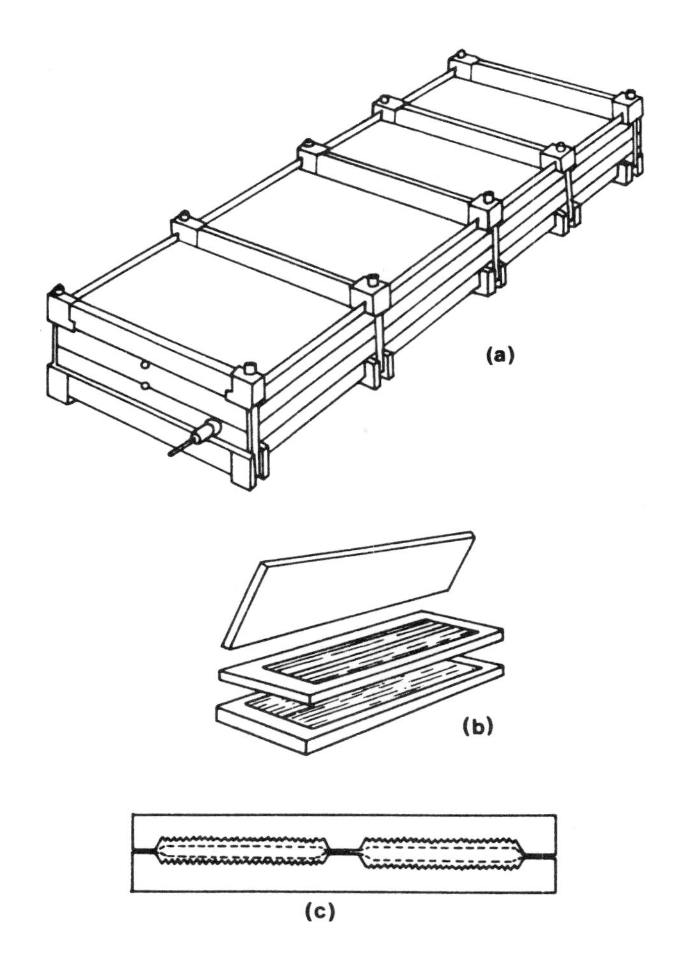

FIG. 9.1. The Kiil kidney (a) assembled, (b) exploded, and (c) cross section.

are flattened, placed on a nylon open-mesh "spacer" material, and rolled into a coil. The coil is then held in a cartridge, 9 in. in diameter by 8 in. high, which is open at each end. Figure 9.2(b) illustrates how the cartridge is normally placed in a large dialysate bath (~100-liter tank) where dialysate is pumped upward through the coil. Flow is therefore "cross flow." A smaller version using two 5.2-m-long tubes, called the Chronic Coil, is also popular, for use with children or for less serious adult renal (kidney) failure. The important operational features of the Kiil and Kolff artificial kidneys are summarized in Table 9.3. These are typical values only. Note that the dialysate flow rates are very much higher for the coil units. This is because the dialysate is recycled over and over through the coil but remains in the 100-liter tank. Since the dialysate bath continually increases in waste concentration, it must be changed every 3 hr or so. Alternatively, continuous bleed and makeup dialysate streams can be installed; flow rates of these are typically about 2 liters/min.

The Kiil devices have much lower blood channel thicknesses than the coil devices (which would develop an intolerably high flow resistance for channel heights as low as 0.3 mm) and thus should have lower resistances to mass transfer on the blood side. However, obtaining uniform blood flow across the entire membrane is a problem, and poor flow distribution tends to increase the blood-side resistance. The overall result is that the Kiil devices are somewhat less efficient than coil devices of comparable area operated at the same blood flow rates. The Kiil devices also require careful time-consuming assembly and sterilization, whereas the coil devices are manufactured in a sterile and ready-to-use form. On the other hand, ultrafiltration is easier to achieve in Kiil units (suction can be applied to the dialysate) and operating costs are generally lower for the Kiil devices. Central dialysate supply tanks feeding several Kiil devices simultaneously on a once-through basis are often economic for large dialysis centers. For small facilities, the convenience of coil dialyzers is to be preferred, even though batch preparation of dialysate (100 liters per batch) is somewhat more expensive.

Figure 9.3 illustrates one type of central dialysate supply system that has been developed, and also shows some of the monitoring equipment needed for safe operation. One must continuously check patient blood pressure and outflow dialysate transparency, so as to detect blood leaks in the system. Dialysate flow, concentration, pressure, and temperature must be checked also. Access to the blood pool of the body is normally made, as this figure shows, by connection to an artery and a vein in the patient's arm. Figure 9.4 shows this in greater detail. The tubes that reside in the artery and vein are called cannulas, and are connected by a shunt when not being used. The development of such permanent indwelling cannulas in 1960 was a major step in the history of artificial kidney treatment.

As a historical note, mention might be made here of a few major developments in artificial kidney devices. Dialysis of dogs using blood flowing through collodion (nitrocellulose) tubes surrounded by saline was first attempted by Abel, Rowntree, and Turner (1914) in the early 1900s. While their experiments were reasonably suc-

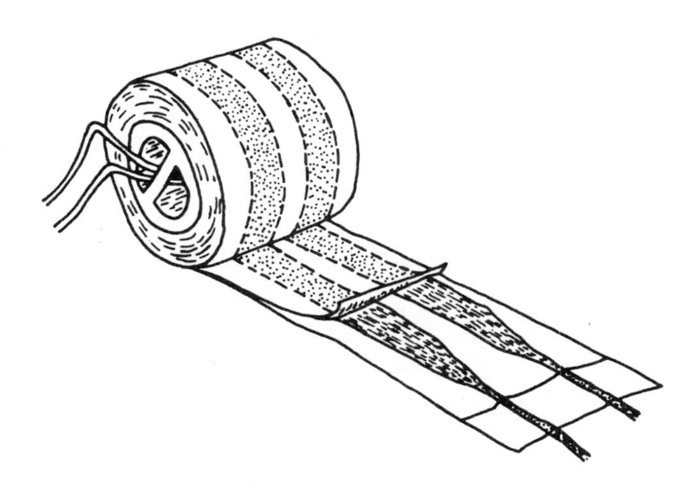

FIG. 9.2a. The Kolff twin coil.

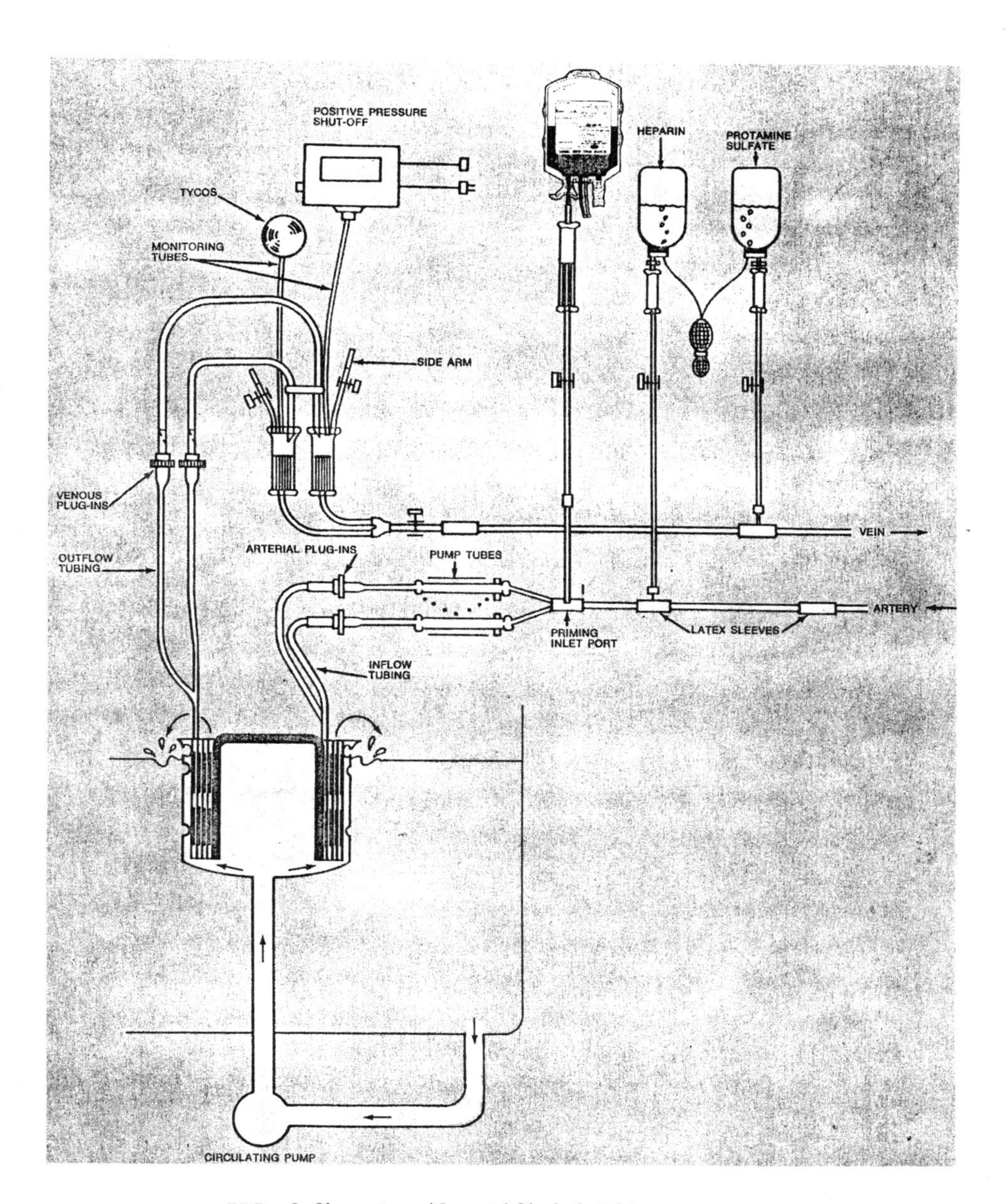

FIG. 9.2b. A coil artificial kidney system.

TABLE 9.3

Comparison of the Kiil and Coil Artificial Kidneys

	Kiil		Twin	Chronic
	Four layer	Two layer	Coil	Coil
Membrane area (m^2)	2.1	1.15	1.9	0.9
Priming volume (ml)	400	130	1000	500
Pump needed?	Yes	No	Yes	No
Blood flow rate (ml/min)	400	140-200	200-300	200
Dialysate flow rate (liters/min)	4.5	2.0	20-30	20-30
Blood channel thickness (mm)	0.3	0.2	1.2	0.8
Treatment time (hr)	6	6-8	6-8	8-10

cessful (actually, their main purpose was to extract certain solutes from the blood, not necessarily metabolites; however, they were aware of their device's potential use for treating renal failure) further development of such devices was very limited until reliable cellophane membranes and effective blood anticoagulants (e.g., heparin, which is used in all present-day hemodialyses) were discovered. In 1943, Kolff developed the first clinically successful dialyzer made of a long tube of cellophane coiled on a drum which was immersed in dialysate. A whole series of designs were generated by others, particularly from 1950 onward. The Kolff Twin Coil appeared in 1956, and the Kiil unit (which evolved from several earlier flat plate devices) was developed in 1960.

C. *Hollow Fiber Devices*

A recent promising type of dialysis unit is the hollow fiber or capillary artificial kidney. This looks like a typical shell-

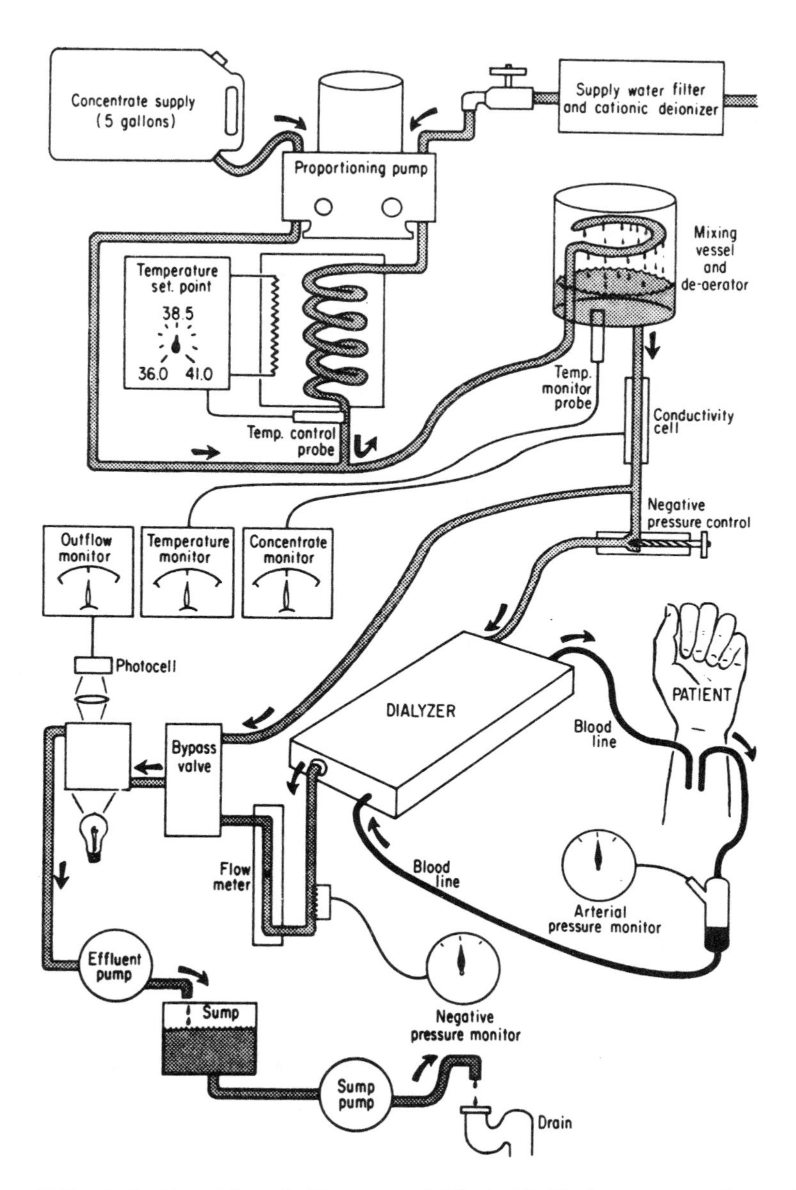

FIG. 9.3. Functional diagram of Mini-II dialysate supply unit. [From Babb et al. (1967).]

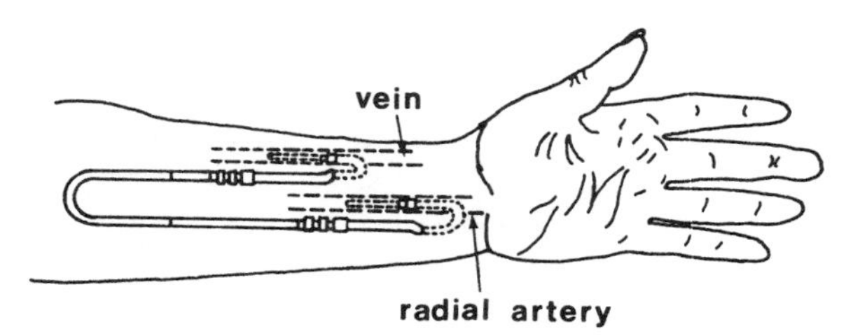

FIG. 9.4. Arteriovenous shunt and typical cannula system.

and-tube heat exchanger (see Figure 9.5) and contains up to 11,000 capillaries made of regenerated cellulose, each one being 13.5 cm long, 225 μm inside diameter, and 30 μm in wall thickness. Total blood priming volume is only 95 ml, and no blood pump is needed. Efficiency is good. In addition, the units are relatively inexpensive, and are disposable and presterilized. This type of device should enjoy growing popularity.

Further data on a whole range of older and newer dialyzers are presented in Table 9.4. The mass transfer figures given in this table are interpreted after a theoretical framework for analyzing mass transfer in dialyzers has been established. This is our next topic.

III. ANALYSIS OF MASS TRANSFER IN DIALYZERS

Mass transfer in dialyzers is normally modeled using a "film theory" approach. This approach assumes that all of the resistance to mass transfer in the flowing fluids (whether dialysate or blood) is localized in stagnant films of thickness δ_D and δ_B (for dialysate and blood, respectively). In reality we know that there do not exist adjacent fully mixed and stagnant fluid regions; rather there is always a general variation of velocity, and of lateral fluid mixing, from a maximum far from any surface to a zero value at the surface. Mass transport far from the wall is large (if turbulence

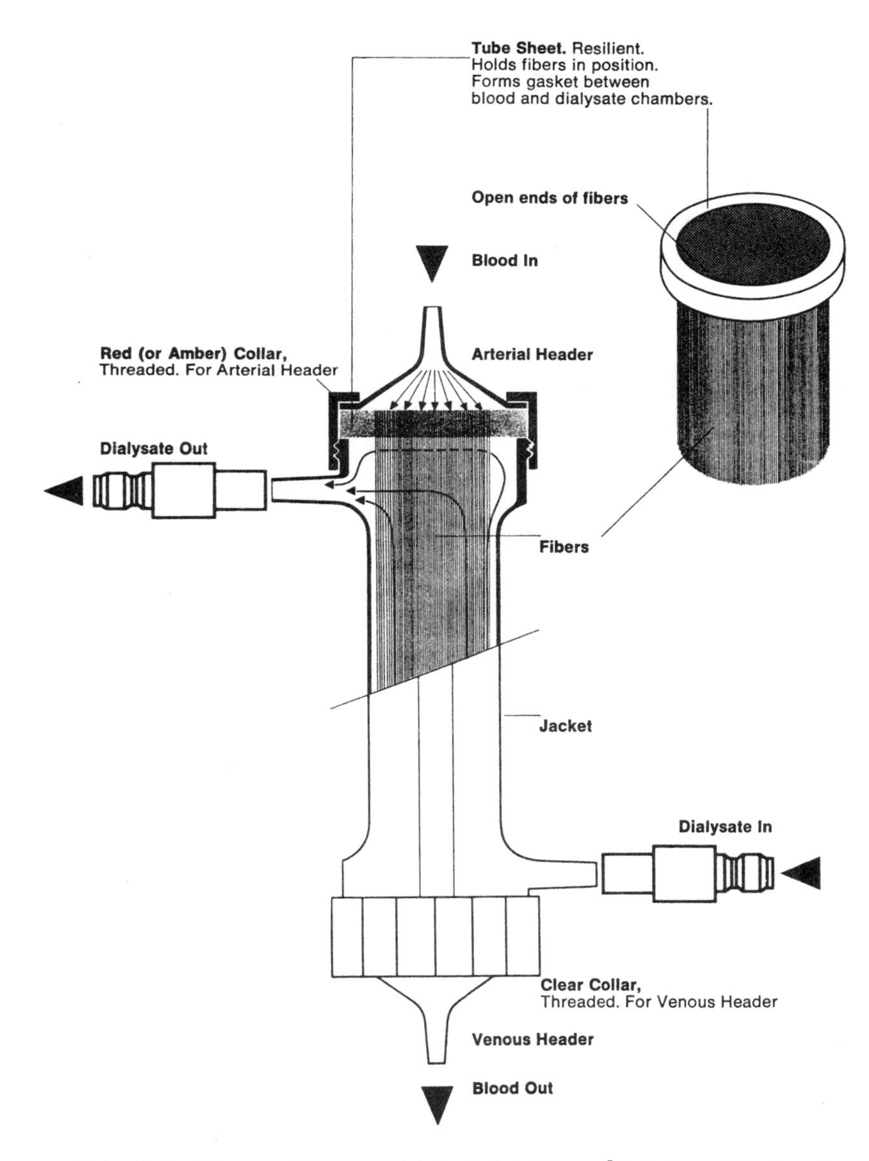

FIG. 9.5. The capillary artificial kidney [8.5 in. (21.6 cm) long by 2.75 in. (6.99 cm) in diameter].

exists) because of fluid mixing, and concentration gradients are therefore small. Very near the wall transfer occurs by molecular diffusion, since no lateral fluid motion exists, and concentration gradients are relatively large. In applying the film theory concept one simply replaces the continuous variation of fluid conditions by an "equivalent" two-zone model of stagnant and fully mixed regions. It is equivalent to the real situation in the sense that the assigned value of the stagnant film thickness δ correctly predicts the overall resistance of the fluid to mass transfer.

Figure 9.6 shows a film-type model of a dialyzer, and typical concentration profiles. Here we assume that the same partition coefficient α can be used on both sides of the membrane, i.e.,

$$\alpha = \frac{C_M'}{C_B'} = \frac{C_M''}{C_D''}$$

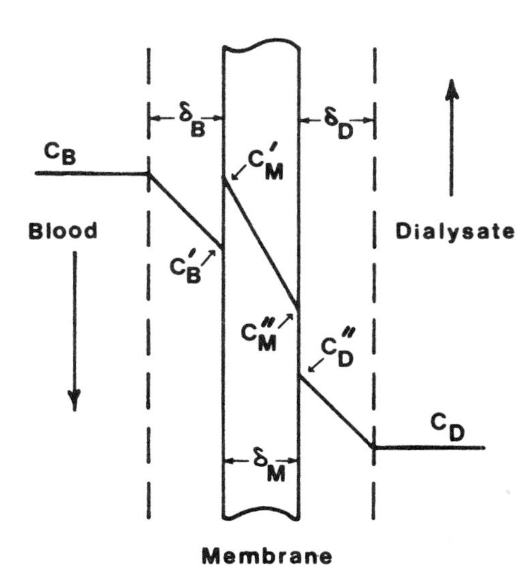

FIG. 9.6. Solute concentrations in the vicinity of a membrane during transport. [From Spaeth (1970).]

At steady state (no accumulation of solute in any region) the fluxes through both fluid films and through the membrane are all equal, so that

$$N = \frac{D_B(C_B - C_B')}{\delta_B} = \frac{D_D(C_D'' - C_D)}{\delta_D} = \frac{D_M(C_M' - C_M'')}{\delta_M} \tag{9.1}$$

where we have assumed (a) linear concentration profiles, (b) zero "bulk flow," (c) no electrical potential gradients, and (d) constant diffusivities. δ_M is the membrane thickness.

Now we can write the overall concentration difference as

$$C_B - C_D = (C_B - C_B') + (C_B' - C_D'') + (C_D'' - C_D)$$

Using the partition coefficient it is clear that

$$N = \frac{D_M\alpha}{\delta_M}\left(\frac{C_M'}{\alpha} - \frac{C_M''}{\alpha}\right) = \frac{D_M\alpha}{\delta_M}(C_B' - C_D'')$$

or $C_B' - C_D'' = \delta_M N/D_M\alpha$. From Equation 9.1 it is also evident that

$$C_B - C_B' = \frac{\delta_B N}{D_B} \text{ and } C_D'' - C_D = \frac{\delta_D N}{D_D}$$

Hence

$$C_B - C_D = \frac{\delta_B N}{D_B} + \frac{\delta_M N}{\alpha D_M} + \frac{\delta_D N}{D_D}$$

or

$$N = K(C_B - C_D)$$

where K, the overall mass transfer coefficient, is given by the expression

$$\frac{1}{K} = R = R_B + R_M + R_D = \frac{\delta_B}{D_B} + \frac{\delta_M}{\alpha D_M} + \frac{\delta_D}{D_D}$$

Here we have indicated that the overall transfer coefficient may be regarded as the inverse of an overall resistance R which in turn is the sum of the blood-side, membrane, and dialysate-side mass transfer resistances. The expression $N = K(C_B - C_D)$ can be regarded as a definition of K. Since C_B and C_D vary with position in actual dialyzers, this equation is valid only for particular localities, and does not characterize the dialyzer on an overall basis. Expressions for total transfer in an entire dialyzer can be derived by applying the flux expression differentially and integrating across the whole dialyzer, as we shall now show.

A. *Expressions for the Overall Mass Transfer Rate*

Consider the cocurrent flow dialyzer shown in Figure 9.7. For any small section of length dx, and associated membrane area dA, the mass transferred, dW, is

$$dW = K(C_B - C_D)\ dA = Q_D\ dC_D = -Q_B\ dC_B$$

Hence,

$$\frac{dC_B}{C_B - C_D} = -\frac{K}{Q_B}\ dA$$

and

$$\frac{dC_D}{C_B - C_D} = \frac{K}{Q_D}\ dA$$

These may be combined to yield

$$-\frac{d(C_B - C_D)}{C_B - C_D} = K\left(\frac{1}{Q_B} + \frac{1}{Q_D}\right) dA$$

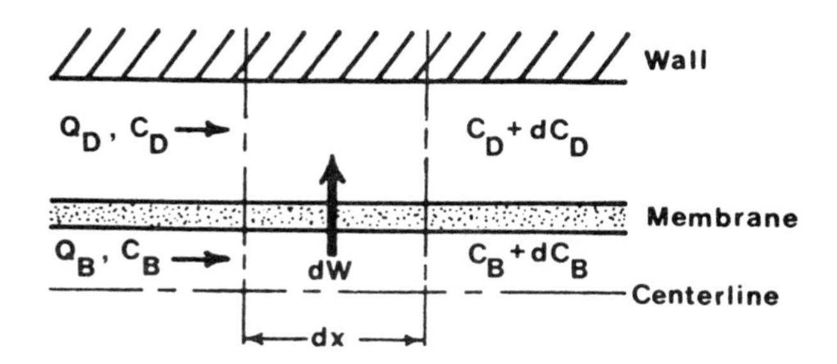

FIG. 9.7. Mass transfer in differential length of a dialyzer. [From Spaeth (1970).]

Integrating from the inlet to the outlet of the dialyzer and use of the proper boundary conditions then gives

$$\ln\left(\frac{C_{Bi} - C_{Di}}{C_{Bo} - C_{Do}}\right) = KA\left(\frac{1}{Q_B} + \frac{1}{Q_D}\right)$$

where the subscripts i and o refer to the dialyzer inlet and outlet, respectively. Now, since the total mass transferred in the dialyzer is

$$W = -Q_B(C_{Bo} - C_{Bi}) = Q_D(C_{Do} - C_{Di}) \tag{9.2}$$

we can write

$$\ln\left(\frac{C_{Bi} - C_{Di}}{C_{Bo} - C_{Do}}\right) = KA\left(\frac{C_{Bi} - C_{Bo}}{W} + \frac{C_{Do} - C_{Di}}{W}\right)$$

or

$$W = KA\left\{\frac{(C_{Bi} - C_{Di}) - (C_{Bo} - C_{Do})}{\ln[(C_{Bi} - C_{Di})/(C_{Bo} - C_{Do})]}\right\} \tag{9.3}$$

i.e.,

$$W = KA(\Delta C)_{\text{log mean}}$$

This demonstrates that the total mass transferred can be characterized by using the log mean concentration driving force. Cocurrent heat exchanger equations are of the same form, only in terms of total heat transferred, an overall heat transfer coefficient, and a log mean temperature difference.

B. *Expressions for Dialysance, Clearance, and Extraction Ratio*

It has been common practice to characterize the performance of dialyzers in terms of a quantity called the dialysance, which is defined as

$$D^* = Q_B \frac{C_{Bi} - C_{Bo}}{C_{Bi} - C_{Di}} = \frac{W}{(C_{Bi} - C_{Di})} \tag{9.4}$$

This is equal to the total mass transferred per unit concentration difference, based on <u>inlet</u> concentrations. The clearance of an artificial kidney device is similarly defined:

$$C^* = \frac{Q_B(C_{Bi} - C_{Bo})}{C_{Bi}} = \frac{W}{C_{Bi}}$$

and represents the equivalent amount of inlet blood (e.g., in milliliters per minute) that would be completely cleared of solute at the prevailing mass transfer rate. Another meaningful performance index, the extraction ratio E, has also been used. This is simply $E = D^*/Q_B$ and represents the amount of solute concentration change achieved relative to what would result from complete equilibrium with a very large supply of dialysate having a concentration C_{Di}. Note that if $C_{Di} = 0$, then $E = 1 - (C_{Bo}/C_{Bi})$, or the fraction of solute removed. As membrane area is increased and the amount of dialysate used is increased, the parameter E approaches unity.

From Equation 9.2 we may write

$$C_{Bo} = -\frac{W}{Q_B} + C_{Bi}, \quad C_{Do} = \frac{W}{Q_D} + C_{Di}$$

For a cocurrent dialyzer we may then rewrite Equation 9.3 as

$$W = KA\frac{(-W/Q_B + C_{Bi} - W/Q_D - C_{Di} - C_{Bi} + C_{Di})}{\ln[(-W/Q_B + C_{Bi} - W/Q_D - C_{Di})/(C_{Bi} - C_{Di})]}$$

$$W = KA\frac{-W(1/Q_B + 1/Q_D)}{\ln\,[-W(1/Q_B + 1/Q_D) + W/D^*]/(W/D^*)}$$

where we have used the relationship $W = D^*(C_{Bi} - C_{Di})$. Upon further manipulation the result just given can be expressed in the form

$$E = \frac{1 - \exp[-(KA/Q_B)(1 + Q_B/Q_D)]}{(1 + Q_B/Q_D)}$$

Defining $N_T = KA/Q_B$ and $Z = Q_B/Q_D$, this becomes

$$E = \frac{1 - \exp[-N_T(1 + Z)]}{1 + Z}$$

The quantity N_T is a dimensionless parameter called the number of mass transfer units of the dialyzer, and it indicates quantitatively the mass transfer capabilities of the dialyzer. Figure 9.8 presents E as a function of Z for various N_T values, for cocurrent or parallel flow. It is clear that E increases as the ratio Q_B/Q_D becomes smaller, as one would expect (less solute to remove, larger amount of dialysate to remove it), and increases as the membrane area and mass transfer coefficient become larger.

One can easily show that the log mean driving force is the proper kind of mean to use in the equation $W = KA\,\Delta C_{mean}$ for two other important cases besides parallel flow. These are (a) countercurrent flow and (b) "mixed dialysate" flow—i.e., where the dialysate is flowing in such large volume and/or is so turbulent that the solute concentration in the dialysate can be assumed to be uniform and not a function of location. This latter type of flow is very closely approached in coil types of dialyzers. For these

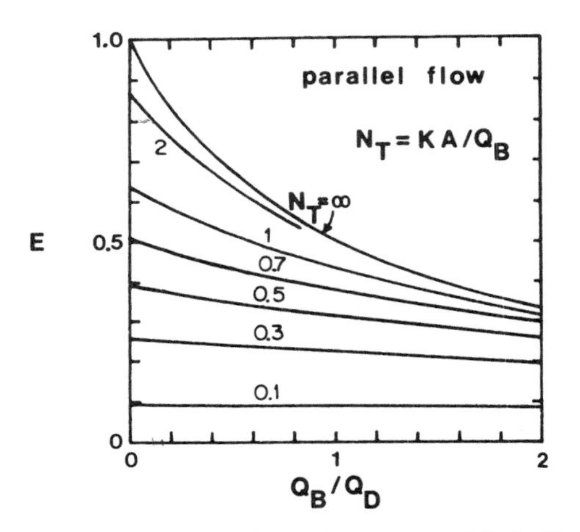

FIG. 9.8. Performance profiles for a parallel-flow dialyzer. [From Michaels (1966).]

two additional cases, Michaels (1966) has shown that the efficiency expressions are

Countercurrent flow: $$E = \frac{1 - \exp[N_T(1 - Z)]}{Z - \exp[N_T(1 - Z)]}$$

or, if Z = 1, $$E = \frac{N_T}{1 + N_T}$$

Mixed dialysate flow: $$E = \frac{1 - \exp(-N_T)}{1 + Z[1 - \exp(-N_T)]}$$

Derivations of these equations are obtained in the same fashion as that for parallel flow, as shown above. Figures 9.9 and 9.10 give E versus Z for various N_T values for these two cases. Comparison of Figures 9.8-9.10 reveals that countercurrent flow is inherently much more efficient than the other two modes (which are, in turn, very similar in efficiency) for high values of $N_T = KA/Q_B$. This is because, at high KA/Q_B values, extraction of solute from blood tends to be limited, not by K or A, but by the fact that solute building up in the dialysate destroys the concentration driving force for

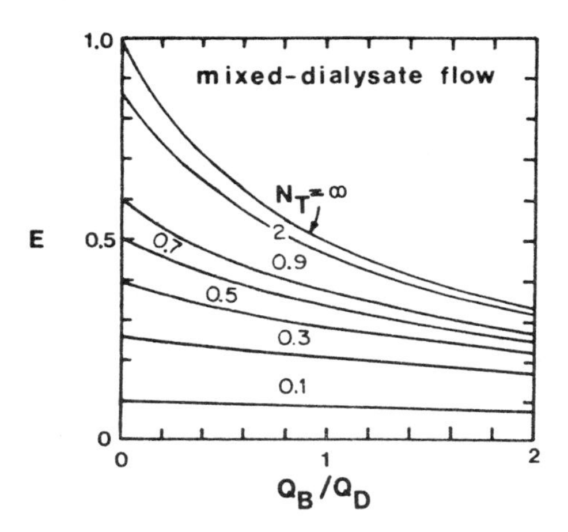

FIG. 9.9. Performance profiles for a mixed-dialysate dialyzer. [From Michaels (1966).]

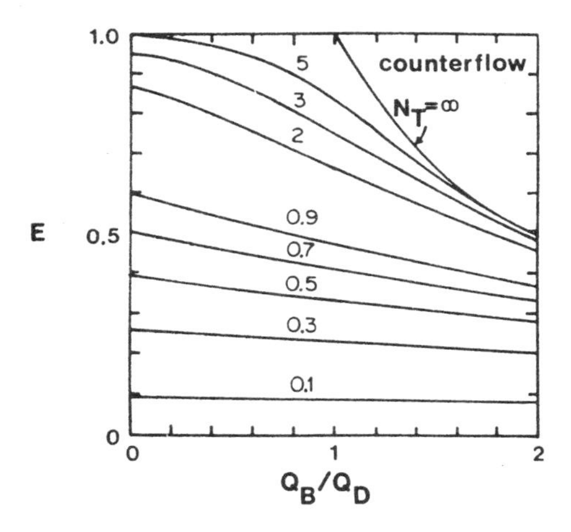

FIG. 9.10. Performance profiles for a counterflow dialyzer. [From Michaels (1966).]

mass transfer. In counterflow operation the concentration driving force stays high throughout the entire dialyzer and this effect is minimized.

Since dialysate flow rates in actual practice are usually kept quite large relative to blood flow rates, to ensure reasonably rapid solute removal, simplified forms of the efficiency equations given above are often adequate for describing hemodialysis operations. For $Q_B/Q_D \cong 0$ we have

$$E \cong 1 - \exp(-N_T)$$

for <u>all</u> three cases discussed. This implies that for any given value of N_T the value at which the curve of E versus Q_B/Q_D intercepts the ordinate should be the same for all three flow arrangements. A look at Figures 9.8-9.10 confirms this. Another limiting case which never really occurs in practice but which can be mathematically defined is that of $Q_B/Q_D \to \infty$. For this situation all efficiency equations become $E = 1/Z = Q_D/Q_B$. This just says that $E \to 0$ as $Q_D/Q_B \to 0$, which is logical. However, it also implies that E for large, but still quite finite, Z values is independent of flow configuration. Again the plotted E curves suggest this is probably approximately true for $Z > 2.0$.

C. Experimental Mass Transfer Resistance Values

Colton (1967) has used the general efficiency equations presented above to determine overall mass transfer coefficient values from published data on clinical and laboratory dialyzers of various types. A summary of the devices, blood flow rates, dialysate flow rates, and derived values of D^*, N_T, K, R, R_M, R_D, and R_B are given in Table 9.4. Colton's general procedure was to determine K (and hence R, the overall resistance) from quoted data on membrane areas, dialysances, D^* (or from given C_{Bo}, C_{Bi}, C_{Do}, and C_{Di} data), and Q_B and Q_D values. He then constructed Wilson plots of overall resistance versus $Q_D^{-0.8}$. This type of plot is based on the fact that

TABLE 9.4

Mass Transfer Characteristics of Hemodialyzers at 37°C[a,b,c]

Type of hemodialyzer	Membrane	Area (m^2)	Solute and fluid	Q_B	Q_D	D*	N_T	$K \times 10^3$	R	R_M	R_D	R_B
Kolff Twin Coil CF	Visking tubing	1.8	Urea-blood (human) in vivo	100	13000	72.5	1.30	7.19	131	23.5	3.5	113
				200	↓	111	0.81	9.0	111	↓	↓	84
				300	↓	121	0.52	8.62	116	↓	↓	89
				400	↓	124	0.45	9.9	101	↓	↓	74
			Uric acid-blood (human) in vivo	100	13000	42	0.64	3.54	274	50.1	6.3	218
				200	↓	75	0.47	5.21	192	↓	↓	136
Mini Coil CF	Visking tubing	0.39	Urea-blood (dog) in vivo	40	167	10	0.29	2.97	328	23.5	22	283
Kolff Twin Coil CF	Visking tubing	1.9	Urea-blood in vitro	100	30000	78.5	1.54	7.32	137	23.5	16	97
				200	↓	120	0.92	8.75	115	↓	↓	75
				400	↓	161	0.52	9.8	101	↓	↓	61
			Creatinine-blood in vitro	100	↓	66.7	1.1	5.25	191	53.0	30	109
				200	↓	84	0.55	5.2	193	↓	↓	110
				400	↓	119	0.35	6.72	149	↓	↓	67

TABLE 9.4 (Cont'd)

Mass Transfer Characteristics of Hemodialyzers at 37°C

Type of hemodialyzer	Membrane	Area (m^2)	Solute and fluid	Q_B	Q_D	D*	N_T	$K \times 10^3$	R	R_M	R_D	R_B
Kolff Chronic Coil CF	Visking tubing	0.9	Urea-blood in vitro	100	30000	60	0.92	10.2	98	23.5		
				200	↓	88.2	0.57	13.0	77	↓		
				300	↓	100	0.41	13.5	74	↓		
Kiil, two layer P	du Pont PD 215	1.15	Urea-blood in vitro	100	2000	77	1.17	10.3	98	24.2		
				200	↓	104	0.77	13.5	74	↓		
				400	↓	116	0.53	13.7	73	↓		
Kiil, four layer P	du Pont PD 215	2.1	Urea-blood in vitro	100	4500	92.5	2.78	13.2	76	24.2		
				200	↓	140	1.42	13.5	74	↓		
				400	↓	219	0.83	15.8	63	↓		
			Creatinine-blood in vitro	100	↓	83.3	1.87	8.9	122	53.0		
				200	↓	122	0.97	9.2	108	↓		
				400	↓	147	0.47	9.0	112	↓		

MacNeill-Collins (flattened tubes) P	Visking tubing	1.0	Urea-blood (dog) in vivo	240	3000	77	0.39	9.3	108	23.5	11.1	72.9
Kiil, two layer P	du Pont PD 215	1.15	Urea-blood (human) in vivo	130	1800	91	1.3	14.7	68	24.2	37°C	
				↓	↓	66	0.73	8.3	122	↓	10°C	
			Creatinine-blood (human) in vivo	130	1800	72	0.84	9.5	106	53.0	37°C	
				↓	↓	50	0.50	5.6	179	↓	10°C	
Modified Kiil, two layer CC	Bemberg PT-150	1.15	Urea-blood in vivo	139	2000	64	0.63	7.65	131	8.3	20°C	
				142	↓	70	0.68	8.25	122	↓	20°C	

[a]Adapted from Colton (1967)

[b]Abbreviations: P, parallel cocurrent flow; CC, countercurrent flow; CF, cross flow. Temperature 37°C unless otherwise indicated.

[c]Q_B, Q_D, D* in ml/min; R, R_M, R_D, R_B in min/cm; K in cm/min.

for a stream in turbulent flow, as the dialysate normally is, the mass transfer coefficient for that stream is proportional to the stream Reynolds number to the 0.8 power. Hence, its resistance is proportional to its flow rate to the -0.8 power. Plotting total resistance versus $Q_D^{-0.8}$ and extrapolating back to zero $Q_D^{-0.8}$ (i.e., infinite Q_D) gives an intercept that should be equal to the sum of the membrane and blood-side resistances only. The membrane resistance was determined by separate data on solute transport through various membranes in standard "diffusion" cells (e.g., two well-stirred compartments separated by a membrane). Knowing R_M + R_B and R_M alone obviously allows one to infer a value for R_B. This whole procedure requires having data on mass transfer for various dialysate rates at a single blood flow rate.

Figure 9.11 shows Colton's calculated results for blood-side resistance as a percentage of total resistance versus blood flow rate, for urea, uric acid, and creatinine removal in a Twin Coil dialyzer. For a typical Q_B of 200 ml/min, the membrane, blood-side, and dialysate-side resistances for urea removal are roughly 20, 70, and 10% of the total, respectively. Table 9.4 indicates that a MacNeill-Collins dialyzer, which is similar to the Kiil type, has membrane, blood, and dialysate resistances of 22, 68 and 10% of the total resistance, respectively, for urea removal from dog blood at typical flow rates. The values for coil and flat plate units therefore seem to be similar. The dialysate is seen to have only about 10% of the total resistance, which is not surprising. While R_B values control mass transfer, higher blood flow rates or smaller blood channel thicknesses, which would decrease blood resistance, are difficult to attain. Blood flow rates are limited either by the flow resistances of the dialyzers themselves, at low or moderate flows (hence smaller channels would greatly raise flow resistances), or by the source (patient) resistance, at higher flows. Increasing Q_B can induce vascular collapse or, at the very least, create extra hemolysis. Blood channels cannot be made much smaller than current values (0.2-1.2 mm), not only because of the increased blood flow

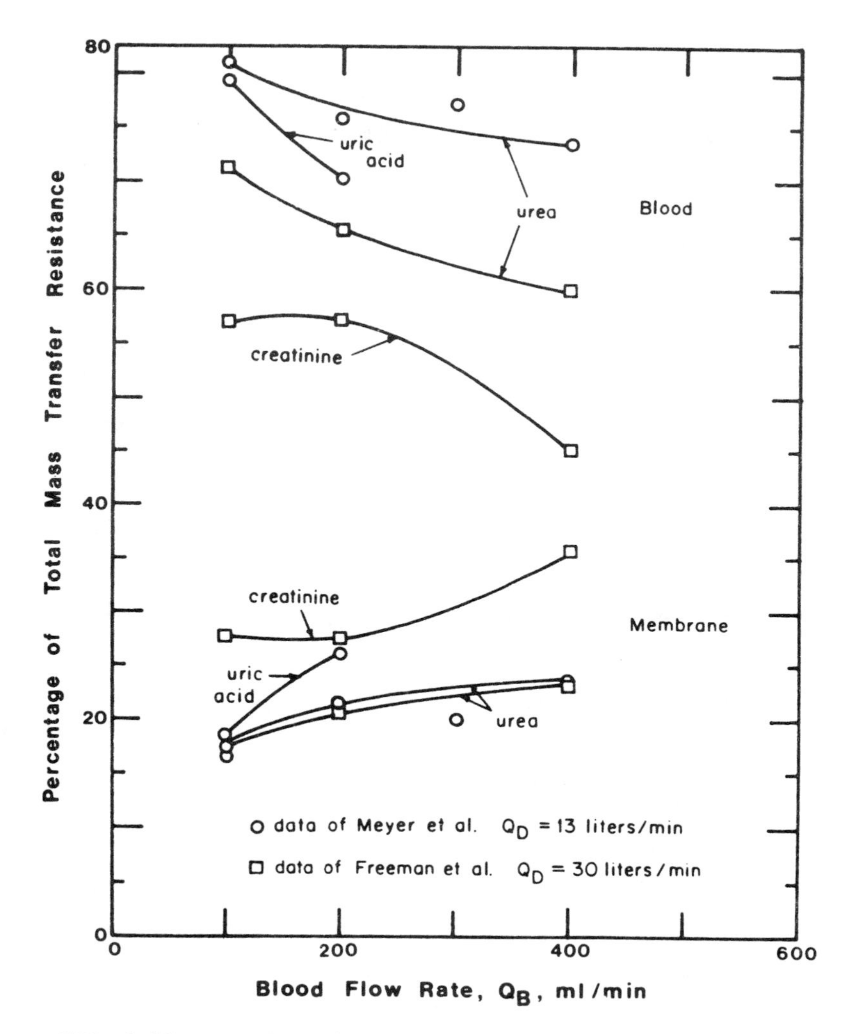

FIG. 9.11. Fraction of total mass transfer resistance for blood and membrane as a function of blood flow rate for a Twin Coil hemodialyzer at 37°C. [From Colton (1967).]

resistance that would occur (this would offset any gains), but because obtaining uniform flow through very thin channels is very difficult. Machining epoxy boards, or wrapping coils, to achieve very small uniform gap heights is quite tricky.

In addition to these considerations, it is also recognized that current mass transfer rates are really high enough and further increases are physiologically undesirable anyway. The reason this is true is that solute (especially urea) transfer from the cerebrospinal fluid (CSF) to the blood is not inherently fast. Hence, removing urea rapidly from blood causes the blood to become hypotonic relative to the CSF. Water therefore shifts osmotically into the CSF, thus causing swelling of the brain, and what is known as the "disequilibrium syndrome" (headache, nausea, etc.). A dialysis treatment in less than about 5 hr time generally causes such effects. Hence, present-day dialyzers are <u>efficient enough</u>; their main drawback is their high cost per treatment [much of the cost is for supervisory personnel (doctors and nurses) and various hospital charges; the disposable cartridge may only be 10% of the total cost].

Table 9.4 indicates that, for the Kolff and Kiil units, the overall transfer resistances R for urea transport between blood and dialysate at 37°C are as follows:

Blood flow rate 200 ml/min		Blood flow rate 400 ml/min	
Kolff Twin Coil	$R \cong 113$ min/cm	Kolff Twin Coil	$R = 101$ min/cm
Kolff Chronic Coil	$R = 77$	Four-layer Kiil	$R = 63$
Four-layer Kiil	$R = 74$		
Two-layer Kiil	$R = 74$		

These figures suggest that the two- and four-layered Kiil and Chronic Coil units all have essentially the same resistances and that the Twin Coil has a significantly higher resistance. One must remember, however, that the normal operating blood flows and areas of these devices all vary and that a better comparison would be in terms of the extraction ratio and clearance values given in Table 9.5. On this basis the four-layer Kiil is best; the Twin Coil and two-layer Kiil units are somewhat lower in mass transfer capability. The Chronic Coil, having a rather small area and operating at a low Q_B, has the lowest transfer rate. Treatment times for patients would vary in the reverse order as the clearance values, assuming a given total mass removal requirement.

TABLE 9.5

Extraction and Clearance Values for Normal Operation

Unit	Normal Q_B (cc/min)	Area (cm^2)	K (cm/min)	N_T	E	C* (cc/min)
Twin Coil	225	19000	1/112	0.75	0.53	119
Chronic Coil	200	9000	1/77	0.58	0.44	89
Four-layer Kiil	400	21000	1/63	0.83	0.57	226
Two-layer Kiil	400	11500	1/63	0.46	0.37	146

Note: Extraction ratio E and clearance C* calculated assuming high dialysate flow rate.

A typical treatment on a totally anuric patient (zero urine production) is done two or three times per week and reduces the blood's metabolites as shown in Table 9.6.

IV. MODELING OF THE PATIENT-ARTIFICIAL KIDNEY SYSTEM

The equation derived for artificial kidney devices at high dialysate flow rates was (for any flow arrangement)

$$E \cong 1 - \exp(-N_T) = 1 - \exp\left(-\frac{KA}{Q_B}\right)$$

E can be written, using concentrations, as

$$E = \frac{D^*}{Q_B} = \frac{Q_B}{Q_B}\left(\frac{C_{Bi} - C_{Bo}}{C_{Bi} - C_{Di}}\right) \cong \frac{C_{Bi} - C_{Bo}}{C_{Bi}} = 1 - \frac{C_{Bo}}{C_{Bi}}$$

where we have assumed that $C_{Di} = 0$, i.e., either the dialysate comes in "fresh" with no solute as in a flat plate dialyzer type of system or, as in a coil dialyzer system, the amount of dialysate makeup is high enough so that $C_{Di} \cong 0$ at all times. Hence

TABLE 9.6

Concentration of Metabolites in the Blood (mg%)

Solute	Predialysis	Postdialysis	Normal
Urea[a]	90	30	15
Uric acid	10	4	1.5
Creatinine	15	7	3

[a]Urea values are BUN (blood urea nitrogen) values which represent only the nitrogen content of urea. Total urea values would be 60/28 or 2.1 times higher. BUNs are normally used because the analysis of urea involves measuring the N_2 released upon chemical treatment of the sample.

$$C_{Bo} = C_{Bi} \exp\left(-\frac{KA}{Q_B}\right)$$

Now, this equation only applies to a certain instant of time, since C_{Bi} varies with time during the course of a treatment. To determine how the solute content in the patient varies over any finite interval of time this equation must be combined with a mass balance for the patient. The simplest model for the patient is a 50-liter well-stirred tank of fluid of uniform concentration, as shown in Figure 9.12. A differential mass balance for the "patient" then takes the form (neglecting solute production by the body)

$$V_{body} \frac{dC_{Bi}}{dt} = Q_B(C_{Bo} - C_{Bi})$$

Substituting $C_{Bo} = C_{Bi} \exp(-\frac{KA}{Q_B})$ and integrating, with the boundary condition that $C_{Bi} = C^0_{Bi}$ at time zero, gives

$$\frac{C_{Bi}}{C^0_{Bi}} = \exp \frac{Q_B(\beta - 1)t}{V}$$

where $\beta = \exp(-KA/Q_B)$. Let us now apply this formula as shown in the following section.

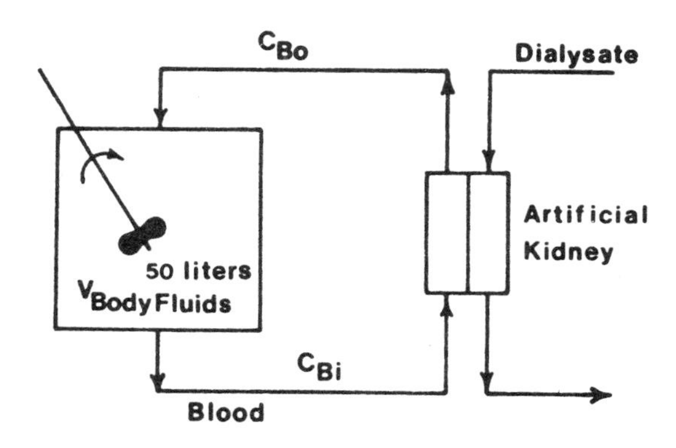

FIG. 9.12. Model of a patient-artificial kidney system.

A. *Prediction of Required Treatment Time*

Consider a flat plate dialyzer with the following specifications:

Q_D = high
Q_B = 200 cc/min
A = 1.0 m^2
R_D = 10% of R
R_B = 70% of R
R_M = 20% of R
R = 60 min/cm

1. When this device is first connected to the patient his BUN (blood urea nitrogen) is 150 mg%. What will the BUN in the blood returning to the patient be at this instant?

$$C_{Bo} = C_{Bi} \exp(-KA/Q_B)$$

Now

$$\frac{KA}{Q_B} = \frac{10{,}000 \text{ cm}^2}{(60 \text{ min/cm})(200 \text{ cc/min})} = 0.833$$

Hence

$$C_{Bo} = 150e^{-0.833} = 150(0.435) = 65.2 \text{ mg\%}$$

2. What is the clearance value for urea in the device, i.e., the mass removal rate expressed as the equivalent cubic centimeters per minute of inlet blood which would be totally cleared of urea?

Clearance is defined as previously shown, by

$$C^* = \frac{Q_B(C_{Bi} - C_{Bo})}{C_{Bi}} = Q_B\left(1 - \frac{C_{Bo}}{C_{Bi}}\right)$$

In this case

$$C^* = Q_B\left[1 - \exp\left(\frac{-KA}{Q_B}\right)\right] = (200)(1 - 0.435) = 113 \text{ cc/min}$$

The dialyzer removes urea at a rate equivalent to completely cleansing 113 cc/min of blood. Note that C^* is independent of time.

3. The treatment is considered complete when the patient's BUN is 50 mg%. If urea production in the body during the dialysis period is neglected, how long will this take?

Since $\exp(-KA/Q_B) = 0.435$, then $\beta = 0.435$. Hence

$$\frac{C_{Bi}}{C_{Bi}^{o}} = \exp\left(\frac{Q_B(\beta - 1)t}{V}\right)$$

gives

$$\frac{50}{150} = \exp\left(\frac{200(-0.565)t}{50000}\right)$$

Solving for t gives t = 486 min, or 8.1 hr.

This agrees with actual clinical treatment times for flat plate dialyzers of 1.0 m^2 urea. It should be noted that the nature of $C_{Bi}(t)$ is an exponential decay.

B. *Babb's Two-Compartment Model*

Babb et al. (1967) have developed a more detailed model for urea removal in a patient-artificial kidney system, in which the patient's body is broken down into two compartments and urea generation by metabolism is accounted for. Figure 9.13 shows their model.

Assuming fresh dialysate is constantly fed to the artificial kidney, the clearance C^* will not change with time and the rate of urea removal from the patient in grams per hour will be C^*C_{Bi}, where C_{Bi} is the grams of urea per milliliter in the blood entering the dialyzer, and C^* is the clearance in milliliters per hour.

Differential mass balances for the intracellular and extracellular fluid pools, which are assumed to be perfectly mixed, are

$$V_1 \frac{dC_1}{dt} = G - k(C_1 - C_2)$$

$$V_2 \frac{dC_2}{dt} = k(C_1 - C_2) - C^*C_2$$

where G represents the grams of urea produced per hour by metabolism, and k is an interpool mass transfer parameter (equal to a mass transfer coefficient times an interfacial area). Note that the clearance term C^*C_{Bi} is written as C^*C_2. Since the extracellular pool includes the blood as well as interstitial fluid, the

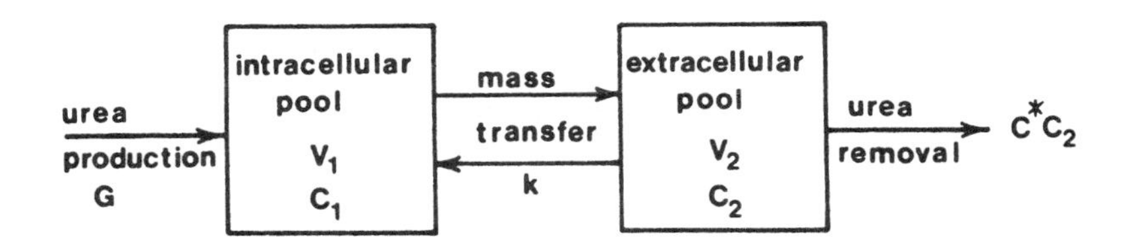

FIG. 9.13. The two-compartment patient model of Babb et al. (1967).

blood urea concentration is the same as that in the extracellular pool as a whole.

Babb et al. (1967) solved the equations just given on an analog computer. The value of G for the patient involved (patient R.H., a 34-year-old, 105-lb male) was determined from BUN measurements on the patient's blood during the periods between dialyses. G was found to be 0.18 g/hr. C* was determined independently for the dialyzer involved (a Kiil type unit) and was found to be 4.6 liters/hr for the blood flow rate used in the study. The total fluid volume in the patient's body was estimated from physiological correlations to be 33.2 liters, and (again from physiological data) V_1 was assumed to be 70% of this and V_2 to be the other 30%. The value of the only remaining parameter, k, was found by comparing the analog computer solution to actual BUN values for the patient, and varying k (by changing a potentiometer setting) until the best match was achieved. The k value obtained this way was 33.1 liters/hr. It should be mentioned that the clearance term, C^*C_2, was set equal to zero for those time periods during which the patient was not undergoing dialysis.

Figure 9.14 shows how well the two-compartment model matches BUN data over a period of more than four days. One may note clearly the exponential type of drop-off of BUN during the 3-hr dialysis periods at the start of each day, the short period of "rebound" (rapid rise of BUN) following dialysis, and the linear buildup of urea during the remainder of the day. The "rebound" effect is due to reequilibration of the blood with the intracellular pool (which is at a higher concentration during dialysis). Overall, it is evident that the relatively simple two-compartment model is an impressively accurate representation of urea dynamics in the dialysis patient.

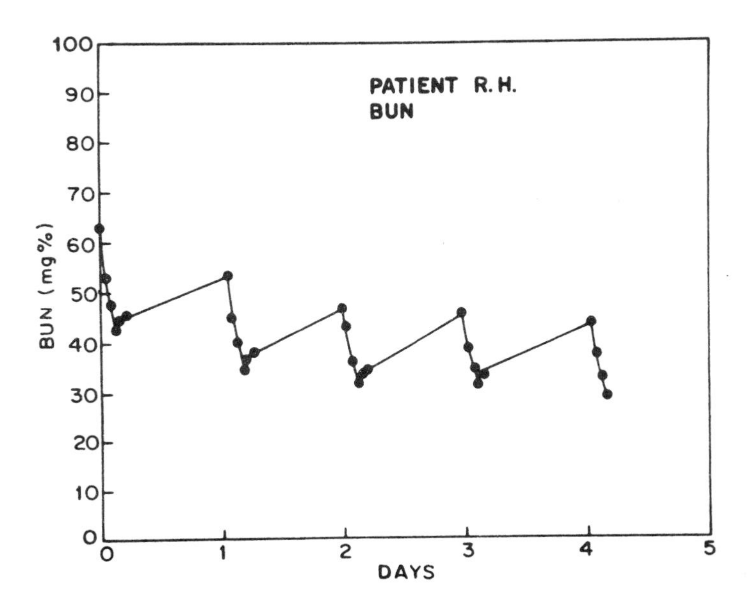

FIG. 9.14. Experimental data (dots) and simulated BUN values (lines) for patient R.H. [From Babb et al. (1967).]

PROBLEMS

1. *Characteristics of a two-layer Kiil unit.* Cooney et al. (1974) have considered the removal of urea in two-layer Kiil dialyzers having 0.54 m^2 of membrane per layer. They indicated that for Q_B = 200 ml/min and Q_D = 1000 ml/min, typical resistances in this device are R_B = 24 min/cm, R_M = 15 min/cm, and R_D = 16 min/cm.

What is the overall mass transfer coefficient K for this unit? What is the value of N_T for this device? What fraction of the urea in the inlet blood would be removed if flow were countercurrent? What would be the fraction for parallel-flow operation? Assume urea-free inlet dialysate for both flow configurations. What would be the clearances for countercurrent and parallel flow?

2. *Required treatment time with the two-layer Kiil unit.* Using the artificial kidney described above, determine how long it would take to lower the BUN value of a patient from 100 to 30 mg%. Assume countercurrent flow and consider the patient's body to be a single well-mixed fluid pool of 50-liters volume for purposes of this computation.

3. *High dialysate flow rate operation (countercurrent flow case).* Assume that if the dialysate flow rate for the Kiil unit described above were doubled (to 2 liters/min), the dialysate-side resistance R_D would be only 9 min/cm. What would be the treatment time determined in the last example? How much time would be saved?

If it costs $30 per hour to treat a person with the Kiil device (a typical figure), and dialysate costs $0.05 per liter, would the high dialysate flow operation result in a net savings?

4. *Low dialysate flow rate operation.* At a dialysate flow rate of 250 ml/min, the value of R_D for the Kiil device mentioned in Problem 1 would probably be about 28 min/cm. What would be the treatment time determined in Problem 2 for a low dialysate flow rate operation? Using the cost figures given in Problem 3, what would be the net saving or loss?

5. *Priming volume.* The Kiil device considered above has two layers; each layer contains a pair of membranes 0.025 cm apart (this gap is where the blood flows). Each membrane is in contact with the blood over an area 30 cm wide by 90 cm long. What is the blood-side priming volume of this device?

REFERENCES

Abel, J. J., Rowntree, L. G., and Turner, B. B., On the removal of diffusible substances from the circulating blood of living animals by dialysis, *J. Pharmacol. Exper. Therap.*, 5, 275 (1914).

Babb, A. L., Grimsrud, L., Bell, R. L., and Layno, S. B., Engineering aspects of artificial kidney systems, *Chemical Engineering in Medicine and Biology*, (D. Hershey, ed.), Plenum, New York, 1967, pp. 289-332.

Colton, C. K., A review of the development and performance of hemodialyzers, Natl. Inst. Arthritis and Metabolic Diseases, N.I.H., U.S.P.H.S., May 1967.

Cooney, D. O., Kim, S. S., and Davis, E. J., Analyses of mass transfer in hemodialyzers for laminar blood flow and homogeneous dialysate, *Chem. Eng. Sci.*, 29, 1731 (1974).

Freeman, R. B., Setter, J. G., Maher, J. F., and Schreiner, G. E., Characteristics and comparative efficiencies of coil and parallel flow hemodialyzers, *Trans. Am. Soc. Artif. Intern. Organs* 10, 174 (1964).

Meyer, R., Straffon, R. A., Rees, S. B., Guild, W. R., and Merrill, J. P., A laboratory and clinical evaluation of the Kolff coil kidney, *J. Lab. Clin. Med.*, 51, 715 (1958).

Michaels, A. S., Operating parameters and performance criteria for hemodialyzers and other membrane-separation devices, *Trans. Am. Soc. Artif. Intern. Organs*, 12, 387 (1966).

Spaeth, E. E., Analysis and optimization of an artificial kidney system, Washington Univ. Design Case Study 9, St. Louis, July 1970.

BIBLIOGRAPHY

Leonard, E. F., and Dedrick, R. L., The artificial kidney: Problems and approaches for the chemical engineer, *Chem. Eng. Prog. Symp. Ser.*, 64, No. 84, 15 (1968).

Lipps, B. J., Stewart, R. D., Perkins, H. A., Holmes, G. W., McLain, E. A., Rolfs, M. A., and Oja, P. D., The hollow fiber artificial kidney, *Trans. Am. Soc. Artif. Intern. Organs*, 13, 200 (1967).

Nosé, Y., The artificial kidney, in *Advances in Biomedical Engineering and Medical Physics*, Vol. 4 (S. N. Levine, ed.), Wiley-Interscience, New York, 1971.

Chapter 10

THE HUMAN LUNGS

The primary functions of the human lungs are obviously to supply oxygen to the blood, which in turn transports it to all of the cells of the body for sustaining metabolic processes, and the removal of carbon dioxide, a primary metabolic end product and a key factor in the acid-base balance of the body. Other functions of the lungs (e.g., to strain out and digest small blood clots) could be described but are not relevant to the present discussion. In this chapter we shall review the elements of respiratory physiology and quantitatively characterize the transport of O_2 and CO_2 between the blood and gas phases in the human lungs.

I. STRUCTURE AND GROSS OPERATIONAL FEATURES OF THE RESPIRATORY SYSTEM

Figure 10.1 shows the gross anatomy of the respiratory system. The upper tracts, which warm, humidify, and cleanse the inspired air (larger particles are removed by impaction and by centrifugal action), are not discussed except to note that they constitute most of the "dead space" region of the lungs, a region of about 150 ml volume where no O_2-CO_2 transfer occurs. The actual transfer of gases occurs in the 250 million or so tiny sacs called alveoli which comprise the terminal ends of the whole branched network of flow passages. These sacs, which are about 0.1 mm (100 μm) in diameter, are illustrated in Figure 10.2.

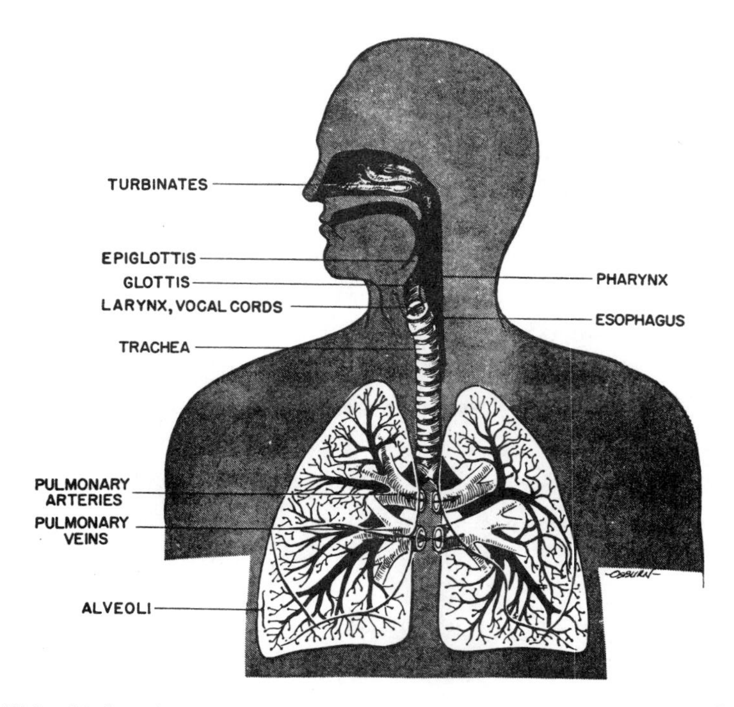

FIG. 10.1. The gross anatomy of the respiratory system. [From Guyton (1971), p. 465.]

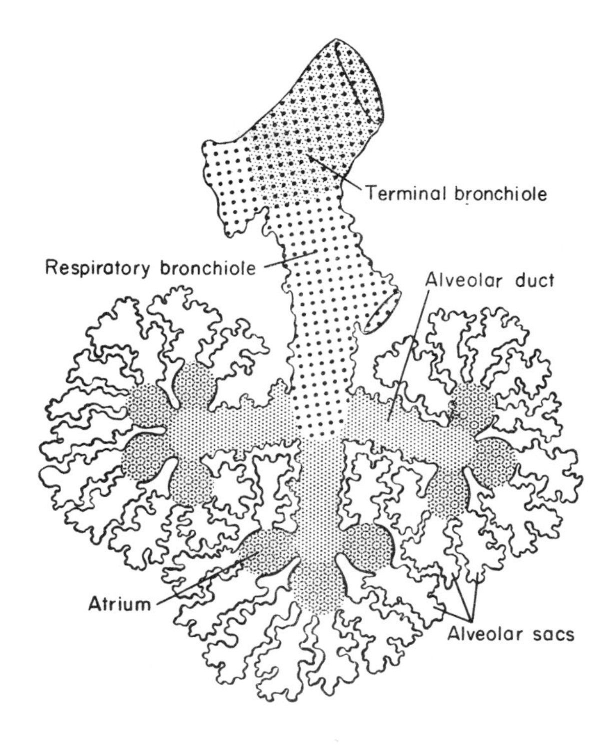

FIG. 10.2. The respiratory lobule. [From Guyton (1971), p.477.]

The microscopic structure of the alveolar region is shown in Figure 10.3. Several layers are seen to exist between the alveolar gas space and the capillary blood. First there are the three layers of the alveolar membrane: a monomolecular layer of surfactants (phospholipids) which reduce the surface tension along the alveolar walls, a thin fluid layer, and a layer of epithelial cells. There is then an intervening space filled with interstitial fluid. Finally, there are two layers comprising the blood capillary walls: a basement membrane and an endothelial cell layer. This whole series of layers separating the alveolar gas space and the blood plasma is collectively called the respiratory membrane and, surprisingly, its overall thickness is only about 0.1-1.0 μm (thickness varies with

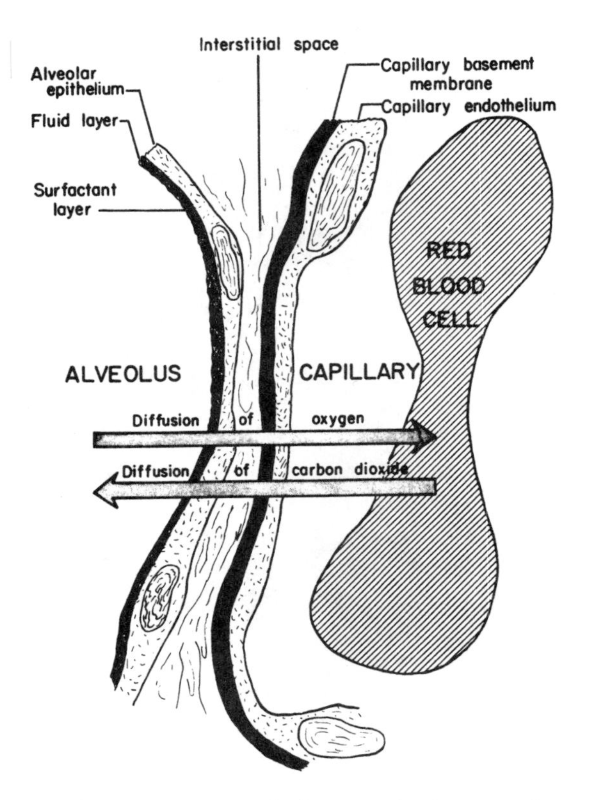

FIG. 10.3. Ultrastructure of the respiratory membrane. [From Guyton (1971), p. 478.]

location). The total surface area of the respiratory membrane is an astonishing 70 m^2 for an average male adult, yet the volume of blood in the lung capillaries at any instant is no more than about 70-100 ml. Lung capillaries average about 7 μm in diameter, and therefore red blood cells are forced to squeeze through. The combination of tremendous blood-side mixing, short diffusion distances, and large membrane area makes the lungs extremely efficient mass transfer devices.

The lungs, under conditions of rest, normally take in and expel 500 ml of air per breath (the tidal volume), varying between roughly 2300 and 2800 ml total gas volume during each cycle. Ordinarily 12 breaths per minute are taken. Therefore, the minute respiratory volume is 6000 ml/min. Since 150 ml of each breath simply moves in and out of the upper dead space region, the alveolar ventilation rate is (12)(500 - 150) = 4200 ml/min. This is the gas from which O_2 is extracted and into which CO_2 is rejected. Under conditions of maximum effort or forced inspiration and expiration lung gas volumes can be varied over a much wider range, from 1200 to 5800 ml (a difference of 4600 ml, or more than nine times normal). Various appellations have been given to these volumes and capacities, as Figure 10.4 indicates.

Gas compositions in the respiratory system for resting conditions are quoted in Table 10.1. Here it is shown how humidification of fairly dry ambient air to a water partial pressure level of 47 mm Hg (value at 37°C) has the effect of diluting the concentra-

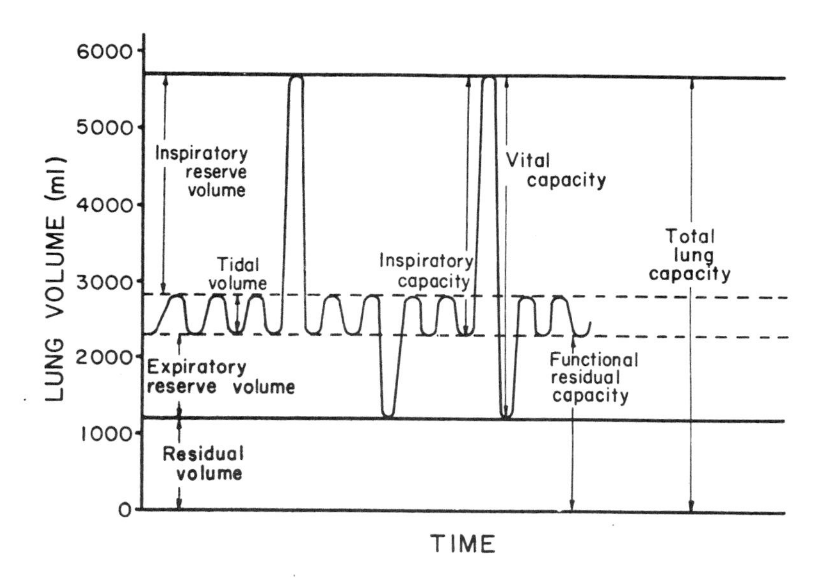

FIG. 10.4. Diagram showing respiratory excursions during normal breathing and during maximal inspiration and maximal expiration. [From Guyton (1971), p. 460.]

TABLE 10.1

Partial Pressures of Respiratory Gases as They Enter and Leave the Lungs (at Sea Level)—Percent Concentrations Are Given in Parentheses[a]

	Atmospheric air[b] (mm Hg)		Humidified air (mm Hg)		Alveolar air (mm Hg)		Expired air (mm Hg)	
N_2	597.0	(78.62%)	563.4	(74.09%)	569.0	(74.9%)	566.0	(74.5%)
O_2	159.0	(20.84%)	149.3	(19.67%)	104.0	(13.6%)	120.0	(15.7%)
CO_2	0.3	(0.04%)	0.3	(0.04%)	40.0	(5.3%)	27.0	(3.6%)
H_2O	3.7	(0.50%)	47.0	(6.20%)	47.0	(6.2%)	47.0	(6.2%)
Total	760.0	(100.0%)	760.0	(100.0%)	760.0	(100.0%)	760.0	(100.0%)

[a] From Guyton (1971), p. 474.

[b] On an average cool, clear day.

tions of the other components. Note that the time-averaged O_2 and CO_2 concentrations in the alveoli are 104 and 40 mm Hg, respectively, versus 149 and 0.3 mm Hg in the humidified air. Also, it is apparent that mixing 150 ml of dead space air with 350 ml of alveolar air results in an expired air having lower CO_2 and higher O_2 concentrations than the alveolar air itself.

Of course the composition of alveolar air (and expired air) will depend on the balance between the rates at which O_2 and CO_2 are being carried in and out by breathing and the rates at which O_2 and CO_2 are consumed and generated by metabolism. Figures 10.5 and 10.6 relate the partial pressures of alveolar O_2 and CO_2 to alveolar ventilation rate and metabolic reaction rates (normal resting O_2 consumption and CO_2 production rates are 250 and 200 ml/min, respectively). Since higher ventilation rates and higher metabolic rates usually occur together, one can deduce that on

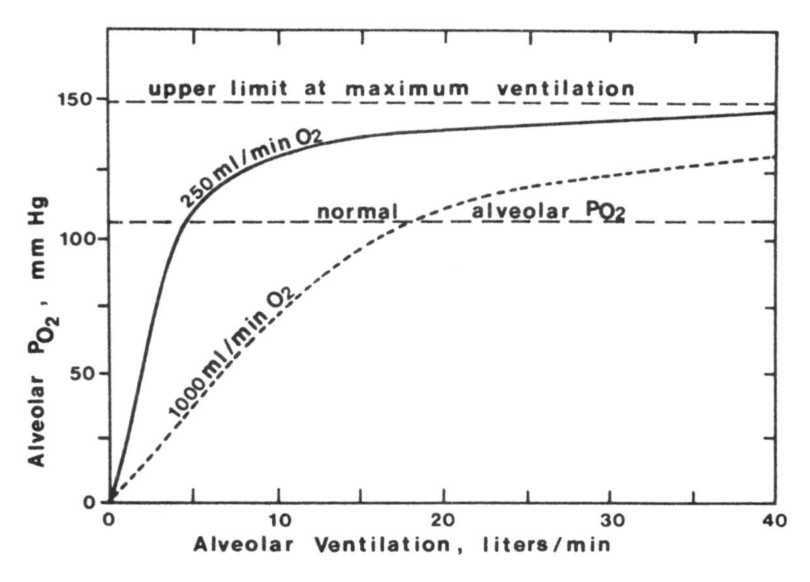

FIG. 10.5. Effect of alveolar ventilation and rate of oxygen absorption from the alveoli on the alveolar P_{O_2}. [From Guyton (1971), p. 476.]

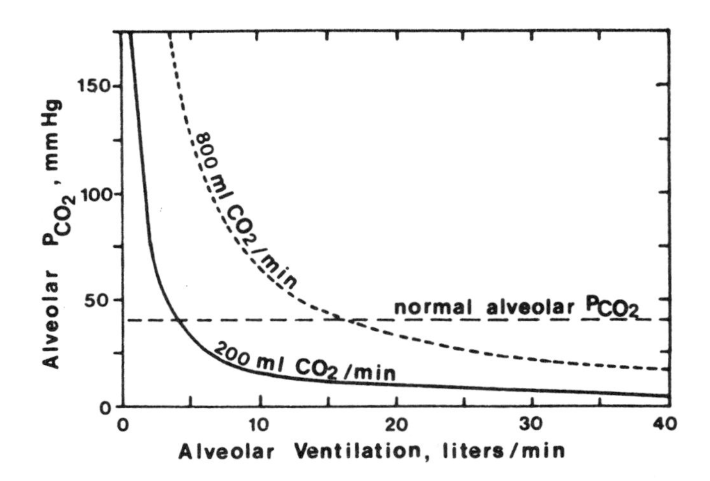

FIG. 10.6. Effect on alveolar P_{CO_2} of alveolar ventilation and rate of carbon dioxide excretion from the blood. [From Guyton (1971), p. 476.]

balance O_2 and CO_2 partial pressures in the alveoli will stay nearly constant over a wide range of conditions.

II. SIMPLE MASS BALANCES ON THE LUNGS

Elementary mass balances can be used to verify some of the composition data presented in Table 10.1 and to compute total consumptions or losses of O_2, CO_2, and H_2O via the lungs (say, in grams per day). Let us assume that the ambient air has the composition shown in Table 10.1. Further, assume the tidal volume is 500 ml per breath, referred to 37°C and 1 atm (BTP, body temperature and pressure); the O_2 metabolic consumption rate is 250 ml/min at STP, or 284 ml/min at BTP; the CO_2 rejection rate is 200 ml/min at STP, or 227 ml/min at BTP; and the number of breaths per minute is 12.

On a per-breath basis the inspired air will contain 393.1 ml N_2, 104.2 ml O_2, 0.2 ml CO_2, and 2.5 ml H_2O. The expired air will contain 393.1 ml N_2 (no N_2 transfer occurs), 104.2 - (284/12) = 104.2 - 23.6 = 80.6 ml O_2, and 0.2 + (227/12) = 0.2 + 18.9 = 19.1 ml CO_2. The total milliliters of dry gas in the expired breath will be 393.1 + 80.6 + 19.1 = 492.8. If we assume the expired air to be fully saturated with water vapor (partial pressure of water at 37°C is 47 mm Hg), then the ratio of water vapor to dry gas in the expired air must be 47/(760 - 47). Thus, the expired air will contain 492.8(47/713) = 32.5 ml water vapor, and the total wet air expired will comprise 492.8 + 32.5 = 525.3 ml. The percentages of the various components in the expired air, as determined by these figures, are N_2 = 74.8%, O_2 = 15.4%, CO_2 = 3.6%, and H_2O = 6.2%. These percentages agree very closely with those given in Table 10.1, indicating our simple calculations are quite valid.

Note that the total volume of air expired exceeds the volume inspired by about 25 ml per breath. These values refer to 1 atm pressure. In the lungs, the actual inspired and expired volumes are equal (they must be if the breathing cycle always returns to the same conditions), and the intrapleural pressure during inspiration is somewhat subatmospheric (by about 10 mm Hg) and is superatmospheric (around 780 mm Hg) during expirations. These pressure variations are, of course, the driving force for air movement. Hence, the actual volumes inspired and expired are identical and are roughly 510 ml per breath.

On a daily basis it is interesting to compute masses lost and gained by the body via respiration. These are easily determined (the reader should check the values given) to be

$$\left.\begin{array}{r}O_2 \text{ gain} = 515 \text{ g/day} \\ CO_2 \text{ loss} = 565 \text{ g/day} \\ H_2O \text{ loss} = 367 \text{ g/day}\end{array}\right\} \quad \begin{array}{l}\text{net loss} = 417 \text{ g/day} \\ \text{(almost a pound!)}\end{array}$$

The water loss is of course strongly dependent on the inspired air humidity. In this case fairly dry air has been assumed (Table 10.1).

As Seagrave (1971) points out, the mass balance analysis can be extended further by taking into account the fact that the expired air actually consists of about 150 ml dead space air, which is humidified but has undergone no O_2 or CO_2 transfer, and about 350 ml of alveolar air. Let us assume that the dead space contains 150 ml worth of inspired air. Breaking this down gives 117.8 ml N_2, 31.3 ml O_2, 0.1 ml CO_2, and 0.8 ml H_2O (total dry gas is 149.2 ml). When this inspired air is fully humidified in the dead space regions, the gas will contain 149.2(47/713) = 9.8 ml water vapor. The total gas volume will then expand to 159.0 ml.

The alveolar gas composition is conveniently determined by simple subtraction of the dead space gas from the overall expired gas quantities, previously computed. Thus, the alveolar gas will therefore contain

$$
\begin{aligned}
N_2 &= 393.1 - 117.8 = 275.3 \text{ ml } (75.1\%) \\
O_2 &= 80.6 - 31.3 = 49.3 \text{ ml } (13.5\%) \\
CO_2 &= 19.1 - 0.1 = 19.0 \text{ ml } (5.2\%) \\
H_2O &= 32.5 - 9.8 = \underline{22.7 \text{ ml}} \ (6.2\%) \\
& \qquad\qquad\qquad 366.3 \text{ ml}
\end{aligned}
$$

The percent composition again agrees extremely well with Table 10.1. Partial pressures of O_2 and CO_2 in the alveolar gas, based on a total time-averaged pressure of 770 mm Hg, are easily calculated to be (49.3/366.3)770 = 104 and (19.0/366.3)770 = 40 mm Hg, respectively. These values are the same as those cited earlier. This shows again that very simple mass balances can be useful in deducing important physiological quantities.

III. GAS TRANSPORT MECHANISMS IN THE LUNGS

The limiting resistance to the transport of O_2 and CO_2 (and other gases such as N_2 and CO, if concentration gradients for these should be created) resides in the aqueous fluid of the interstitial layer of the respiratory membrane and in the blood plasma. All common gases have very high lipid solubilities compared to aqueous solubilities and thus move through the various epithelial and endothelial layers quite easily. Transport of gases can be characterized by the passive transport flux equations presented in Chapter 7, i.e.,

$$N_i - X_i \Sigma N_j = -D_i \frac{dC_i}{dz}$$

where C_i is the molar concentration of i <u>in the respiratory membrane</u>. It is common practice to neglect the bulk flow term since the flux of O_2 in one direction is at least 80% counterbalanced by the flux of CO_2 in the opposite direction. And, since X_i values are much less than unity, the term $X_i \Sigma N_j$ is therefore small relative to N_i. Additionally, it is usually assumed that the concentration gradient is linear ($dC_i/dz = \Delta C/\delta$) and to then replace ΔC_i by $K_{Di}\ \Delta P_i$, where ΔP is a partial pressure difference and K_{Di} is a solubility coefficient. Thus,

$$N_i = -\frac{D_i K_{Di}}{\delta} \Delta P_i$$

Although the blood side is liquid and no partial pressure of a gaseous species really is present on that side, there certainly exists a gas partial pressure that <u>would be in equilibrium</u> with the blood at its prevailing composition. This equilibrium partial pressure is the value used when computing ΔP for transport between alveolar gas and blood.

Since fluid resistances predominate, K_{Di} represents the gas species solubility in aqueous fluid. For reasonably low partial pressures (e.g., 200 mm Hg or less) the gas solubility coefficients (or Henry's law coefficients, since Henry's law is $C_i = K_{Di} P_i$) are constant and concentration independent. For some common gases values at 37°C in units of milliliters of gas per milliliter of fluid per atmosphere of partial pressure are

Gas	K_D
O_2	0.024
CO_2	0.570
CO	0.018
N_2	0.012
He	0.008

The solubility of CO_2 is strikingly high, and is in fact 24 times that of O_2.

The rate of solute transport by diffusion also depends on molecular size, to the extent that D_i values in liquids (as well as in gases) follow Graham's law, i.e., D_i is proportional to $(\text{mol wt})^{-1/2}$. Taking this into account, the gases listed above have D_iK_{Di} product values, and hence transport rates, as shown below (normalized to a figure of 1.0 for O_2):

Gas	DK_D
O_2	1.0
CO_2	20.3
CO	0.81
N_2	0.53
He	0.95

This suggests that CO_2 should transport 20 times faster than O_2 (for the same ΔP driving force) through the respiratory membrane, and experiments have indeed confirmed this.

If one wishes to represent the total amount of gas transported per unit time, one simply multiplies the flux by the mass transfer area A, to obtain

$$W = -\frac{D_iK_{Di}A}{\delta} \Delta P_i = -D_{Li} \Delta P_i$$

The parameters A and δ are very difficult to determine accurately and it is therefore standard practice to lump all of the parameters which multiply ΔP_i into a single quantity called the diffusing capacity, D_{Li}. Because W is usually measured as milliliters per minute, the units of D_L are generally reported as milliliters of i transferred per minute for each millimeter of mercury of partial pressure driving force. Under resting conditions the diffusing capacity of O_2 is about 21 ml/min-mm Hg and that of CO_2 is 400-450 ml/min-mm Hg.

Figures 10.7 and 10.8 show typical curves of blood O_2 content and blood CO_2 content versus distance in a lung capillary, under resting conditions. Note that the concentration of O_2 in blood entering the capillary is equivalent to an O_2 partial pressure of about 40 mm Hg. The inlet ΔP is thus 104-40, or 64. Because the blood leaves essentially in equilibrium with the alveolar gas, the exit ΔP is very close to zero. Although the arithmetic average ΔP is therefore 32, the time-averaged ΔP obtained as follows (blood flow rate assumed constant)

$$\Delta P_{av} = \frac{1}{L}\int_0^L \Delta P \, dx$$

is roughly 12 mm Hg. Here L is the total capillary length. Therefore, the total O_2 transferred would be (21)(12) = 252 ml/min, which agrees with the figure previously quoted. For CO_2, the total transfer rate is about 200 ml/min. Because its D_L value is 400-450 (say 425), the time-averaged ΔP for CO_2 must be approximately 0.47 mm Hg. One must _infer_ this value because physiological measurements accurate enough to confirm it have not been achieved. Figure 10.8 indicates the inlet ΔP for CO_2 is about 5 mm Hg and the outlet $\Delta P \cong 0$, for an arithmetic average of 2.5 mm Hg (more than five times the more meaningful time average). Because of the high aqueous solubility of CO_2 relative to O_2 (and hence high D_L), the partial pressure differences needed to cause CO_2 to transfer are much lower than those needed for O_2 transfer.

Because O_2 and CO_2 transfer is essentially completed in only about a third of the capillary under resting conditions, it is evident that under exercise conditions where the cardiac output may be tripled, a close approach to equilibrium between the outlet

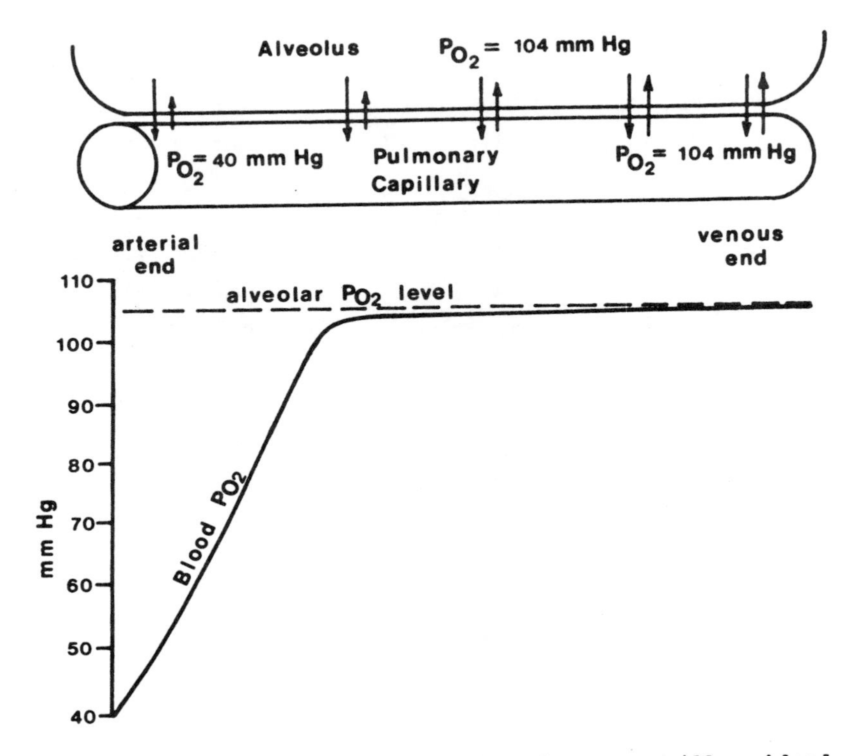

FIG. 10.7. Uptake of oxygen by the pulmonary capillary blood. [From Guyton (1971), p. 482.]

blood and the alveolar gas will still be achieved. Additionally, more capillaries open up under exercise conditions, so good transfer actually exists for cardiac outputs as high as six times the resting value.

IV. OXYGEN TRANSPORT IN THE BLOOD

As suggested by the K_D value quoted above for O_2, the solubility of O_2 in aqueous solutions is rather poor. If transport of O_2 as dissolved gas were the only means for bringing O_2 to cells,

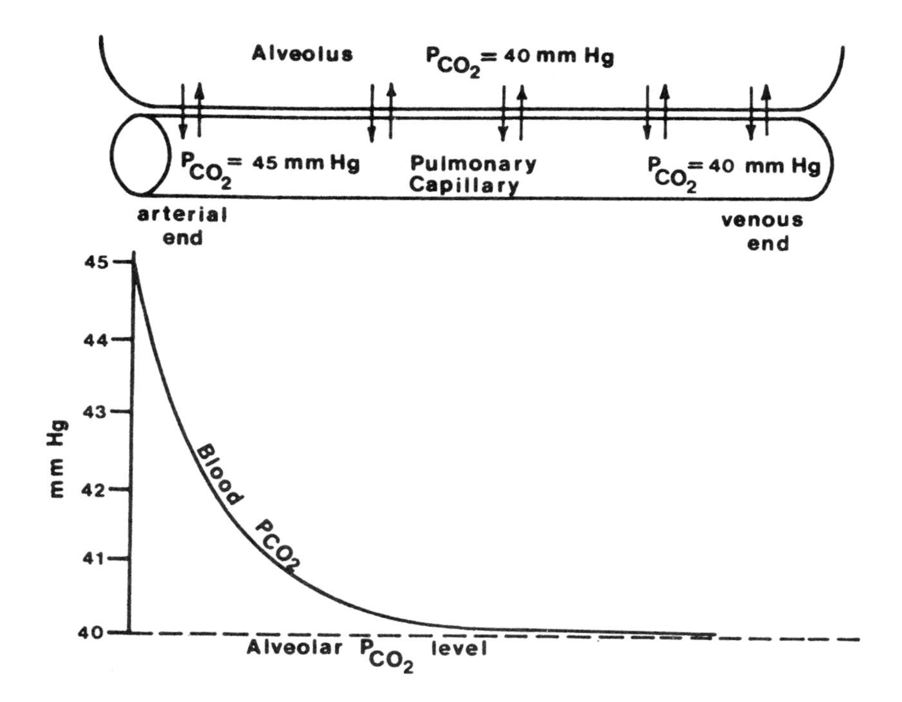

FIG. 10.8. Diffusion of carbon dioxide from the pulmonary blood into the alveolus. [From Guyton (1971), p. 485.]

life would be impossible for all but very small organisms. Fortunately, blood contains large amounts of hemoglobin which can reversibly bind O_2 (and CO_2) in significant quantity. The reactions between hemoglobin and O_2 are properly represented as

$$Hb_4 + O_2 \underset{k_1'}{\overset{k_1}{\rightleftharpoons}} Hb_4O_2$$

$$Hb_4O_2 + O_2 \underset{k_2'}{\overset{k_2}{\rightleftharpoons}} Hb_4(O_2)_2$$

$$Hb_4(O_2)_2 + O_2 \underset{k_3'}{\overset{k_3}{\rightleftharpoons}} Hb_4(O_2)_3$$

$$Hb_4(O_2)_3 + O_2 \underset{k'_4}{\overset{k_4}{\rightleftharpoons}} Hb_4(O_2)_4$$

The hemoglobin molecule contains four heme groups (here represented as Hb), each one of which can bind a molecule of O_2.

For a complex reaction sequence such as this the overall equilibrium relationship expressing the percent saturation of hemoglobin (i.e., amount of O_2 bound to Hb relative to the maximum amount that could be bound) versus O_2 partial pressure can be represented graphically, as shown in Figure 10.9. Note that the equilibrium relation is quite nonlinear and is a function of the amount of CO_2 present and blood pH (however, these are often related). Temperature also affects the equilibrium.

This oxyhemoglobin dissociation curve can be well represented by the so-called Hill equation

$$\psi = \frac{(P/P_0)^n}{1 + (P/P_0)^n}$$

where ψ is the fractional saturation. This is based on modeling the reaction as

$$Hb_n + nO_2 \rightleftharpoons (HbO_2)_n$$

Empirically it has been found that $n \cong 2.7$ and P_0 (the partial pressure for 50% saturation) is about 27.2 mm Hg, for normal blood at 37°C and pH 7.4.

Figure 10.10 compares the amount of O_2 bound to hemoglobin to the amount of O_2 dissolved in blood as a function of partial pressure. Clearly, the dissolved O_2 is minor. Under normal conditions, in fact, only about 1.5% of the O_2 in arterial blood exists as dissolved gas; the other 98.5% is bound to hemoglobin.

The Adair intermediate-compound theory can be used to develop a more theoretically based relation between ψ and P. If one defines equilibrium constants for each of the four reaction steps as $K = k/k'$, then

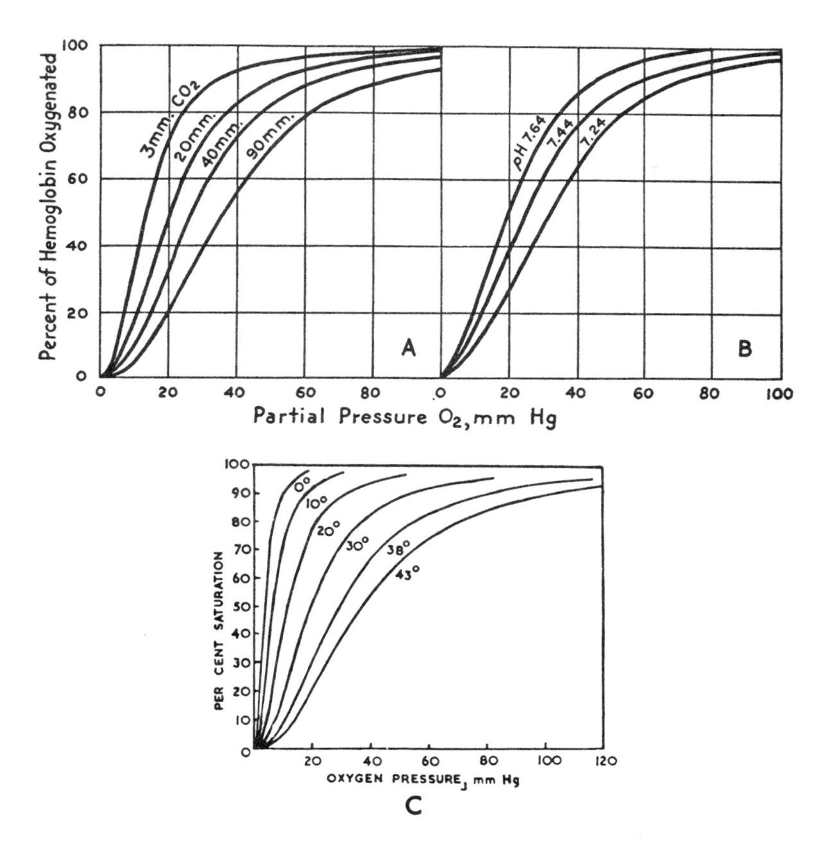

FIG. 10.9. (A) Effect of CO_2 on oxygen dissociation curve of whole blood. (B) Effect of acidity on oxygen dissociation curve of blood. (C) Effect of temperature on oxygen dissociation curve of blood. [From Ruch and Patton (1965), p. 765.]

$$[Hb_4O_2] = K_1P[Hb_4]$$

$$[Hb_4O_4] = K_2P[Hb_4O_2] = K_1K_2P^2[Hb_4]$$

$$[Hb_4O_6] = K_3P[Hb_4O_4] = K_1K_2K_3P^3[Hb_4]$$

$$[Hb_4O_8] = K_4P[Hb_4O_6] = K_1K_2K_3K_4P^4[Hb_4]$$

Now, since the oxygen combined with blood for any arbitrary state equals

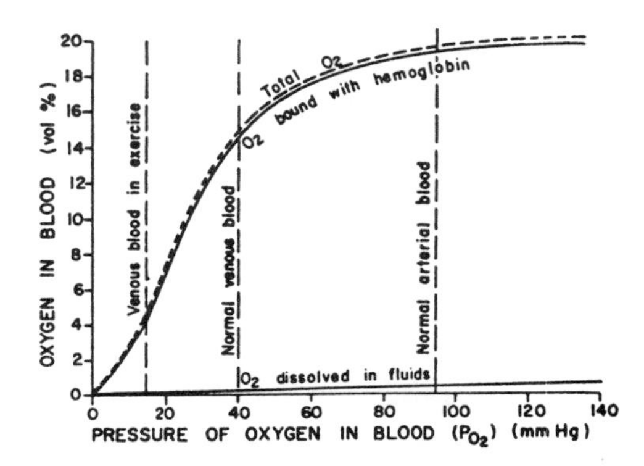

FIG. 10.10. Curves showing the total oxygen in each 100 ml of normal blood, the portion bound to hemoglobin, and the portion dissolved in the water of the blood. [From Guyton (1971), p. 485.]

$$[Hb_4O_2] + 2[Hb_4O_4] + 3[Hb_4O_6] + 4[Hb_4O_8]$$

and the oxygen capacity of blood equals

$$4([Hb_4] + [Hb_4O_2] + [Hb_4O_4] + [Hb_4O_6] + [Hb_4O_8])$$

i.e., four times the moles of iron present in the hemoglobin (concentrations here are in moles per liter), then one can readily show that

$$\psi = \frac{K_1P + 2K_1K_2P^2 + 3K_1K_2K_3P^3 + 4K_1K_2K_3K_4P^4}{4(1 + K_1P + K_1K_2P^2 + K_1K_2K_3P^3 + K_1K_2K_3K_4P^4)}$$

or

$$\psi = \frac{A_1P + 2A_2P^2 + 3A_3P^3 + 4A_4P^4}{4(1 + A_1P + A_2P^2 + A_3P^3 + A_4P^4)}$$

where A_1, A_2, A_3, and A_4 are composite constants. In practice severe problems are encountered in trying to determine these constants. At very low P, this result reduces to

$$\psi \cong \frac{A_1 P}{4}$$

Thus, data obtained at low P can be used to estimate A_1. Likewise, at high P, the equation simplifies to

$$\psi \cong \frac{4A_4 P}{A_3 + 4A_4 P}$$

Data at high oxygen pressures therefore give one the ratio A_4/A_3. Besides these approaches, very little can be done except to find the best statistical fit to the general equation. Roughton (1964) discusses this problem in some detail.

If one assumes that the rate constants for the forward reactions are proportional to the number of uncombined iron atoms (i.e., $k_1:k_2:k_3 = 4:3:2$) and by similar reasoning that $k_1':k_2':k_3' = 1:2:3$, then $K_1:K_2:K_3 = 4:(3/2):(2/3)$. The constant k_4 is considered to be very large, since occupation of three iron atoms is presumed to make the fourth iron atom very reactive. Hence, K_4 is also very large. Under these conditions, the general Adair equation reduces to

$$\psi = \frac{K_1 P[1 + (K_1 P/4)]^3 + K_1^3 K_4 P^4/4}{4[1 + (K_1 P/4)]^4 + K_1^3 K_4 P^4/4}$$

This turns out to fit much available data quite well, e.g., for dilute sheep blood it is accurate to within 1.5% in ψ if K_1 is set at 0.32 mm Hg^{-1} and K_4 at 8.8 mm Hg^{-1}. More detailed work on sheep blood at pH 9.1 has indicated that k_4' is very small compared to k_1', k_2', and k_3'; i.e., the dissociation of $Hb_4(O_2)_4$ strongly controls the overall reverse reaction sequence. In addition, k_1 and k_4 have been estimated and it appears that $k_1:k_4$ is about 1:3. These data _do_ support the idea that K_4 is large—but not because k_4 is huge (as assumed above), but rather because k_4' is small. Much experimental work is needed before additional conclusions can be stated with any confidence.

V. CARBON DIOXIDE TRANSPORT IN THE BLOOD

CO_2 is also bound reversibly to hemoglobin, at different sites than those where O_2 is bound, and therefore is transported by this means. Since CO_2 has a good solubility in aqueous solutions, a fair amount also is carried as dissolved gas. However, the major share of CO_2 is not transported in either of these forms but in the form of bicarbonate ions, which are generated by the reaction

$$CO_2 + H_2O \rightleftharpoons H_2CO_3 \rightleftharpoons HCO_3^- + H^+$$

The formation of the intermediate carbonic acid occurs very slowly unless catalyzed by the enzyme carbonic anhydrase, an enzyme found in red blood cells but not in plasma. Thus, as depicted in Figure 10.11, CO_2 must first diffuse into a red blood cell and then react. The equilibrium and rate constants for the second step strongly favor rapid and extensive dissociation, so that 99.9% of the H_2CO_3 splits almost instantaneously into bicarbonate ion and H^+ (which then tends to bind with hemoglobin). Overall, about 7% of CO_2 is transported as dissolved gas, about 63% transports as HCO_3^-, and essentially all of the remainder (30%) is carried as $HbCO_2$. One can represent the total amount of CO_2 present in all of these forms in blood as a function of CO_2 partial pressure, as shown in Figure 10.12. This carbon dioxide dissociation curve is different from the HbO_2 dissociation curve in the lack of a sigmoid shape at low partial pressures and the absence of an asymptote at high partial pressures.

Table 10.2 lists the gas contents of arterial and venous blood under resting conditions. Note that venous blood enters the lungs with 75% of the hemoglobin saturated with O_2 and leaves 97% satu-

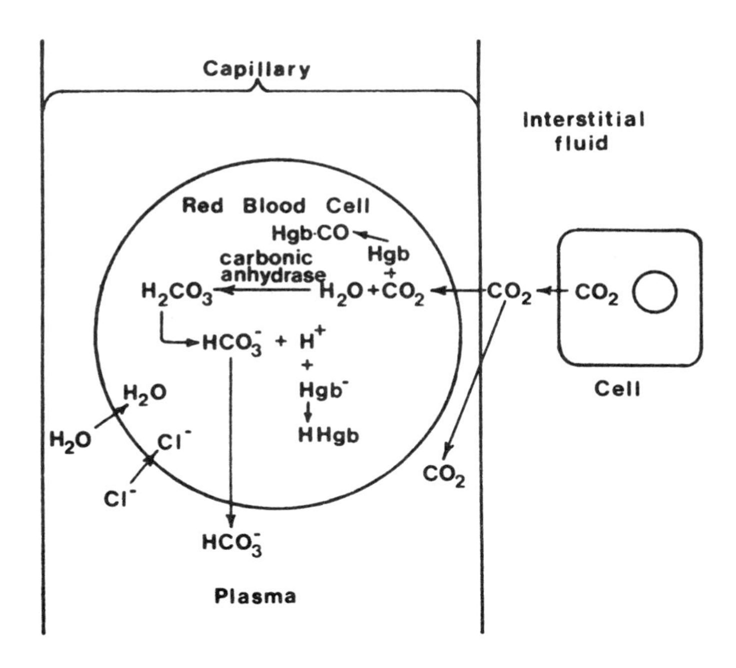

FIG. 10.11. Transport of carbon dioxide in the blood. [From Guyton (1971), p. 491.]

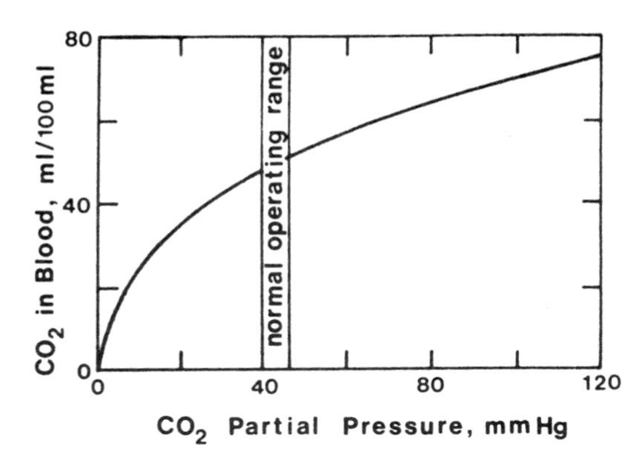

FIG. 10.12. The carbon dioxide dissociation curve. [From Guyton (1971), p. 491.]

TABLE 10.2

Gas Content of Blood

	ml/100 ml of blood containing 15 g hemoglobin			
	Arterial blood[a]		Venous blood[b]	
Gas	Dissolved	Combined	Dissolved	Combined
O_2	0.3	19.2	0.1	14.4
CO_2	2.6	46.6	2.9	50.3
N_2	1.04	0	1.04	0

[a] P_{O_2} 95 mm Hg; P_{CO_2} 40 mm Hg; Hb 97% saturated.

[b] P_{O_2} 40 mm Hg; P_{CO_2} 46 mm Hg; Hb 75% saturated.

rated (because of the shape of the HbO_2 dissociation curve the percentage of change in P_{O_2} is much greater). CO_2 contents are considerably higher than O_2 contents, and vary much less from the arterial to venous side. Finally, the minor contributions of dissolved O_2 and CO_2 are apparent. (It is interesting to note that the O_2 content of arterial blood is, on the basis of milliliters of gas per milliliter of blood, essentially the same as the O_2 concentration in air—about 20 ml O_2/ml fluid.)

VI. OXYGEN AND CARBON DIOXIDE TRANSFER FROM TISSUES

It should be pointed out briefly that what occurs in the tissue capillaries (e.g., liver, brain, muscle, etc.) is basically the reverse of what occurs in the lung capillaries, and that profiles of blood O_2 and CO_2 versus distance have the same general shapes as those shown in Figures 10.7 and 10.8 (except that one must, of course, relabel the ordinate scales appropriately).

We are not concerned here with modeling capillary-tissue transport, and therefore will only summarize figures indicating the sizes of the partial pressures in a typical tissue region:

Arterial blood: P_{O_2} = 95 mm Hg, P_{CO_2} = 40 mm Hg

Venous blood: P_{O_2} = 40 mm Hg, P_{CO_2} = 45 mm Hg

Interstitial fluid: P_{O_2} = 40 mm Hg, P_{CO_2} = 45 mm Hg

Intracellular fluid: P_{O_2} = 6 mm Hg, P_{CO_2} = 46 mm Hg

The ΔP for transport of O_2 out of the cells is seen to be 40-6 or 34 mm Hg, versus a ΔP of about 1 mm Hg for CO_2. Again, the inherently larger transport rate for CO_2 as compared to O_2 is evident. Note that the venous blood leaves in equilibrium with the interstitial fluid, as one would expect. Finally, one might wonder why the arterial blood P_{O_2} is only 95 mm Hg, since a figure of 104 mm Hg was given earlier for the P_{O_2} of blood leaving the pulmonary capillaries. This comes about because some venous blood flows through pulmonary shunts which bypass the lungs. Upon mixing this shunted blood with blood at P_{O_2} = 104, the end result is blood at P_{O_2} = 95 mm Hg. Although the amount of shunted blood is small (1 or 2% of the total) and although it has little effect on the total quantity of O_2 carried by the blood, the flat nature of the oxyhemoglobin dissociation curve at high P_{O_2} values causes it to have a significant effect on the blood's P_{O_2}.

VII. MASS TRANSFER RESISTANCES IN THE RESPIRATORY SYSTEM

The preceding discussion characterized mass transfer in the lungs in terms of a single parameter, the diffusing capacity D_L. It should be pointed out that this single coefficient really accounts for the overall operation of a whole series of mass transfer steps. Transport of a gas species from the alveolar region to the interior of a red blood cell involves (see Figure 10.13) diffusion or transport through:

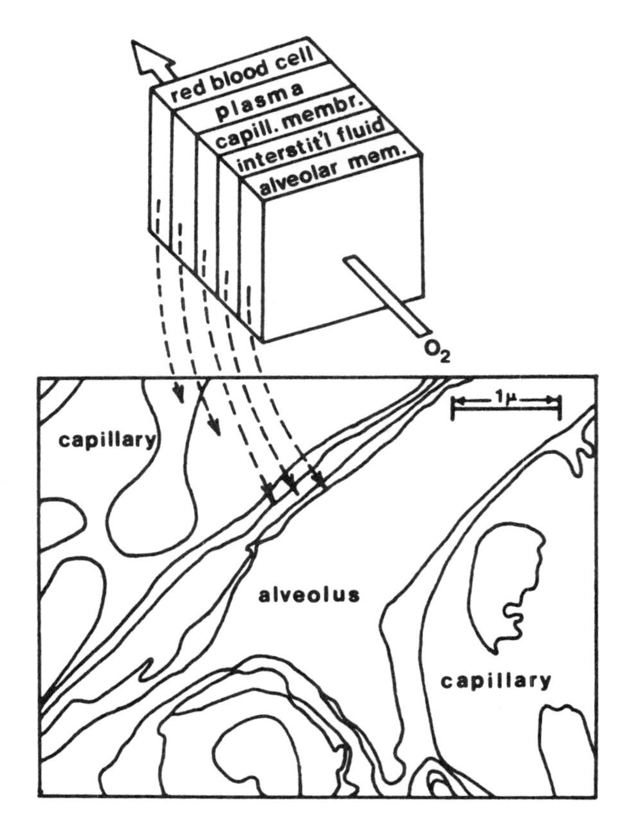

FIG. 10.13. Anatomy of alveoli and capillaries.

1. the alveolar gas phase (or, equivalently, through a stagnant gas film next to the alveolar membrane)

2. the alveolar membrane

3. the interstitial fluid

4. the capillary wall

5. the blood plasma (note that the thickness of this region depends on how close the red cell is to the capillary wall)

6. the red blood cell membrane

7. the interior of the red blood cell (concentrated Hb solution)

followed by an eighth step, chemical reaction with hemoglobin (for some species no reaction occurs).

Simple computations can be done to prove that, for normal physiological states, the diffusional resistance in the alveolar gas phase is extremely small, so that the gas composition is essentially uniform everywhere (including the region adjacent to the alveolar membrane). It is common practice to lump items 2, 3, and 4 together, as "diffusion through the respiratory membrane." As previously stated, however, the interstitial fluid transport resistance is by far the most important one of the three. Experimental evidence suggests that the other items (5-8) are all important enough so that none can be neglected. However, it is nearly impossible to perform measurements that can isolate the effects of any single transport resistance, and so the precise importance of these various steps is an unsolved question at present.

Let us consider the transport of oxygen as an example. Assuming steady-state conditions we may characterize the O_2 transport (W^*, moles/min-cc) through the respiratory membrane as

$$W^* = -D_M \frac{\Delta P_M}{\delta_M} K_D A_M$$

W^* can be conveniently defined on the basis of moles per minute <u>per unit volume of capillary blood</u>, for instance (other bases could be used if desired). Here we have assumed (a) that bulk flow can be neglected (or at least accounted for by the effective diffusion coefficient), (b) that dP/dz can be represented by $\Delta P_M/\delta_M$ (i.e., a linear P versus z profile exists across the membrane), and (c) that Henry's law, $C = K_D P$, characterizes the solubility of O_2 in the respiratory membrane. Now, it is also usual to assume that δ_M is the total respiratory membrane thickness, even though only the central interstitial fluid layer controls diffusion (it is very difficult to measure any thickness with accuracy), and to consider K_D as being the solubility in aqueous solution (again, since the interstitial fluid controls) rather than an average solubility for the whole membrane. All errors involved with the assumptions are "absorbed" into D_M, the effective diffusivity, which is determined by establishing values for all of the other quantities in the equation. ΔP_M is the O_2 partial pressure difference across the membrane only, and A_M is an effective membrane area per unit volume of capillary blood.

At steady-state it must also be true that

$$W^* = -D_B \frac{\Delta P_B}{\delta_B} K_D A_B$$

where ΔP_B is the P_{O_2} difference across a blood plasma gap having an effective thickness of δ_B, and K_D is the solubility of O_2 in plasma (note that the cells are excluded). Experimental measurements have confirmed that the K_D value here, in plasma, is essentially the same as that in the respiratory membrane. A_B is again an effective transport area, not necessarily equal to A_M. D_B is some effective diffusivity which accounts for the transport resistances of the stagnant film next to the respiratory membrane, the bulk of the plasma, and the stagnant film adjacent to the red blood cell membrane.

For the red blood cell membrane we may write

$$W^* = -D_{CM} \frac{\Delta P_{CM}}{\delta_{CM}} K_{D_{CM}} A_{CM}$$

where the subscript CM stands for cell membrane. A_{CM} is the area of the red cell membranes per unit blood volume. Likewise, for the red cell interior we can set down the expression

$$W^* = -D_{CI} \frac{\Delta P_{CI}}{\delta_{CI}} \alpha_{CI} A_{CI}$$

where CI means cell interior. ΔP_{CI} is the difference between the partial pressures just inside the red blood cell membrane and at the site at which the reaction $Hb + O_2 \rightleftharpoons HbO_2$ is occurring. δ_{CI} is the effective diffusion path length between the cell membrane and the reaction site. Note that δ_{CI} is therefore really a function of time, or of the extent of reaction (however, we shall ignore this dependence). A_{CI} is some effective area for transport (difficult to define for something having the shape of a red blood cell). The item α_{CI} represents the solubility of O_2 in the cell interior, which is roughly a 35 wt% hemoglobin solution, and D_{CI} is the oxygen diffusivity in the cell interior. Note that facilitated transport of O_2, in the form of HbO_2, has been neglected here. It is assumed (although not yet proved) that HbO_2 diffuses too slowly to aid O_2 transport significantly.

The chemical reaction of O_2 can be modeled using the rate law

$$W^* = kP_{RS}(Hb) - k'(HbO_2)$$

where k and k' are rate constants, (Hb) and (HbO_2) are concentrations, and P_{RS} is the oxygen partial pressure <u>at</u> the reaction site. This equation simply says that at steady state oxygen reacts and disappears at the same rate at which it is conveyed to the reaction sites. It may also be written in the form $W^* = k(Hb)[P_{RS} - P_{eq}]$

where P_{eq} is the value of P_{RS} which _would be_ in equilibrium with the prevailing HbO_2 concentration, _if_ equilibrium existed. P_{eq} is given by

$$P_{eq} = \frac{k'(HbO_2)}{k(Hb)}$$

As discussed earlier with respect to heat transport through a series of resistances, one may characterize transport using any of these equations _alone_ or in _combination_—it all depends on which ΔP is desired. For example, if one _knows_ the P_{O_2} in the alveoli and the P_{O_2} in the plasma, one would want to write

$$\Delta P_M = -\frac{\delta_M W^*}{D_M K_D A_M}$$

$$\Delta P_B = -\frac{\delta_B W^*}{D_B K_D A_B}$$

and, since $\Delta P_{MB} = P_{alv} - P_{plasma} = \Delta P_M + \Delta P_B$,

$$W^* = -\left(\frac{\delta_M}{D_M K_D A_M} + \frac{\delta_B}{D_B K_D A_B}\right)^{-1} \Delta P_{MB}$$

Clearly, one could extend this idea to writing the expression for W^* in terms of the _whole_ P_{O_2} difference between the alveoli and that corresponding to equilibrium with the prevailing HbO_2, i.e., $\Delta P_{tot} = P_{alv} - P_{eq}$:

$$W^* = -\left[\frac{\delta_M}{D_M K_D A_M} + \frac{\delta_B}{D_B K_D A_B} + \frac{\delta_{CM}}{D_{CM} K_{D_{CM}} A_{CM}} + \frac{\delta_{CI}}{D_{CI} \alpha_{CI} A_{CI}} + \frac{1}{k(Hb)}\right]^{-1} \Delta P_{tot}$$

In practice, nearly all of the parameters defined in this analysis are either difficult or impossible to measure, and models of this complexity are of no utility. Forster (1964a) has, however, made extensive application of a gross two-resistance model expressed by the relationships

$$\frac{W}{-\Delta P} = \frac{\text{ml species i}}{\text{min-mm Hg}} = D_L = \text{diffusing capacity of i}$$

$$\frac{1}{D_L} = \frac{1}{D'_M} + \frac{1}{\theta V_C}$$

where $-\Delta P$ is the alveolar partial pressure of the species less that corresponding to the reacted state such as HbO_2, $HbCO_2$, HbCO, etc. That is, the reacted state partial pressure of, say, O_2 would be the P_{O_2} that would be in equilibrium with the prevailing HbO_2 concentration, if equilibrium were to exist. D_L is the overall diffusing capacity or conductance described earlier, and it is assumed, when written as a resistance $(1/D_L)$, to be composed of a membrane resistance $1/D'_M$ and a red blood cell resistance $1/(\theta V_c)$.

D'_M, the membrane diffusing capacity, characterizes transport through the respiratory membrane and through the blood plasma (its name is misleading in that the plasma region appears not to be included in the D'_M term). θV_c represents the diffusing capacity or rate of species uptake of all of the red blood cells in the capillaries at any time, θ being the rate of uptake in ml i/min-mm Hg-cc blood and V_c being the cubic centimeters of blood in the capillaries. The quantity $1/(\theta V_c)$ represents the transport resistance of the red cell membrane, the internal hemoglobin solution, and the chemical reaction.

VIII. MEASUREMENT OF θV_c

For species that do react with hemoglobin (CO, CO_2, O_2), the rate of diffusional and reactional uptake of the species by red blood cells can be measured conveniently in the rapid-reaction apparatus developed by Hartridge and Roughton (1923), shown in Figure 10.14.

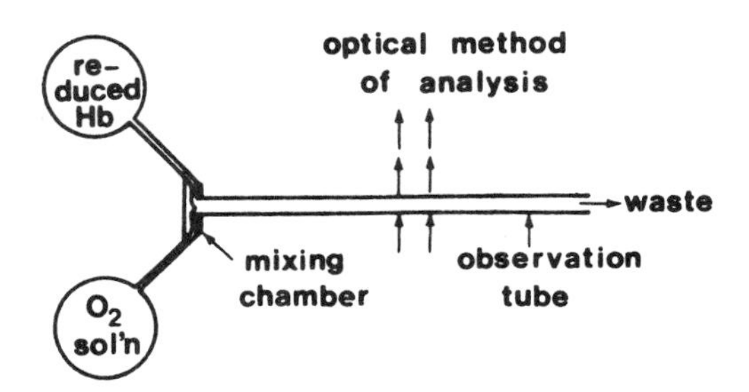

FIG. 10.14. The Hartridge-Roughton method for measuring the velocity of rapid chemical reactions, for the particular case of the reaction $Hb + O_2 \rightarrow HbO_2$. [From Roughton (1964).]

A suspension of red blood cells is mixed rapidly (in less than ∿0.001 sec) with a buffered solution of, say, oxygen, and the mixture then passes down an observation tube. At various points in the tube HbO_2 concentrations are monitored by colorimetry, or by other techniques. From the flow rate, the time of travel to any point is easily calculated. One thus obtains a record of HbO_2 concentration versus time. Because no respiratory membrane exists here, and because the plasma mixing is intense, causing the plasma mass transfer resistance to be very small, $D_L \cong \theta V_c$ for this apparatus.

Figure 10.15 shows data for θ versus HbO_2 concentration for CO and O_2. At high HbO_2 concentrations, the amount of unreacted Hb present falls off sharply, causing the θ values also to decrease sharply. Note that the uptake rates for O_2 are nearly three times as large as those for CO.

The same apparatus has been used to study the rates of reactions of various gases with Hb in free solution, i.e., without a red cell membrane barrier. Table 10.3 gives typical results, which show that reaction rates are generally higher when free Hb is employed (however, if the reaction is slow enough, there ceases to be much difference). Clearly, the data indicate that diffusion through the red blood cell membrane and through the red blood cell interior offers a significant mass transfer resistance. Detailed models for the diffusion and reaction of a gas in the red cell membrane and interior have been developed. In the following section, some of them are discussed.

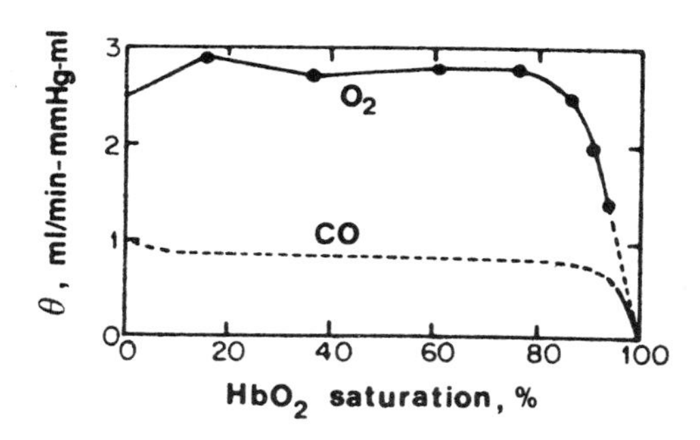

FIG. 10.15. Rate of uptake of O_2 and CO at 37°C by normal human blood, as a function of HbO_2 saturation. [From Forster (1964b).]

IX. THEORETICAL MODELS FOR OXYGEN UPTAKE BY RED BLOOD CELLS

Nicholson and Roughton (1951) have successfully modeled the initial stages of O_2 uptake by red blood cells by starting with a flat layer model of a cell, as depicted in Figure 10.16. Because a red blood cell is much larger in diameter than in thickness, such a representation, which neglects gas transfer through the ends and which also neglects the curvature of the cell's surfaces (b_1 is some effective thickness), turns out to be surprisingly good.

The equations describing O_2 transport through the membrane and the simultaneous diffusion and reaction processes in the cell interior are

$$\text{Membrane:} \quad \frac{\partial c'}{\partial t} = D_2 \frac{\partial^2 c'}{\partial x^2}$$

$$\text{Cell interior:} \quad \frac{\partial c}{\partial t} = D_1 \frac{\partial^2 c}{\partial x^2} + k'(y_0 - y) - kcy$$

$$\frac{\partial y}{\partial t} = D_{Hb} \frac{\partial^2 y}{\partial x^2} + k'(y_0 - y) - kcy$$

TABLE 10.3

Rates of Reactions of Hemoglobin in Solution and in Red Cell Suspension (at pH ∿ 7.2)[a]

Process	Species	Temperature (°C)	Half-time (sec)		Ratio
			Solution	Cell suspension	
I. $Hb + O_2 \rightarrow HbO_2$	Sheep	15	0.004	0.050	1:12.5
Initial (O_2) 1.5 ×		37	0.004	0.050	1:12.5
10^{-4}M (equivalent to an oxygen gas pressure of 75 mm Hg)	Man	37	0.002	0.071	1:36
II. $Hb + CO \rightarrow HbCO$	Sheep	15	0.033	0.072	1:2.2
Initial (CO) 1.5 ×		37	0.007		
10^{-4}M	Man	15	0.040		
		37	0.013	0.084	1:6.5
III. $HbO_2 \rightarrow Hb + O_2$	Sheep	15	0.035	0.16	1:4.5
		37	0.004	0.03	1:7.5
	Man	15	0.026	0.20	1:7.7
		37	0.004	0.038	1:9.5

IV. $Hb_4(CO)_4 \rightarrow$	Sheep	15	60	60	1:1
$Hb_4(CO)_3 + CO$		37	3.4		
followed by	Man	37	8.2	8.2	1:1
$O_2 + Hb_4(CO)_3 \rightarrow$					
$Hb_4(CO)_3O_2$					
or					
$NO + Hb_4(CO)_3 \rightarrow$					
$Hb_4(CO)_3NO$					
V. $HbO_2 + CO \rightarrow$	Sheep	15	0.37		
$HbCO + O_2$	Man	37	0.047	0.10	1:2.1

[a]Hemoglobin concentrations 0.01-0.4 g/100 ml. Red cell suspensions—whole blood diluted 1/40 to 1/100 in 1% NaCl solution or Ringer-Tyrode solution. [From Roughton (1964).]

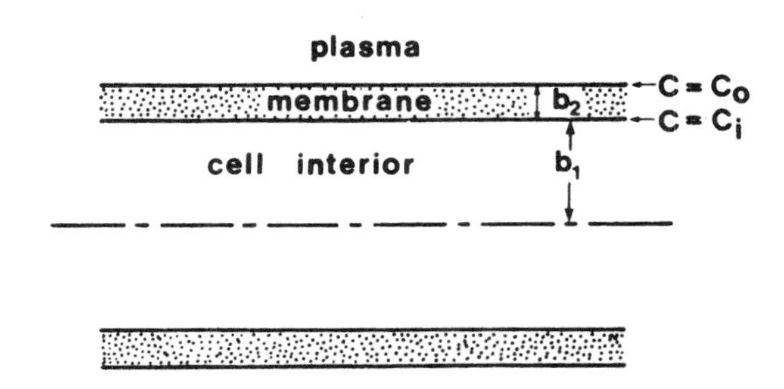

FIG. 10.16. Planar model of red cell, for modeling diffusion and reaction. [From Middleman (1972), p. 59.]

where c and c' are O_2 concentrations in the cell and membrane, respectively; y is the hemoglobin concentration in the cell (the membrane is assumed to be devoid of hemoglobin); y_0 is the initial concentration of hemoglobin (so that $y_o - y$ represents the concentration of oxyhemoglobin at any instant); and k and k' are forward and reverse reaction rate constants for the reaction $O_2 + Hb \rightleftharpoons HbO_2$.

Extensive calculations have revealed that during the gas uptake period, gas diffuses into the membrane and cell very quickly until a quasi-steady-state condition is established, in which the O_2 supplied to any local region by diffusion is exactly balanced by the O_2 loss from the region by chemical reaction. In this quasi-steady-state situation the terms $\partial c/\partial t$ and $\partial c'/\partial t$ are essentially zero. What is striking about this process is that the transient period required to reach the quasi-steady-state condition is extremely brief (in general less than 0.001 sec) <u>and</u> during all of this the concentration of hemoglobin has not changed significantly (i.e., $y \cong y_o$). For purposes of modeling the initial uptake of O_2 by blood one can therefore assume that $\partial c/\partial t = \partial c'/\partial t \cong 0$ and one can neglect any effect of the backreaction term $k'(y_o - y)$. With these assumptions, plus the assumption that $D_{Hb} \cong 0$ (since hemoglobin is so large it diffuses very slowly), the equations for the system reduce to

$$D_2 \frac{\partial^2 c'}{\partial x^2} = 0$$

$$D_1 \frac{\partial^2 c}{\partial x^2} = kcy$$

$$\frac{\partial y}{\partial t} = -kcy$$

The equation for the membrane implies that dc'/dx is a constant; i.e., the concentration profile is linear. Therefore, one can show that

$$c' = \frac{(c_o - c_i)(x - b_1)}{b_2} + c_i$$

where c_i is the O_2 concentration _in_ the membrane at the boundary where the membrane and cell interior meet, and c_o is the O_2 concentration _in_ the membrane at the boundary where the membrane and the surrounding fluid (plasma) meet.

The boundary conditions needed for solving the system equations are

1. c and c' = 0 at t = 0 (although any uniform initial concentration can be handled)
2. $y = y_o$ at t = 0 in the cell interior
3. $c' = c_o$ at t = 0 at $x = b_1 + b_2$, as discussed above
4. $\partial c/\partial x = 0$ at x = 0 at all times (symmetry)
5. $c' = \alpha c$ at $x = b_1$ at all times
6. $D_2\, \partial c'/\partial x = \alpha D_1\, \partial c/\partial x$ at $x = b_1$ at all times

The last two conditions take into account the possibility that the solubilities of O_2 in the membrane and in the internal hemoglobin solution may be different, so that they are related by a partition coefficient α, which is not equal to one. Experimental data suggest, however, that $\alpha \cong 1$ and so we shall proceed on this basis (one _could_ carry α along in the analysis with no difficulty).

From the known solution for $c'(x)$, we can rewrite the sixth boundary condition as

$$\frac{\partial c}{\partial x} = \frac{D_2}{D_1 b_2}(c_o - c_i) \quad \text{at } x = b_1, \quad \text{at all times}$$

Now we define the following dimensionless variables

$$\eta = \frac{x}{b_1}$$

$$C = \frac{c}{c_o}$$

$$Y = \frac{y}{y_o}$$

$$\tau = \frac{tD_1}{b_1^2}$$

$$\omega^2 = \frac{y_o k b_1^2}{D_1}$$

$$\gamma = \frac{c_o k b_1^2}{D_1}$$

Our equations for the cell interior, rewritten in terms of these variables, become

$$\frac{\partial^2 C}{\partial \eta^2} = \omega^2 CY, \quad \frac{\partial Y}{\partial \tau} = -\gamma CY$$

and the boundary conditions transform to

$$C = 0 \quad \text{at } \tau = 0 \text{ (all } \eta)$$

$$Y = 1 \quad \text{at } \tau = 0 \ (\eta \leq 1)$$

$$\frac{\partial C}{\partial \eta} = 0 \quad \text{at } \eta = 0 \text{ (all } \tau)$$

$$\frac{\partial C}{\partial \eta} = \lambda(1 - C) \quad \text{at } \eta = 1 \text{ (all } \tau)$$

where $\lambda = (b_1/D_1)/(b_2/D_2)$. It might be mentioned here that for systems in which the membrane resistance is likely to be unimportant, one would use the same equations just presented. However, the last boundary condition would have the form $C = 1$ at $\eta = 1$ (all τ) instead of the one given above (note that $\lambda = \infty$ for such a case, so that C must equal one, if $\partial C/\partial\eta$ is to be finite).

Nicholson and Roughton (1951) have presented the following analytical solution to this problem

$$C = \frac{\cosh \omega\eta}{\cosh \omega + (1/\lambda) \sinh \omega}$$

The rate of O_2 uptake, R_{O_2} (say moles per second), may be written as (note that the flux is in the -x direction)

$$R_{O_2} = +AD_1 \left.\frac{\partial c}{\partial x}\right|_{x=b_1} \quad \text{or} \quad R_{O_2} = \frac{+AD_1 c_o}{b_1} \left.\frac{\partial C}{\partial \eta}\right|_{\eta=1}$$

where A is the area of the interface through which mass transport is occurring. Evaluating $\partial C/\partial\eta$ at $\eta = 1$ from the solution cited above leads to

$$R_{O_2} = \frac{(AD_1 c_o/b_1)\ \omega \tanh \omega}{1 + (1/\lambda) \tanh \omega}$$

Now since 1 mole of hemoglobin disappears for each mole of O_2 that reacts, it is clear that

$$R_{O_2} = -b_1 A \frac{d\bar{y}}{dt} = \frac{-D_1 A y_0}{b_1} \frac{d\bar{Y}}{d\tau}$$

where $\bar{y}$ is the average hemoglobin concentration in the cell interior. It therefore follows that

$$\frac{d\bar{Y}}{d\tau} = - \frac{c_o}{y_o}\ \omega \frac{\tanh \omega}{1 + (1/\lambda) \tanh \omega}$$

Since $c_o/y_0 = \gamma/\omega^2$, we get (let us integrate also, with the condition that $\bar{Y} = 1$ at $\tau = 0$)

$$\bar{Y} = 1 - \frac{\gamma \tanh \omega}{\omega} \frac{1}{1 + (1/\lambda) \tanh \omega} \tau$$

Experimentally, one usually measures the fractional saturation of hemoglobin, Ψ, which can be expressed as $\Psi = 1 - \bar{Y}$. Therefore, the predicted dependence of Ψ on time is

$$\Psi = 1 - \bar{Y} = \frac{\gamma \tanh \omega}{\omega} \frac{1}{1 + (1/\lambda) \tanh \omega} \tau$$

Certain special cases of this result may be identified. When the membrane resistance is very low, the parameter

$$\lambda = \frac{b_1/D_1}{b_2/D_2} = \frac{\text{cell interior diffusion resistance}}{\text{membrane diffusion resistance}}$$

tends to infinity. The factor $1 + (1/\lambda)\tanh \omega$ then becomes unity and

$$\Psi = \frac{\gamma \tanh \omega}{\omega} = \omega \frac{c_o}{y_o} \tanh \omega$$

The data in Table 10.4 indicate that λ can be taken as ∞ (i.e., the membrane resistance neglected) only for reactions that are intrinsically slow. For fast reactions, neglect of the membrane leads to predicted initial uptake rates that are as much as 5.5 times too high, as shown in the table.

The parameter ω, equal to $b_1(y_0 k/D_1)^{1/2}$, may be viewed as representing the ratio of the reaction rate to the intracellular diffusion rate, or, in terms of resistances,

$$\omega = \frac{\text{diffusion resistance inside cell}}{\text{reaction resistance inside cell}}$$

For $\omega = 0$, we have a situation where the chemical reaction rate completely controls O_2 uptake (i.e., diffusion is so fast that it does not slow up the process).

Figure 10.17 shows Ψ versus real time for cases such as $\omega = 0$; ω finite but $\lambda = \infty$; ω and λ both finite. The dashed lines are plots of the solutions presented here. The curved lines are solu-

TABLE 10.4

Comparison of Calculated Initial Rate of Gas Exchange of an Infinite Layer of Hemoglobin Solution and Experimentally Determined Initial Rate of Gas Exchange of Human Red Cell Suspension, at 37°C[a]

Reaction	Initial reaction (%/sec)		Calculated initial rate divided by the experimental initial rate
	Calculated	Experimental	
Hb + NO → HbNO	7150	2640	2.7
Hb + O_2 → HbO_2	5350	970	5.5
HbO_2 → Hb + O_2	2500	1800	1.4
Hb + CO → HbCO	2260	790	2.9
HbO_2 + CO → HbCO + O_2	175	118	1.5
$Hb_4(CO)_4$ → CO + $Hb_4(CO)_3$	6.6	6.6	1

[a]Calculated values obtained assuming $\lambda = \infty$ (zero membrane resistance). Experimental data obtained for a dilute cell suspension in 1% NaCl solution. [From Forster (1964b).]

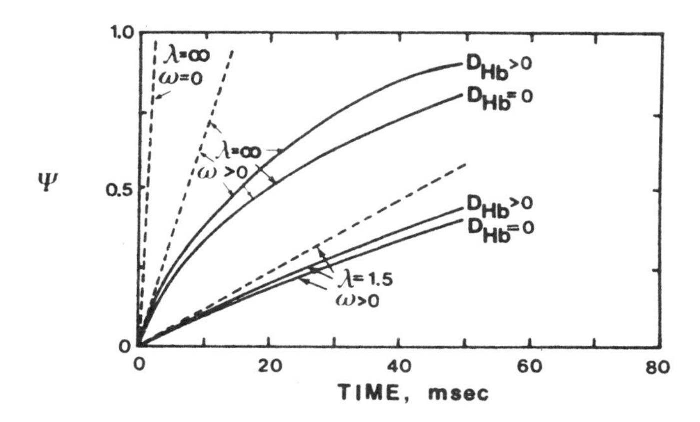

FIG. 10.17. Oxygen uptake by hemoglobin. Note: Case $\omega = 0$, $\lambda = \infty$ corresponds to free hemoglobin in solution; $\omega = 0$ means zero diffusion resistance inside the cell interior; and $\lambda = \infty$ means zero resistance inside the cell membrane. [From Middleman (1972), p. 66.]

tions obtained from the original, general differential equations without the quasi-steady-state assumption and without the neglect of backreaction [see Moll (1968) and Kutchai (1970)]. One can see that these assumptions are good for perhaps only 5-20 msec, depending on conditions. This same figure shows curves obtained from the original differential equations without the assumption that $D_{Hb} \cong 0$. Letting D_{Hb} have its proper value of roughly 4.5×10^{-8} cm²/sec is seen to have a significant effect on O_2 uptake (it enhances the rate of uptake), but only at longer times.

The question now arises as to what parameter values (ω, λ) are required to match experimental data. For O_2 uptake, Forster (1964b) has shown that $\omega \cong 5$ and $\lambda \cong 1.5$ give good agreement between theory and experiment. The fact that $\lambda = 1.5$ indicates a significant membrane resistance. Middleman (1972) summarizes the arguments of other investigators, which suggest that the red blood cell membrane really has negligible resistance. The finding of a membrane resistance is ascribed to the original investigators having worked with cells that were partially dehydrated, through contact with a hyperosmotic medium. This would raise the hemoglobin content of the interior and increase the overall diffusion resistance.

Let us assume for the moment that the value of $\lambda \cong 1.5$ is correct. Since, for O_2, the quantity $D_{CI} \cong 7.6 \times 10^{-6}$ cm^2/sec at 37°C, $\delta_{CM} \cong 100$ Å, and b_1 can be estimated as roughly 0.8 μm (half the average thickness of the biconcave red cell), then

$$D_{CM} \cong (1.5)\, \frac{100 \times 10^{-8}}{0.8 \times 10^{-4}}\, (7.6 \times 10^{-6})$$

$$= 0.14 \times 10^{-6}$$

Therefore, the apparent diffusivity of O_2 (and other gases) through the cell membrane is about 1/50 of the diffusivity in the internal 35 wt% Hb solution. This is a surprisingly low diffusivity and is logically open to question (however, we shall not explore the point further here).

It might also be mentioned in regard to this topic that some additional numerical calculations by Forster (1964b) have indicated that the shape of the red blood cell has only a minor effect on gas uptake; i.e., a flat disc of uniform thickness has essentially the same uptake rate as a biconcave cell having the same volume. Hence, the planar model originally assumed is not a bad approximation.

X. MEASUREMENT OF D_L

If a human subject breathes air containing a small amount of carbon monoxide, for which hemoglobin has a very great affinity, his blood will quickly and nearly irreversibly react with the CO according to the reaction Hb + CO → HbCO. For low alveolar air CO concentrations, and hence low HbCO concentrations, the reverse reaction is negligible and the quantity $P_{eq} \cong 0$. The overall partial pressure difference ΔP_{tot} therefore is equal to P_{alv} (alveolar CO partial pressure) alone. This quantity as well as the total CO uptake in milliliters per minute can be determined by monitoring inspired and expired air CO concentrations during various types of experiments. One therefore can determine D_L directly by dividing the uptake rate in milliliters per minute by the value of P_{alv} in millimeters of mercury. Table 10.5 shows D_L values for CO (plus one value for O_2) for several types of techniques. The most reliable D_L values are those near the bottom.

For O_2 this approach must be altered. The affinity of Hb for O_2 is much less, and therefore the backpressure of the dissociation reaction $HbO_2 \rightarrow Hb + O_2$ along the capillary must be taken into account. That is, $\Delta P_{tot} = P_{alv} - P_{eq}$ will vary because P_{eq} will be significant and of increasing importance along the capillary. If one assumes chemical reaction equilibrium always exists (a reasonable assumption since the reaction $Hb + O_2 \rightleftharpoons HbO_2$ is known to be very fast, both ways), then ΔP will equal $P_{alv} - P_{CI}$ where P_{CI} is the oxygen partial

TABLE 10.5

Values of Diffusing Capacity of Lung Obtained by Various Techniques[a]

Method	Average value in normal subject at rest (ml CO/min-mm Hg)
O_2 steady state	>15
CO steady state physiological dead space	16.9, 23.5
CO steady state end-tidal sample	17.6
CO equilibration	29.2
CO rebreathing	25.3
CO breath holding	27.1

[a]Average alveolar P_{O_2} = 100 mm Hg. Inspired CO < 0.5%. Adult subjects with unspecified body surface area, except for breath-holding measurement, in which surface area was 1.8 m^2.[From Forster (1964a).]

pressure in the interior Hb solution. This quantity is related to HbO_2 concentration by the oxyhemoglobin dissociation curve.

If one assumes that D'_M and θV_c are essentially constant along the capillary, then the rate of uptake will be proportional to $P_{alv} - P_{CI}$. In any differential length of a capillary

$$D_L(P_{alv} - P_{CI}) = Q_B \, dC_{O_2}$$

where Q_B is the blood flow rate in the capillary and dC_{O_2} is the change in the oxygen content of the blood along the differential length (in milliliters of O_2 per milliliter of blood). Hence, for the whole capillary

$$D_L = Q_B \int_a^b \frac{dC_{O_2}}{P_{alv} - P_{CI}}$$

where a is inlet C_{O_2} and b is outlet C_{O_2}. If one assumes that P_{alv} is constant at all locations and if one uses the relation $P_{CI} = f[C_{O_2}]$ given by the oxyhemoglobin dissociation curve, then the equation just displayed can be numerically integrated to give D_L as a function of the inlet and outlet blood C_{O_2} concentrations. These concentrations also allow one to calculate the total O_2 uptake in milliliters per minute. Thus, if one can manage to take arterial and venous blood samples (accounting for the effect of shunted blood) to determine the C_{O_2} values and can estimate P_{alv} for O_2, one can estimate D_{L,O_2}. This is difficult, and the best values obtained to date suggest that D_L is somewhat greater than 15 ml/min-mm Hg for O_2.

XI. DETERMINATION OF D_M'

One way to estimate D_M', the respiratory membrane plus plasma diffusing capacity, is to plot $1/D_L$ versus $1/\theta$, these values having been determined for various alveolar O_2 partial pressures. A plot for CO is shown in Figure 10.18. The intercept equals $1/D_M'$ and the slope is $1/V_c$. Note that $V_c \cong 100$ ml and $D'_{M_{CO}} \cong 60$ ml/min-mm Hg. These values both agree with estimates obtained by other methods.

Table 10.6 summarizes typical values of D_L, D_M', and V_c for CO transport as determined by three different experimental procedures. The bottom set of numbers indicates that $1/D_L = 0.0333$ and $1/D_M' = 0.0175$; hence, $1/(\theta V_c)$ must equal 0.0158 (therefore, $\theta V_c = 63.3$ and $\theta = 63.3/79 = 0.80$). The fraction of the resistance, and therefore of the overall ΔP, which resides in the red blood cell membrane, cell interior, and in the chemical reaction step is therefore

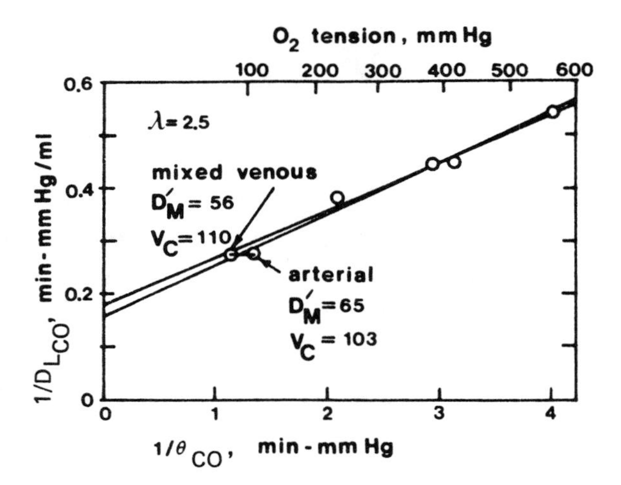

FIG. 10.18. A graph of $1/D_{L_{CO}}$ versus $1/\theta_{CO}$. The value for $D_{L_{CO}}$ at the lowest alveolar O_2 tension is plotted against the value of $1/\theta$ corresponding to the HbO_2 at the beginning (mixed venous) and at the end (arterial) of the capillary, because the correct value must lie in between. [From Forster (1964a).]

TABLE 10.6

Estimations of D_L, D'_M, and V_c in Man at Rest[a]

	$D_{L_{CO}}$[b]	D'_M[b]	V_c (ml)	% Total diffusion resistance in blood
Steady state:				
end-tidal sample	15	26	73	42
Rebreathing method	27	40	110	32
Breath-holding method	30	57	79	48

[a]From Forster (1964a).

[b]In units of ml/min-mm Hg.

0.0158/0.033 = 0.475. That is, nearly half of the mass transfer resistance is associated with the red cells themselves.

For O_2, D'_M may be estimated as

$$D'_{M,O_2} = D'_{M,CO}\left[\frac{28}{32}\right]^{1/2} \frac{0.024}{0.018}$$

$$= 1.24D'_{M,CO}$$

where the factors involved are molecular weight and aqueous solubility ratios. Hence, if D_L for O_2 is, say, 20 and $D'_M = 1.24(57) = 71$, then

$$\frac{1}{\theta V_c} = \frac{1}{20} - \frac{1}{71} = 0.0500 - 0.0141 = 0.0359$$

or $\theta V_c = 28$. Since $V_c \cong 79$, $\theta \cong 0.35$. Figure 10.15 shows that for low HbO_2 saturation, θ is much larger than this. However, for typical capillary conditions where the HbO_2 saturation is high and varies strongly along the capillary, the average θ may indeed be this low. If so, then we can say that about two-thirds or more of the mass transfer resistance to O_2 resides in the red blood cells themselves. It must be emphasized that accurate data on these phenomena are sorely lacking.

XII. MEASUREMENT OF D_L FOR CARBON MONOXIDE BY THE BREATH-HOLDING TECHNIQUE

Several methods exist that will yield experimental estimates of D_L for a gas such as CO, which reacts so fast and strongly with hemoglobin that its partial pressure inside red blood cells can be assumed to be zero (for CO, the inspired air must contain less than ~0.5% CO for this to be true). One simple method, called the breath-holding technique, involves having a subject inspire a large single breath of a gas mixture containing about 0.4% CO and 10% helium.

After holding his breath for any desired time up to about 60 sec, the subject expires forcefully. A sample of the expired gas is taken near the end of the expiration, and this sample is assumed to be part of the alveolar gas (the dead space gas having been expired prior to the time of sampling).

If F_{ACO} is the concentration of carbon monoxide in the expired alveolar gas, in milliliters of CO per milliliter of dry gas, then one can easily derive the rate equation

$$V_A \frac{dF_{ACO}}{dt} = D_{LCO}(P_T - 47)F_{ACO}$$

where the pressure term is the total millimeters of mercury pressure of the alveolar gas minus the partial pressure of water vapor (because the F_{ACO}'s are traditionally expressed on a dry basis), and V_A is the total alveolar volume. This can be integrated to give

$$F_{ACO} = F^0_{ACO} \exp\left[- \frac{D_{LCO}(P_T - 47)t}{V_A}\right]$$

where F^0_{ACO} is the value of F_{ACO} at time zero. This quantity is of course not equal to the concentration in the inspired gas, since the inspired gas becomes diluted with considerable residual lung gas as it is taken in. It can be conveniently determined, however, by using helium, a gas that does not transfer very strongly to the blood or tissues, in the inspired gas. Then, one computes F^0_{ACO} from the inspired gas compositions (F_{ICO}, F_{IHe}) and the measured value of helium in the expired gas sample (F_{AHe}). That is,

$$F^0_{ACO} = F_{ICO} \frac{F_{AHe}}{F_{IHe}}$$

This assumes that CO and He are equally diluted when inspired gas is taken in (this seems reasonable). Alveolar volume must be measured by independent methods, not discussed here.

Since the development given above indicates that

$$\ln \frac{F_{ACO}}{F^0_{ACO}} = -\left[\frac{D_{LCO}(P_T - 47)}{V_A}\right] t$$

plotting data as shown in Figure 10.19 would be expected to yield reasonably linear trends, and indeed this is clearly the case. From the slopes of lines drawn through these data one can calculate D_{LCO} for various kinds of gas mixtures (high O_2, low O_2, etc.), since the slopes equal $-D_{LCO}(P_T - 47)/V_A$. Forster (1964a) gives a very detailed account of this method and discusses in particular some of the practical problems involved in carrying out this procedure, in obtaining values for V_A, and so forth.

XIII. MODELING OXYGEN UPTAKE IN THE PULMONARY CAPILLARIES

The axial O_2 concentration profile in a pulmonary capillary, presented in Figure 10.7, can be determined approximately by the following analytical procedure.

Assume the following values for a normal state of activity:

Average capillary diameter, 7 μm

Number of open lung capillaries, 2.8×10^9

Length of each capillary, 650 μm

Total capillary blood volume in lungs, 70 cc

Blood flow rate to lungs, 6000 cc/min

Oxygen diffusing capacity, 20 ml O_2/min-mm Hg

Alveolar P_{O_2}, 104 mm Hg

Inlet blood P_{O_2}, 40 mm Hg

Since the diffusing capacity is based on the total area for transfer and we will want to make a mass balance on a differential length of

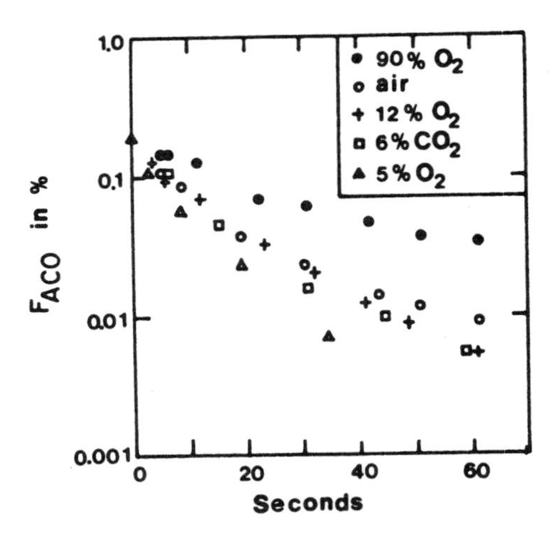

FIG. 10.19. A graph of expired alveolar CO concentration F_{ACO} against time of breath holding in a normal seated subject at various alveolar O_2 and CO_2 concentrations. [From Forster (1964a).]

a capillary containing a differential mass transfer area, we must first determine the value of the diffusing capacity per unit transfer area.

$$\frac{D_L}{A} = \frac{20}{n\pi DL} = \frac{20}{(2.8 \times 10^9)(3.14)(7 \times 10^{-4})(650 \times 10^{-4})}$$

$$= 5 \times 10^{-5} \text{ ml } O_2/\text{min-mm Hg-cm}^2$$

A mass balance on oxygen over a differential length dz of a capillary then yields

$$Q_B \, dC = \frac{D_L}{A} (P_{alv} - P)(\pi D \, dz)$$

where Q_B is the blood flow rate to a single capillary, C is the oxygen concentration in the blood in milliliters of O_2 per cubic centimeter of blood, P_{alv} is alveolar P_{O_2} (104 mm Hg), and P is P_{O_2} in the blood. Now we must relate C to P in order to rewrite the mass balance entirely in terms of P, so that it can be integrated. The relation between C and P is the one shown graphically in Figure 10.10. Since this is a highly nonlinear relationship, let us assume as an approximation that we can express

$$\frac{dC}{dP} = \alpha$$

where α is the slope of a line connecting the points on the hemoglobin saturation curve corresponding to $P_{O_2} = 40$ mm Hg (inlet value) and $P_{O_2} \cong 104$ mm Hg (presumed outlet value, which will be shown later to be correct). That is, from Figure 10.10 (or Table 10.2)

$$\frac{dC}{dP} = \frac{0.195 - 0.145}{104 - 40} = \frac{0.05}{64} = 0.78 \times 10^{-3}$$

Hence,

$$\frac{dP}{104 - P} = \frac{(5 \times 10^{-5})(3.14)(7 \times 10^{-4})}{(6000/2.8 \times 10^{9})(0.78 \times 10^{-3})} \, dz$$

or

$$\frac{dP}{104 - P} = 65.7 \, dz$$

Integrating, and using the inlet boundary condition ($P_{O_2} = 40$ at $z = 0$) gives the final result

$$P = 104 - 64 \exp[-65.7z]$$

Figure 10.20 shows this approximate result graphically along with the exact solution. Comparison of the two solutions indicates that the use of an average slope for dC/dP causes the predicted profile to be much too steep initially and much too broad further down the capillary.

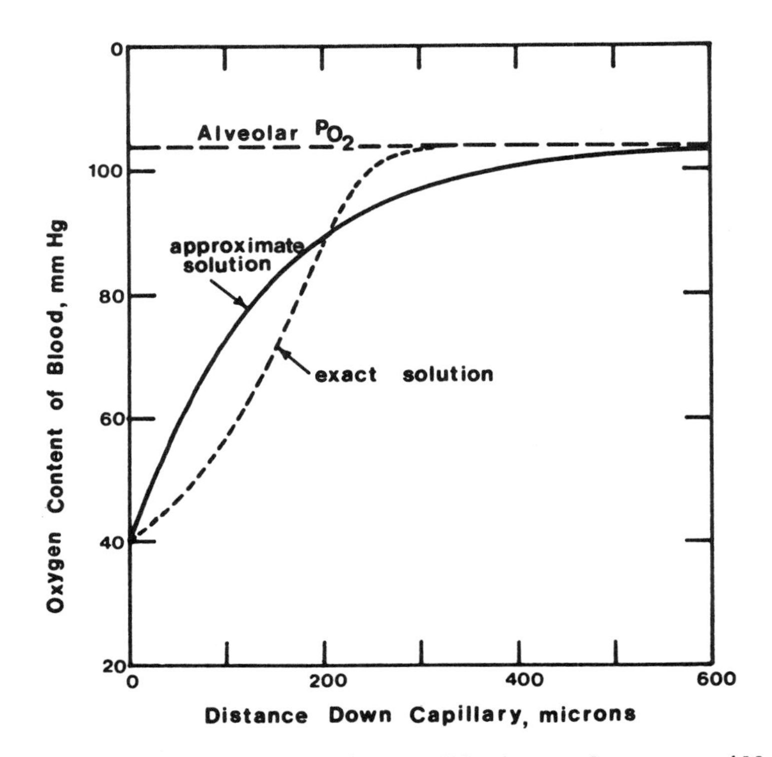

FIG. 10.20. Oxygen concentration profile in a pulmonary capillary.

The exact solution was obtained using Hill's equation, i.e.,

$$\psi = \frac{C}{C_{sat}} = \frac{(P/27.2)^{2.7}}{1 + (P/27.2)^{2.7}}$$

for which

$$\frac{dC}{dP} = \frac{(2.7C_{sat}/27.2)(P/27.2)^{1.7}}{[1 + (P/27.2)^{2.7}]^2}$$

where C_{sat} is the O_2 concentration in blood corresponding to complete saturation of hemoglobin (~0.201 ml O_2/ml blood). Combining this with the mass balance yields a differential equation for P which is easily integrated numerically by standard procedures.

XIV. INERT GAS UPTAKE IN THE PULMONARY CAPILLARIES

The theoretical treatment of inert gas uptake in pulmonary blood is quite simple and leads to useful information, and so we present an analysis here. By inert gases we mean those gases that do not combine chemically with any component of the blood (e.g., hemoglobin) and which only dissolve physically. Such gases include nitrogen, helium, argon, and nitrous oxide (in fact, almost any ordinary gas except O_2, CO_2, and CO).

For inert gases a mass balance on a differential capillary section gives (as shown before)

$$Q_B \, dC = \frac{D_L}{A} (P_{alv} - P)(\pi D \, dz)$$

This can be rewritten, using Henry's law ($C = K_D P$), as

$$\frac{dP}{P_{alv} - P} = \frac{D_L \pi D}{A K_D Q_B} dz$$

Integrating for constant alveolar partial pressure P_{alv}, and using the initial condition that $P = P^0$ at $z = 0$, gives

$$\frac{P_{alv} - P}{P_{alv} - P^0} = \exp\left[- \frac{D_L \pi D}{A K_D Q_B} z\right] = \exp\left[- \frac{D_L}{K_D Q_{tot}} \frac{z}{L}\right]$$

where we have used the fact that $A = n\pi DL$ and Q_{tot}, the total blood flow rate to the lungs, equals the number of capillaries (n) times the blood flow rate per capillary (Q_B).

A sample computation for, say, nitrogen reveals how quickly inert gases tend to equilibrate with blood. For nitrogen, $K_D = 0.012$ ml N_2/ml blood-atm at 37°C. D_L for nitrogen is equal to D'_M for nitrogen, since no chemical reaction occurs. D'_M can be estimated from the known value of D'_M for CO in normal man of 63.5 ml/min-mm Hg (Forster, 1964a) as follows:

$$D'_{M,N_2} = 63.5\frac{0.012}{0.018}\left[\frac{28}{28}\right]^{1/2} = 42.3$$

where the factors employed are those for solubility and molecular weight. Taking Q_{tot} = 6000 cc/min we have

$$\frac{P_{alv} - P}{P_{alv} - P^0} = \exp\{-[(42.3)(760)][(6000)(0.012)]\frac{z}{L}\}$$

$$= \exp(-447)\frac{z}{L}$$

For 99% equilibration, i.e., $(P_{alv} - P)/(P_{alv} - P^0) = 0.01$, a value of $z/L = 0.0103$ is obtained. In other words, 99% equilibration is attained in the first 1% of travel down the capillary. Since the residence time of blood in a single capillary is about 0.7 sec for normal resting conditions, the time required for 99% equilibration is only 0.007 sec, less than a hundredth of a second.

Since inert gas uptake is blood flow limited rather than diffusion limited, inert gases are useful for estimating pulmonary blood flow rates. That is, if one is certain that equilibration with blood is complete within the capillaries, then clearly the uptake rate of inert gas from the alveolar gas will equal the total pulmonary capillary blood flow rate times the product of solubility and alveolar partial pressure. Since measurements of inspired and expired gas compositions and flow rates are relatively easily carried out, one can assess the total uptake from the alveoli in ml gas/min-mm Hg. Division by the solubility gives the blood flow rate. This method is most easily applied if an inert gas that is not normally found in the blood is used. Then the amount of inert gas in the blood going to the lungs may be essentially zero during the course of the experiment, and blood samples need not be taken to establish the alveolar-capillary ΔP.

D_L (or D'_M in this case) cannot, however, be conveniently determined with inert gases because the effective alveolar-capillary ΔP differences are so small that they cannot be estimated.

PROBLEMS

1. *Measurement of functional residual capacity.* At the end of a normal expiration, a subject suddenly switches from breathing air to breathing pure oxygen. During the next few minutes all the N_2 in his lungs is washed out in the expired air. If the expired air collected during this time is found to contain 1720 ml of N_2, and if it is known (by other measurements) that the normal percentage of N_2 in the gas in the lungs is around 75% (see Table 10.1), what is the subject's functional residual capacity?

2. *Washout of gas from the lungs.* Suppose a person were to take a breathful (500 ml) of a gas such as helium, which is not absorbed into the bloodstream. Assume that the lungs contain 2300 ml of gas at the start of inspiration, and that the 500 ml of inspired gas mixes perfectly with all of this 2300 ml of initial gas.

On expiration after breathing the helium, what fraction of the original helium will still be in the lungs? Repeat your computations up to a total of five expirations.

3. *Speed of equilibration of gas in alveoli.* The great quickness with which nonuniformities of gas composition are damped out in alveoli is suggested by the following computation. Consider a spherical alveolus (diameter 0.1 mm) containing a gas mixture such as nitrogen and oxygen. The oxygen concentration is uniform at a value C_1. Now imagine that at a certain instant (time zero) the concentration of oxygen at the walls is raised to a value of C_o and maintained at this value. An approximate equation describing how the concentration C at the center of the alveolus rises with time is given by the equation

$$\frac{C - C_1}{C_o - C_1} \cong 1 - 2\exp\left(-\frac{4D\pi^2 t}{R^2}\right)$$

where D is the diffusivity of O_2 in air (0.18 cm^2/sec), and R is the alveolar radius.

Use this equation to estimate how much time will be needed for the center concentration to attain 99% equilibration, i.e., for $(C - C_1)/(C_o - C_1)$ to equal 0.99. While the equation given above is not a good approximation for early stages of the process, it is very accurate for the extent of equilibration being considered here.

4. *Oxygen P_{O_2} and arterial saturation at high altitudes.* At the top of Mt. Everest (29,028 ft), the barometric pressure is around 235 mm Hg and the oxygen partial pressure in the air is 49 mm Hg. Under these conditions, the O_2 partial pressure in the alveolar gas is about 23 mm Hg. Using the Hill equation, estimate the arterial blood saturation value (ψ) corresponding to this alveolar P_{O_2}. Compare it to the normal value. It should be mentioned that a completely unacclimatized person will lose consciousness if his arterial saturation falls below 40 to 50% (would he do so on Mt. Everest?).

5. *Need for pressurization in jet aircraft.* Assume you are in a commercial jetliner at 40,000 ft (barometric pressure 141 mm Hg). If the cabin were not pressurized, what would your alveolar P_{O_2} be? Your alveolar gas will, as usual, have a P_{H_2O} of 47 mm Hg (this is simply determined by body temperature). Assume the proportion of O_2 in the remaining "dry" gas is the same as normally. What would be the corresponding arterial saturation (ψ) value?

Even neglecting the intolerably low P_{O_2}, there would also be the problem that very rapid breathing would be needed in order to move air in and out of the lungs at a mass flow rate comparable to normal values. What would the breathing rate have to be at 141 mm Hg?

6. *Deep-sea diving.* Compute the volume (in liters, referred to BTP) of N_2 dissolved in a diver's body fluids at a pressure equivalent to that at a depth of 300 ft in the ocean. The total N_2 will actually be about double this, since N_2 has a high solubility in fatty tissues (about five times the solubility in water) and fat can comprise as

much as 20 vol% of the body. What will happen if the diver ascends too rapidly? What are some other lung problems related to deep-sea diving?

7. *Carbon monoxide poisoning.* Carbon monoxide binds to hemoglobin around 210 times more readily than does O_2. CO and O_2 compete, since they bind at the same sites on the hemoglobin molecule. A person will suffer lethal asphyxia if the CO in his inspired air is 0.1 vol%. At this concentration estimate what fraction of the available sites on the hemoglobin molecules will be occupied by CO.

8. *Capillary concentration profiles during exercise.* Compute the type of concentration profile shown in Figure 10.20 using the approximate (linearized) model, for a flow rate three times normal. Take the alveolar P_{O_2} to be 104 mm Hg, as before. From the outlet P_{O_2} value, estimate the fractional saturation value (ψ) and compare this to the value one would have at normal resting blood flow rates.

DISCUSSION QUESTION

Find out about the following lung diseases or abnormalities and determine the specific reasons why each interferes with normal lung performance:

Pulmonary edema

Atelectasis

(a) from airway obstruction

(b) from external compression

(c) as in hyaline membrane disease

Bronchial asthma

Chronic emphysema

Tuberculosis

Pneumonia

REFERENCES

Forster, R. E., Diffusion of gases, Chapter 33 in *Handbook of Physiology*, Section 3, *Respiration*, Vol. 1 (W. O. Fenn and H. Rahn, eds.), Am. Physiol. Soc., Washington, D. C., 1964a.

Forster, R. E., Rate of gas uptake by red cells, Chapter 32 in *Handbook of Physiology*, Section 3, *Respiration*, Vol. 1 (W. O. Fenn and H. Rahn, eds.), Am. Physiol. Soc., Washington, D. C., 1964b.

Guyton, A. C., *Textbook of Medical Physiology*, 4th ed., Saunders, Philadelphia, Pennsylvania, 1971.

Hartridge, H., and Roughton, F. J. W., A method of measuring the velocity of very rapid chemical reactions, *Proc. Roy. Soc. London, Ser. A*, 104, 376 (1923).

Kutchai, H., Numerical study of oxygen uptake by layers of hemoglobin solution, *Respir. Physiol.*, 10, 273 (1970).

Middleman, S., *Transport Phenomena in the Cardiovascular System*, Wiley-Interscience, New York, 1972.

Moll, W., The influence of hemoglobin diffusion on oxygen uptake and release by red cells, *Respir. Physiol.*, 6, 1 (1968).

Nicholson, P., and Roughton, F. J. W., A theoretical study of the influence of diffusion and chemical reaction velocity on the rate of exchange of carbon monoxide and oxygen between the red blood corpuscle and surrounding fluid, *Proc. Roy. Soc. London, Ser. B*, 138, 241 (1951).

Roughton, F. J. W., Transport of oxygen and carbon dioxide, Chapter 31 in *Handbook of Physiology*, Section 3, *Respiration*, Vol. 1 (W. O. Fenn and H. Rahn, eds.), Am. Physiol. Soc., Washington, D. C., 1964.

Ruch, T. C., and Patton, H. D., *Physiology and Biophysics*, 19th ed., Saunders, Philadelphia, Pennsylvania, 1965.

Seagrave, R. C., *Biomedical Applications of Heat and Mass Transfer*, Iowa State Univ. Press, Ames, 1971.

BIBLIOGRAPHY

Adair, G. S., The hemoglobin system. VI. The oxygen dissociation curve of hemoglobin, *J. Biol. Chem.*, 63, 529 (1925).

Comroe, J. H., Jr., *Physiology of Respiration*, Yearbook Med. Publ., Chicago, Illinois, 1965.

Kreuzer, F., and Yahr, W. Z., Influence of the red cell membrane on diffusion of oxygen, *J. Appl. Physiol.*, 15, 1117 (1960).

Staub, N. C., Bishop, J. M., and Forster, R. E., Velocity of O_2 uptake by human red blood cells, *J. Appl. Physiol.*, 16, 511 (1961).

Chapter 11

ARTIFICIAL HEART-LUNG DEVICES

Artificial devices for the oxygenation of blood outside of the body (and for simultaneous removal of carbon dioxide) have been developed intensively during recent years. Their primary application has been in cardiac surgery, where it is advantageous to bypass blood not only around the heart but around the lungs as well. Every heart-lung machine thus consists of a blood pump, to replace the heart's function, and a gas exchange device, to substitute for the natural lungs. Figure 11.1 depicts the basic features of such a system, and indicates how the blood is normally collected from the large systemic veins (venae cavae) by a mechanical pump, which sends it to an oxygenating device. A second pump returns the blood to a branch of the aorta (the aortic valves are closed by backpressure of the blood). The venae cavae are temporarily tied shut with snares between the heart and the points at which the blood is drained off. Hence, no

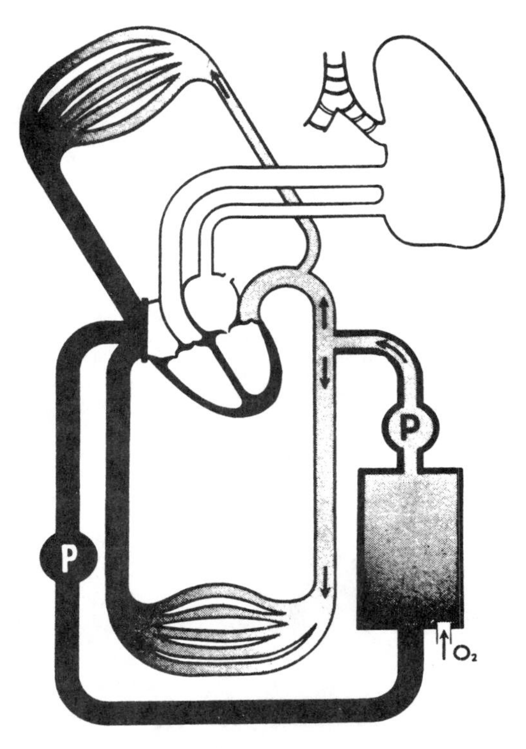

FIG. 11.1. Artificial maintenance of cardiorespiratory function, or "total heart-lung bypass." The entire systemic venous blood is prevented from entering the right heart cavities. Instead it is drained by a mechanical pump (P) into an artificial circuit outside the body, and oxygenated in an artificial gas exchange device (right lower part of figure). The arterialized blood is returned by another pump (P) to the systemic arterial system through a cannula in a branch of the aorta. It then perfuses the various capillary beds, but is prevented from entering the left heart cavities by the closed aortic valves. The extracorporeal circuits are represented by heavy lines. White areas in the figure are those excluded from the circulation and intended to be bloodless. Depending on the site of infusion, the direction of arterial blood flow may be reversed in some areas of the body (indicated by arrows). [From Galletti and Brecher (1962), p. 7.]

blood can enter the heart, and one therefore has a dry bloodless field for cardiac surgery.

Dennis, in 1950, was the first to attempt heart surgery using a pump-oxygenator system. The first successful operation was performed in 1953, by Gibbon. By 1955, the technique began to be used to a significant degree. By the middle 1960s thousands of patients had been treated, and open-heart surgery became common, if not routine. Since that time developments have been more in the nature of refinements rather than breakthroughs; however, new devices are continually being proposed and tested.

In this chapter we shall consider the design and operation of the most successful heart-lung machines developed to date, focusing primarily on the gas exchange parts of such systems. Then we will quantitatively analyze and model O_2 and CO_2 transfer in several types of gas exchangers and show which physical parameters are of most importance.

I. USE OF THE PATIENT'S LUNGS FOR GAS EXCHANGE

One might first ask why an artificial lung is needed at all if one's objective is really just to bypass the heart. Why not provide only a pump and use the patient's own lungs for gas exchange, as shown in Figure 11.2? This idea has been tried many times and has been found to involve certain disadvantages, such as the need to cannulate and later to repair the relatively thin-walled pulmonary arteries and veins (difficult and time-consuming). Problems created in pumping and draining blood from the very delicate lung circulatory system also arise; e.g., if the two blood pumps are not precisely balanced, unusual pressure or suction will occur which can cause vasomotor reactions such as the collection of fluid in the alveolar sacs.

Advantages of using the natural lungs are that less trauma is inflicted on the blood, the extracorporeal circuits are shorter and much simpler, blood priming volume is much less than usual, and gas exchange is excellent. For these reasons, this approach is now being strongly reconsidered. Gravity venous drainage from the lungs is now highly preferred over the use of pump suction.

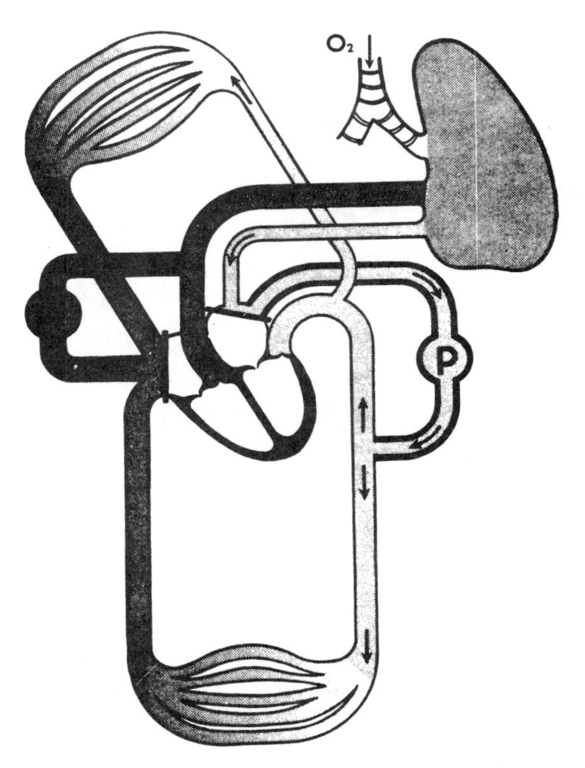

FIG. 11.2. Autogenous lung oxygenation. Through a combination of right and left heart bypass, the lungs of the patient are still able to provide regular gas exchange. Right and left heart cavities are clamped off at atrial or veno-atrial levels and are bloodless. [From Galletti and Brecher (1962), p. 31.]

II. THE IDEAL HEART-LUNG DEVICE

The ideal pump-oxygenator should be efficient in gas exchange and gentle to blood. More specifically, it should

1. Oxygenate up to 5 liters/min of venous blood to 95-100% hemoglobin saturation for, say, 20 min to perhaps several hours.

2. Simultaneously remove enough CO_2 to avoid respiratory acidosis (acidic blood) but not so much that respiratory alkalosis

(alkaline blood) occurs. An outlet P_{CO_2} of about 40 mm Hg is preferred.

3. Have a reasonable priming volume (say 1-4 liters of blood at most).

4. Be gentle enough to avoid intolerable levels of hemolysis and protein denaturation.

5. Be simple, dependable, safe, easily cleaned and assembled, easily sterilized, and conveniently, quickly, and smoothly connected to and disconnected from the patient.

Experience has shown that the surfaces which seem to do the least damage to blood cells and proteins are those that are chemically inert, smooth, have a low wettability (low surface energy), and which possess a negative surface charge. Cellophanes, Teflon, silicone rubber, and Dacron are a few of the better biomaterials.

Blood priming volumes greater than 4 liters are too costly, and volumes less than 1 liter unsafe in the sense that, should blood flow into the device be interrupted for some reason, a minimum of about 20 sec of blood supply should be available to keep blood flowing back to the patient.

III. COMPARISON OF NATURAL AND ARTIFICIAL LUNGS

Table 11.1 compares normal human lungs with typical artificial gas exchange devices. Whereas the natural lungs expose a very thin (5-10 μm) blood layer to a gas containing 100 mm Hg oxygen partial pressure for only 0.1-0.3 sec, the artificial devices have much thicker blood films (100-300 μm) and are thus forced to rely on much longer exposure times and use of a very oxygen-rich gas (about 700 mm Hg oxygen partial pressure). Note that artificial lungs have exchange areas that are much lower than those of the natural lungs. If one assumes that the amount of oxygen transferred is proportional

TABLE 11.1

Mechanical and Chemical Characteristics of Natural Versus Artificial Lung[a]

	Natural lung	Artificial lung
Pulmonary flow	5 liters/min	5 liters/min
Head of pressure	12 mm Hg	0-200 mm Hg
Pulmonary blood volume	1 liter	1-4 liters
Blood transit time	0.1-0.3 sec	3-30 sec
Blood film thickness	0.005-0.010 mm	0.1-0.3 mm
Length of capillary	0.1 mm	2-20 cm
Pulmonary ventilation	7 liters/min	2-10 liters/min
Exchange surface	50-100 m^2	2-10 m^2
Veno-alveolar O_2 gradient	40-50 mm Hg	650 mm Hg
Veno-alveolar CO_2 gradient	3-5 mm Hg	30-50 mm Hg

[a]From Galletti (1968).

to area, ΔP_{O_2}, exposure time, and inversely related to film thickness, then these figures give

$$\text{amount } O_2 \text{ transferred} \propto \frac{(75\ m^2)(11\ mm\ Hg)(0.2\ sec)}{0.0075\ mm} = 2.2 \times 10^3$$

for the natural lungs, where we have used arithmetic averages for all figures quoted as ranges in Table 11.1, except for ΔP_{O_2}, where we have used a more approrriate time-averaged value (see Chapter 10). For the artificial lungs the same calculation gives

$$\text{amount } O_2 \text{ transferred} \propto \frac{(6\ m^2)(650\ mm\ Hg)(16.5\ sec)}{0.2\ mm} = 3.2 \times 10^3$$

These results are very close considering that arithmetic averages of widely ranging values were taken. Also, since the dependence of the amount transferred on blood film thickness is probably stronger than assumed, these results should probably be even more nearly equal. What is clearly shown here is how the net interplay of various factors can produce artificial lung performance which is close to that of the natural lungs.

The natural lung data are for resting conditions. Under exercise situations the natural lungs can dramatically increase O_2 and CO_2 transfer to amounts much larger than reasonable artificial lungs could ever produce. Thus, artificial devices approximate natural lung performance only for resting conditions—but then this is all they are required to do.

IV. BASIC TYPES OF OXYGENATORS

Gas exchange in artificial devices relies mainly on the creation of a large interfacial blood-gas contact area, across which equilibration can occur. This area can be generated by dispersing the gas phase as bubbles in a pool of blood; by spreading blood in a thin film on a stationary or moving solid plate, screen, etc.; by dispersion of blood into a gas phase via foaming or spraying; by flowing blood and gas on opposite sides of a large semipermeable membrane; and so forth. In some units blood flow is single pass, whereas in others a recirculation pump is used to prolong the net contact time by continually recycling some blood from the outlet end to the inlet end of the device. Blood-side mixing, which promotes gas transfer, is achieved by various means: direct mechanical stirring, turbulent gas flow, or moving or rotating the solid surfaces on which the blood films are created.

We will discuss here only the three most successful types of artificial lungs: the bubble, film, and membrane oxygenators illustrated in Figure 11.3 (some devices exhibit features of more than one basic type, so this classification is somewhat arbitrary).

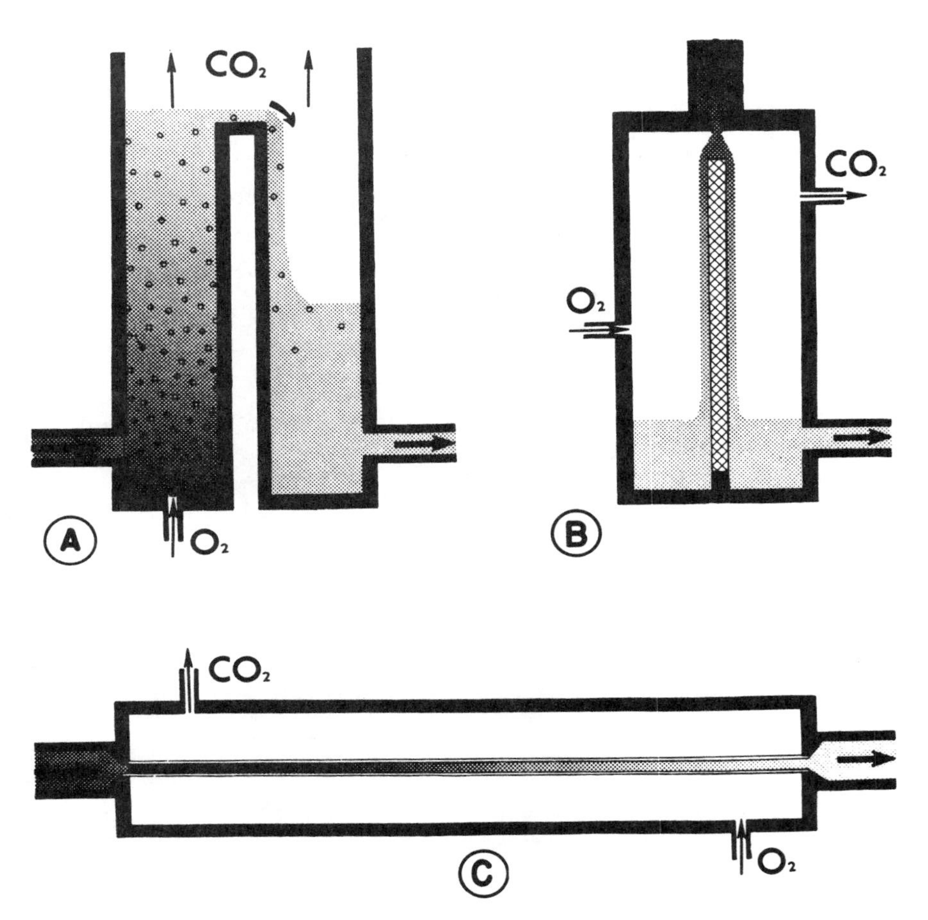

FIG. 11.3. The three basic classes of artificial lungs: (A) bubble, (B) film, (C) membrane. [From Galletti and Brecher (1962), p. 59.]

A. *Bubble Oxygenators*

Bubble oxygenators utilize the fact that gas broken into a large number of small bubbles can provide an extensive interfacial transfer area (e.g., 100 ml of gas dispersed as 1-mm-diameter bubbles contains about 5000 cm^2 of area). Very tiny bubbles (e.g., 0.1 mm diameter), though possessing a great surface area per unit volume, are difficult to remove from the blood. Yet, they must be eliminated. Thus, in practical operation, bubbles of moderate size (say 5 mm) are found to optimize both area and ease of removal. Bubble devices usually contain a bubble chimney, where the gas is mixed with venous blood, and defoaming-settling chambers where gas-blood separation takes place (see Figure 11.3). While bubble oxygenators were invented nearly 100 years ago, satisfactory removal of gas bubbles from blood was not achieved until 1950, when silicone compounds coated onto the contacting surfaces were discovered to be excellent defoaming agents. Besides bursting the bubbles which tend to collect as foam at the top of the blood, these compounds are nontoxic.

One popular oxygenator of the bubble type is that developed by DeWall (Figure 11.4). Here oxygen-rich gas is bubbled through a column of venous blood. The resulting foam flows across an inclined defoaming surface containing conelike projections. This surface is

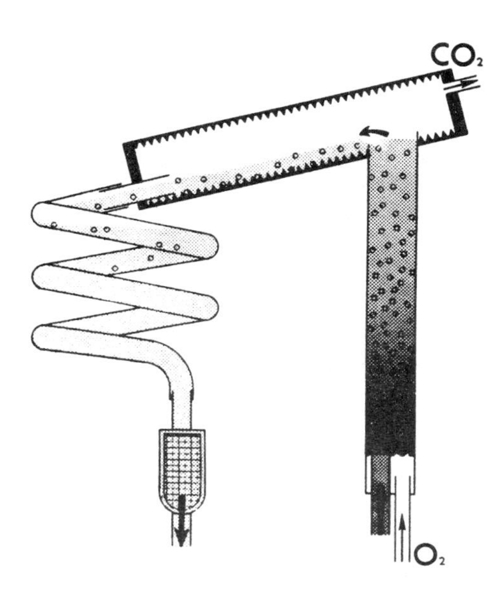

FIG. 11.4. DeWall oxygenator. [From Galletti and Brecher (1962), p. 64.]

coated with silicone compounds (which stick well and do not wash away very appreciably). The blood then flows through a long helical settling chamber from which any remaining bubbles are removed by buoyant rising. A filter at the bottom prevents fibrin strands and other debris from being returned in the arterialized blood. The DeWall unit is normally run with a blood flow of 2 liters/min, and a gas flow (97-98% O_2, 2-3% CO_2) of about three times the blood flow. Priming volume is 3 liters.

B. *Film Oxygenators*

Film-type devices usually have a solid vertical stationary support over which venous blood is spread in a thin film and then runs downward into a settling chamber region (see Figure 11.3). Films have been produced on a hanging plate, a cloth curtain, a metal screen, and a pile of glass beads. Other variations of film oxygenators include those where blood is spread over <u>moving</u> supports, such as spinning cylinders or spinning discs.

With stationary supports, it has been found that smooth surfaces provide very little sidewise mixing in the blood layer, so that the inner parts of the blood layer achieve very poor equilibration with the gas phase. Irregular surfaces, like corrugated materials or screens, promote significant lateral mixing, however, and greatly overcome this problem. Alternatively, pulsatile blood flow can be used to create a wavy film.

Thin films, which equilibrate much more readily with the gas phase than do thick films, can be generated by spreading the blood over a rotating surface. As rotation speed is increased the blood film thins out and mass transfer efficiency increases. Although thinning out the film means that less blood is on the surface at any instant, the increased rotational speed means that the film is renewed more often. On balance, the total amount of blood exposed to gas per unit time is roughly constant. Once the rotational speed exceeds a certain minimum level, however, further increases in speed do not appreciably increase total gas transfer rates. Rotating film devices are smaller in size and require less priming volume than stationary film devices, but incur the possibility of causing excessive hemolysis and protein denaturation.

Devices using stainless steel screens of 0.7-mm-diameter wire, oriented with the wires running 45 degrees to horizontal, are typical of stationary film oxygenators. Larger wire sizes create excessive blood film volume and smaller wire sizes fail to produce enough lateral mixing action in the film (a smooth plate gives only one-eighth the gas transfer of 0.7-mm wires).

So-called sponge oxygenators have also been developed which use thick stationary porous materials (polyurethane). Blood flows by gravity down through the porous material, whose many pores simulate alveoli. Such devices have a large contact area, are efficient, and have very small priming volumes. However, some difficulties have been noted with foaming.

The rotating disc oxygenator, one example of which is shown in Figure 11.5, consists of a horizontal cylinder partly filled with blood and a central shaft on which are mounted many discs. As the shaft is rotated, films of blood are formed on the discs and are exposed to the gas phase in the upper part of the unit. The original Kay-Cross oxygenator, the first of this type, was developed in 1957 and consisted of a Pyrex cylinder 33 cm long by 13.3 cm in diameter. Fifty-nine stainless steel siliconized (or Teflon-coated) discs

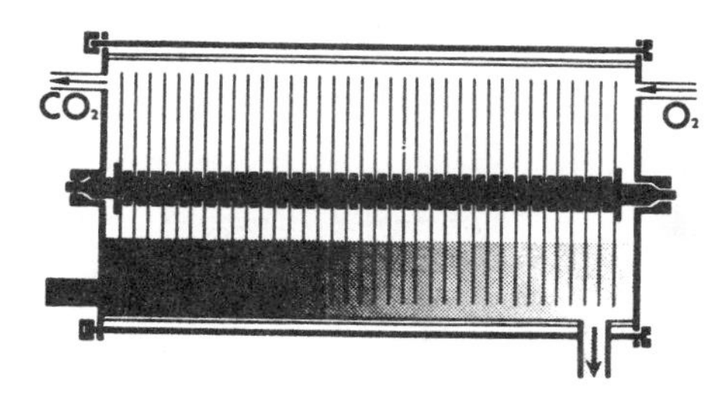

FIG. 11.5. Kay-Cross rotating disc oxygenator. [From Galletti and Brecher (1962), p. 98.]

0.4 mm thick and 12.2 cm in diameter were mounted 0.5 cm apart using spacers on the shaft. When filled with 1.4 liters of blood, the blood level is about one-third from the bottom to the top. At 120 rpm, a film of roughly 0.8 m^2 is generated. This is sufficient to fully arterialize 2 liters of blood per minute. The newer models of this oxygenator are quite similar to the original one, and they are among the most widely used oxygenators in clinical practice. The number of discs on the shaft and/or the rotation speed are conveniently changed to match the particular gas transfer rates required (e.g., reduced for infants).

C. Membrane Oxygenators

Many of the early difficulties encountered in using oxygenators involved froth formation, fibrin deposition, protein denaturation, and hemolysis resulting from the direct contact of blood and gas. To avoid blood trauma, devices were proposed in which a membrane separates the two phases. Several of these oxygenators are almost identical to the coil, flat plate, and capillary artificial kidneys discussed in Chapter 9; the main difference is that the membranes (silicone rubber, Teflon) are essentially permeable to gases only and not to liquids (as in artificial kidneys).

By interposing a membrane between blood and gas, one obviously adds a mass transfer resistance to the system. Whether or not the membrane seriously impedes O_2 and/or CO_2 transport depends on the nature of the membrane, particularly the solubility of O_2 and CO_2 in the membrane. It should be noted that, unlike in the human lungs, the partial pressure driving force for O_2 transport in artificial lungs is very large: about 670 mm Hg inlet ΔP if pure O_2 is used ($670 \cong 760$ total pressure - 50 water partial pressure - 40 inlet venous O_2 partial pressure). The inlet CO_2 partial pressure difference (45 mm Hg) is also much higher than in the human lungs. Hence, the driving force for O_2 transport is 15 times that for CO_2 in artificial lungs. In the natural lungs the ratio is about (104 - 40)/(45 - 40) $\cong$ 13, or quite similar. But the natural respiratory membrane is more than 20 times more permeable to CO_2 than to O_2, as discussed in Chapter 10. Synthetic membranes favor CO_2 over O_2 by only about 2.5:1 (Teflon) or 5:1 (silicone rubber), as shown by Table 11.2. Therefore, membrane artificial lungs must usually be designed for CO_2 transfer as the key consideration. In general, one can state that CO_2 transfer in membrane devices is primarily determined by the synthetic membrane barrier, and O_2 transfer is controlled

TABLE 11.2

Gas Permeability of Teflon and Silicone Rubber Membranes[a]

Membrane	Thickness (mil)	Oxygen	Carbon dioxide	Nitrogen	Helium
Teflon	1/8	239	645	106	1425
	1/4	117	302	56	730
	3/8	77	181	35	430
	1/2	61	126	30	345
	3/4	41	86	23	240
	1	29			
Silicone rubber	3	391	2072	184	224
	4	306	1605	159	187
	5	206	1112	105	133
	7	159	802	81	94
	12	93	425	48	51
	20	59	279	31	43

[a]Permeation rates of oxygen, carbon dioxide, nitrogen, and helium across Teflon and silicone rubber membranes of a given thickness, in ml/min-m^2-atm (STP). [From Galletti (1968).]

primarily by the blood film resistance (as is urea transport in artificial kidneys).

Although silicone rubber is roughly 40 times more permeable to O_2 and 80 times more permeable to CO_2 for the same thickness, the ability to manufacture Teflon membranes about 20 times thinner than silicone rubber (as suggested by Table 11.2) reduces this advantage. Silicone rubber is thus better than Teflon by about 2:1 for O_2 and 4:1 for CO_2 transport. Since CO_2 transport often determines the required membrane area, as discussed above, silicone rubber is much to be preferred over Teflon. Membrane devices offer the advantages of gentle blood handling, avoidance of gas or fibrin emboli, disposability of the parts which contact the blood, and simplicity of control of blood volume in the patient (a very critical aspect). Since the blood-side compartment is geometrically well constrained, significant accumulation or depletion of blood in the heart-lung device (and thus the reverse effect in the patient) is easy to avoid. The membrane units are, however, bulky (hard to fit into sterilizers) and difficult (thus costly) to assemble.

D. *Comparison of Oxygenators*

Table 11.3 compares the most popular heart-lung devices in terms of various crucial items. It should be noted that the flow rate of blood that can be satisfactorily arterialized tends to be low for membrane devices, unless a rather large membrane area is used. Also, it is clear that no single type of unit is decidedly better than the others. Thus, all varieties listed are in widespread use today.

V. TEMPERATURE MAINTENANCE

A few °C drop in body core temperature is not harmful during connection to a heart-lung device. In fact, deliberate cooling (induced hypothermia) is often employed to reduce the metabolic O_2

TABLE 11.3

Comparison of Pump-Oxygenator Systems[a]

	Bubble oxygenator	Film oxygenator	Disc oxygenator	Membrane oxygenator
Flow capacity	Medium	High	High	Low
Priming volume	Medium	Large	Large	Small
Initial cost	Low	High	High	Medium
Maintenance cost	High	Medium	Low	High
Blood trauma	Moderate	Moderate	High	Minimal
Main drawback	Defoaming	Cleaning	Cleaning	Assembly

[a]From Galletti (1968).

requirement of the patient, especially the O_2 needed by the major organs, and thus make prolonged heart-lung bypass safer. Nevertheless, if minimizing the heat loss from the body is desired, it is easily accomplished by (a) placing the heart-lung unit in a temperature-controlled water bath, (b) circulating warm air around the unit, (c) wrapping heating wires around the oxygenator, or (d) shining heat lamps on the device. The only restriction is that surfaces in direct contact with blood should be lower than 43°-45°C to prevent trauma (<39°C if in contact with foam).

VI. GAS FLOW RATE REQUIREMENTS FOR ARTIFICIAL LUNGS

Let us assume, for resting conditions, that a patient has a cardiac output of 5000 cc/min, an O_2 consumption of 250 cc(STP)/min, and a CO_2 production of 200 cc(STP)/min. These last two figures become 284 and 227 cc/min, respectively, when adjusted to body temperature (37°C). This implies an O_2 difference at STP of

5.0 ml O_2/100 ml blood and a CO_2 difference of 4.0 ml CO_2/100 ml blood, between arterial and venous blood (or 5.7 and 4.5 ml/100 ml at 37°C).

If 5 ml of pure O_2 is used for each 100 ml of blood, in a bubble type of heart-lung machine, and if equilibration is achieved, then complete arterialization of the blood will occur. However, all of the gas phase will be consumed, and no gas will exist into which CO_2 can be eliminated. Hence, no CO_2 removal will be possible. This leads to the following problem.

Example 11.1: Gas Rate Needed for CO_2 Removal. Assume that the blood leaving the bubble oxygenator should have a P_{CO_2} of 40 mm Hg maximum. Hence the gas leaving the unit must have a P_{CO_2} of 40 mm Hg maximum (assuming equilibration; in practice it should be lower). If the inlet gas has no CO_2, what ratio of gas to blood flow will be required?

Assume a blood flow rate of 100 ml/min and a temperature of 37°C. The rate of CO_2 removal from the blood will be 4.5 ml/min. Hence, if Q_G is the total outlet gas flow rate, and the partial pressure of CO_2 at the outlet is 40 mm Hg, then

$$\frac{4.5 \text{ ml/min}}{Q_G \text{ ml/min}} = \frac{40 \text{ mm Hg}}{760 \text{ mm Hg}}$$

or Q_G = 85.5 ml/min [the inlet gas rate is therefore 85.5 + 5.7 - 4.5 = 86.7 ml/min if N_2 transfer is neglected (probably not a good assumption)]. A gas-to-blood flow rate ratio of 87/100 or about 1:1 is therefore minimum, if proper CO_2 removal is to be possible. In practice, ratios of 2 or 3:1 are needed. Even ratios of 5 or 10:1 are not rare, but these tend to cause any foam that is generated to be very "dry," which is undesirable, and they also cause increased blood trauma. High gas flows can sometimes remove too much CO_2, creating hypocapnia and undesirably alkaline blood. To avoid this problem it is common practice to use gases containing 2-5% CO_2 (P_{CO_2} = 15-38 mm Hg) in heart-lung machines. Note that even at a 1:1 gas/blood ratio the amount of O_2 available is 18 times the amount required for saturating the blood. Hence, in a bubble oxygenator, very tiny bubbles are not needed for efficient O_2 transfer; in fact, tiny bubbles have low buoyancy, are hard to remove from the blood, and have poor ability to carry away CO_2. Large bubbles are desirable for CO_2 removal. In practice, bubble devices are often equipped with two inlet gas distributors, one of which makes reasonably small bubbles (for better O_2 transfer) and one of which makes fairly large bubbles (for CO_2 removal). The same principles regarding the minimum and best gas/blood flow rate ratios apply of course to all heart-lung devices, not just to the "bubblers."

It should also be evident that using superatmospheric conditions in heart-lung units would be of little benefit. While somewhat enhancing O_2 transfer, it would have no effect on removal of CO_2 from the blood. Worse than this, reducing the blood to atmospheric conditions prior to, or upon, reentry to the patient would cause dangerous gas bubbles to form in the blood (such emboli can block blood vessels in the body and cause tissues to die).

VII. AREA REQUIREMENT FOR MEMBRANE OXYGENATORS

By analogy to the developments of Chapter 9 for artificial kidney devices, it is evident that membrane oxygenators may be described by the equation

$$dW = K(P_G - P_B)\ dA$$

where dW is the milliliters of i transferred to the blood per minute, K is a mass transfer coefficient (ml i/m^2-min-mm Hg), P_B is the partial pressure of i in the blood (millimeters of mercury), P_G is the partial pressure of i in the gas (millimeters of mercury), and dA is the area of the membrane (square meters). This equation applies locally for any differential section of the artificial lung, but may be integrated, as was done in Chapter 9, to yield

$$W = KA(P_G - P_B)_{\text{log mean}}$$

Example 11.2: Area Estimation for a Silicone Rubber Membrane Lung. Let us assume 100% O_2 gas (water saturated) is fed to the membrane unit which is maintained at 37°C and that

Q_B = 4000 cc/min

Q_G = 10000 cc/min (at inlet and at 37°C)

$P_{G,in}$ = 0 mm Hg, for CO_2

$P_{G,in}$ = 760 - 47 mm Hg (water) = 713 mm Hg, for O_2

$P_{B,in}$ = 40 mm Hg for O_2

$P_{B,in}$ = 46 mm Hg for CO_2

O_2 transferred = 5.7 ml/100 ml blood at 37°C

CO_2 transferred = 4.5 ml/100 ml blood at 37°C

$P_{B,out}$ = 95 mm Hg, for O_2

$P_{B,out}$ = 40 mm Hg, for CO_2

The total O_2 consumed is (5.7)(40) = 230 ml/min, and the CO_2 removed is (4.5)(40) = 180 ml/min. Hence, the gas leaving the system totals 9950 ml/min. Therefore,

$$P_{G,out} = \frac{180}{9950} 760 = 13.7 \text{ mm Hg, for } CO_2$$

$$P_{G,out} = \frac{[(713/760)(10000) - 230]}{9950}(760) = 699.0 \text{ mm Hg, for } O_2$$

Thus, for CO_2 (assuming cocurrent flow)

$$\text{log mean } \Delta P = \frac{(46 - 0) - (40 - 13.7)}{\ln[(46 - 0)/(40 - 13.7)]} = 35.3 \text{ mm Hg}$$

and, for O_2 (again, for cocurrent flow)

$$\text{log mean } \Delta P = \frac{(713 - 40) - (699 - 95)}{\ln[(713 - 40)/(699 - 95)]} = 638 \text{ mm Hg}$$

Further, let us assume that the membrane is a 3-mil silicone rubber membrane, for which the O_2 permeability is about 390 ml/min-m^2-atm and the CO_2 permeability is about 2070 ml/min-m^2-atm (Table 11.2). These values become 0.51 and 2.72, respectively, when converted to ml/min-m^2-mm Hg.

Now, _if_ the membrane resistance strongly controls mass transfer, then we may determine the required membrane area in terms of both O_2 and CO_2 transport using the equation

$$A = \frac{W}{K(\Delta P)_{\text{log mean}}}$$

where K is the _membrane_ permeability alone. Since the K values in Table 11.2 refer to STP, the O_2 and CO_2 transport rates given above must be converted to STP, using the absolute temperature ratio 273°K/310°K. Thus, for O_2

$$A = \frac{230\ (273/310)}{(0.51)(638)} = 0.62\ m^2$$

and for CO_2

$$A = \frac{180\ (273/310)}{(2.72)(35.3)} = 1.65\ m^2$$

The required area is about 1.7 m^2 (compare with artificial kidneys). For O_2, the membrane resistance is really only a fraction of the total mass transfer resistance, the blood-side resistance being almost certainly even greater than the membrane resistance. However, even if the blood-side resistance is 65% of the total, 1.7 m^2 will still suffice for satisfactory O_2 transfer.

CO_2 is known to transport well through plasma because of its high aqueous solubility. Since gas-side resistances are surely small for all species, one can conclude that the membrane resistance will dominate CO_2 transport. However, the diffusion and reaction of CO_2 _inside_ red blood cells are not necessarily fast steps, and may offer appreciable resistance. Additionally, uniform blood and gas flow patterns are often difficult to achieve in flat plate mass transfer devices, especially if priming volumes (hence channel heights) are small. Overall, then, one might guess that the 1.7-m^2 area could prove to be too small, and that 2.5 m^2 or so would be a better choice.

VIII. THEORETICAL MODELS FOR BLOOD OXYGENATION

A. *The Advancing Front Theory of Blood-Gas Reactions*

When the rate of chemical reaction between a gas and hemoglobin is very large relative to the rate of diffusion of the gas through the red blood cell membrane and interior, then one may assume the reaction to be instantaneous as an approximation. That is, one assumes that reaction equilibrium prevails everywhere in the blood. If, in addition, the reaction is nearly irreversible, one can view the process of gas uptake by blood as the movement of a sharp boundary, or "front," through the blood. This front separates a totally reacted zone (behind the front) from a completely unreacted zone; e.g., for the case of O_2 uptake the front would separate a zone having much HbO_2 and zero Hb from a zone having much Hb but no HbO_2.

Viewing the gas uptake process in this manner is advantageous, as has been shown by Forster (1964), because it permits simple expressions for describing the process to be written. However, not all gas species react as fast as this theory requires (the reaction of NO and Hb is probably an exception; see Table 10.4). Moreover, the reactions of gases with Hb are not irreversible. One can see for the reaction between O_2 and HbO_2 that the equilibrium curve (Figure 10.10) is quite steep and thus the reaction does simulate irreversible behavior to an extent, but the curve still is far from a pure step function. For reasonably high gas phase oxygen contents (say P_{O_2} of 100 mm Hg or above), the profile of (Hb) versus distance in the blood will be like that shown in Figure 11.6. The (HbO_2) profile would be of the reverse shape (rotate top to bottom). Clearly the situation is somewhat close to that assumed by the advancing front theory. When the gas phase O_2 concentration is low, however, the (Hb) profile will be quite curved and nonzero over most of the reacted zone thickness, and conditions would thus be far from those of the simplified theory.

Taking the necessary assumptions to be valid to at least a first approximation, let us develop gas uptake equations for the

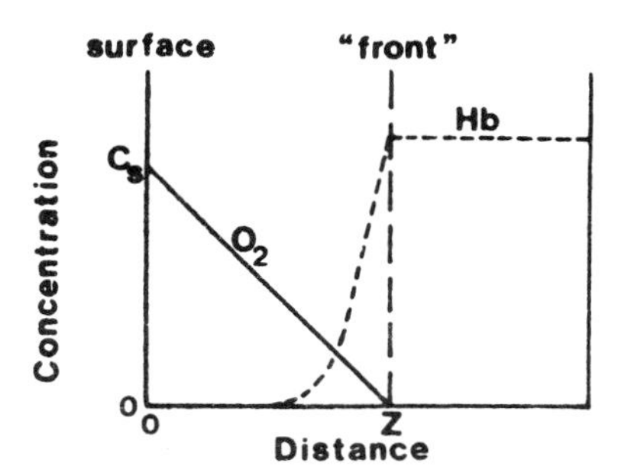

FIG. 11.6. O_2 penetration into blood.

$Hb + O_2 \rightarrow HbO_2$ reaction as an example. If we also assume that the O_2 profile will be nearly linear, then from Fick's law

$$\frac{\text{moles } O_2 \text{ reaching front}}{\text{second}} = -DA\,\frac{dC}{dz} = \frac{DAC_s}{Z}$$

where C_s is the O_2 concentration in the blood at the gas-blood interface, A is the area of the blood layer under consideration (arbitrary), Z is the location of the front, and D is the diffusivity of O_2 in the blood. [The assumption of a linear profile is strictly correct only when the ratio of (Hb) to C_s is large enough so that the front does not move very fast. For fast frontal movement the O_2 profile is "pulled" out of a linear shape and follows a concave type of pattern.] During any time period dt, during which the front will travel a distance dz

$$\text{moles } O_2 \text{ which reached the front} = \text{moles Hb which reacted}$$

or

$$\frac{DC_sA\,dt}{Z} = (Hb)A\,dZ$$

Hence, $dZ/dt = DC_s/[(Hb)Z]$. Integrating and noting that $Z = 0$ at $t = 0$ yields

$$Z = \left[\frac{2DC_s t}{(Hb)}\right]^{1/2}$$

which indicates that the position of the advancing front varies with the square root of time.

We now write

$$\frac{\text{moles of } O_2 \text{ reacted}}{\text{cm}^2\text{-sec}} = \frac{DC_s}{Z} = \left[\frac{DC_s(Hb)}{2t}\right]^{1/2}$$

Therefore, the moles of O_2 consumed between t = 0 and any time t will be

$$O_2 \ (\text{moles/cm}^2) = \int_0^t \left[\frac{DC_s(Hb)}{2t}\right]^{1/2} dt = [2DC_s(Hb)t]^{1/2}$$

For the following parameter values

$(Hb) = 8.8 \times 10^{-3}$ moles/liter (whole blood, as Hb not Hb_4)

$D_{O_2} = 1.2 \times 10^{-5}$ cm^2/sec

$C_{s_{O_2}} = 0.20 \times 10^{-3}$ moles/liter (gas phase, air, 37°C)

the predicted Z versus t relation becomes

$$Z = \left[\frac{2DC_s t}{(Hb)}\right]^{1/2} = 7.4 \times 10^{-4}\sqrt{t} \text{ cm}$$

According to this result, the advancing front will be about 0.0074 cm (74 μm) from the surface after 100 sec.

A major advantage of the advancing front theory is that it predicts the entire time course of the gas uptake, whereas more detailed theories have analytical solutions only for very short initial periods (as we discussed earlier). In that this theory represents the limiting rate of gas uptake as reaction rate becomes very large, this approach is also useful for estimating upper bounds on gas uptake rates and for checking the reasonableness of computations made using more complex analyses.

B. *A More Exact Treatment of Advancing Fronts*

The preceding analysis assumes in essence that the $(Hb)/C_s$ ratio is so large that the frontal movement rate is very low, and thus one can neglect the term $\partial C_{O_2}/\partial t$ in the O_2 mass balance for the reacted zone, which is

$$\frac{\partial C_{O_2}}{\partial t} = D \frac{\partial^2 C_{O_2}}{\partial z^2}$$

(no reaction term appears because the zone behind the front is fully reacted). Clearly the neglect of $\partial C_{O_2}/\partial t$ implies the linear O_2 profile that we assumed earlier. However, one can easily include time dependence. Defining dimensionless variables

$$X = 1 - \frac{C}{C_s}, \qquad \zeta = \frac{z}{(4Dt)^{1/2}}$$

the equation given above becomes

$$-2\zeta \frac{dX}{d\zeta} = \frac{d^2X}{d\zeta^2}$$

Since substitution of $p = dX/d\zeta$ reduces this to

$$-2\zeta p = \frac{dp}{d\zeta}$$

which is easily separated and solved to give (where A is a constant)

$$p = Ae^{-\zeta^2}$$

it is apparent that the solution to the original equation must therefore be

$$X = \frac{\int_0^{\zeta} e^{-y^2}\, dy}{\int_0^{\zeta'} e^{-y^2}\, dy} = \frac{\text{erf } \zeta}{\text{erf } \zeta'}$$

Here we have made use of the boundary conditions

$$X = 0 \text{ at } \zeta = 0 \quad \text{and} \quad X = 1 \text{ at } \zeta = \zeta' \text{ (the "front")}$$

The position of the front with respect to time can be determined via a mass balance on the front:

$$-D \left.\frac{\partial C_{O_2}}{\partial z}\right|_{z=z'} = (\text{Hb}) \frac{dz'}{dt}$$

or, in dimensionless terms,

$$\left.\frac{dX}{d\zeta}\right|_{\zeta=\zeta'} = \frac{2\zeta'(\text{Hb})}{C_s}$$

Evaluation of $dX/d\zeta$ at $\zeta = \zeta'$ from the solution just obtained yields

$$\frac{\sqrt{\pi}(\text{Hb})}{C_s} \zeta' \exp(\zeta'^2) \text{ erf } \zeta' = 1$$

which requires trial and error solution for ζ'. For large $(\text{Hb})/C_s$ ratios, however, one can argue that the penetration depth will be very small for a long time, i.e., $\zeta' << 1$, for which

$$\exp(\zeta'^2) \cong 1 \text{ and erf } \zeta' = \frac{2\zeta'}{\sqrt{\pi}}$$

(this is easily deduced from the series expressions for e^x and erf x). The ζ' relation then reduces to

$$\zeta' = \left[\frac{C_s}{2(\text{Hb})}\right]^{1/2} \text{ or } z' = \left[\frac{2DtC_s}{(\text{Hb})}\right]^{1/2}$$

which is exactly what the simpler advancing front theory predicted. This agreement is of course expected.

The rate at which oxygen enters the blood can be written as:

$$\text{Flux at surface} = -D \left.\frac{\partial C_{O_2}}{\partial z}\right|_{z=0} = C_s \left[\frac{D}{4t}\right]^{1/2} \left.\frac{dX}{d\zeta}\right|_{\zeta=0} = C_s \frac{(D/\pi t)^{1/2}}{\text{erf } \zeta'}$$

For $\zeta' << 1$, the flux equals roughly $C_s(D/4t)^{1/2}/\zeta'$ or, substituting for ζ' from above, $[C_s D(Hb)/2t]^{1/2}$.

C. A Theory for Reversible Reactions

A similar development for the case of a reversible reaction is useful because it can be used in conjunction with the previous analysis to bracket the behavior of a system such as the $Hb\text{-}O_2\text{-}HbO_2$ one, as shown in Figure 11.7. Since reaction will be occurring in the zone behind the advancing front in this case (although limited by diffusion, not kinetics: we shall assume instantaneous reactions) our analysis must begin with the equations

$$\frac{\partial C_{O_2}}{\partial t} = D \frac{\partial^2 C_{O_2}}{\partial z^2} + R_{O_2}$$

$$\frac{\partial C_{HbO_2}}{\partial t} = D_{HbO_2} \frac{\partial^2 C_{HbO_2}}{\partial z^2} + R_{HbO_2}$$

If we write these in terms of moles and add them, the sum of the molar reaction rates, $R_{O_2} + R_{HbO_2}$, drops out, as it is zero. Further, assuming that $D_{HbO_2} \cong 0$ (because of the large size of HbO_2), we obtain

$$\frac{\partial C_{O_2}}{\partial t} (1 + m) = D \frac{\partial^2 C_{O_2}}{\partial z^2}$$

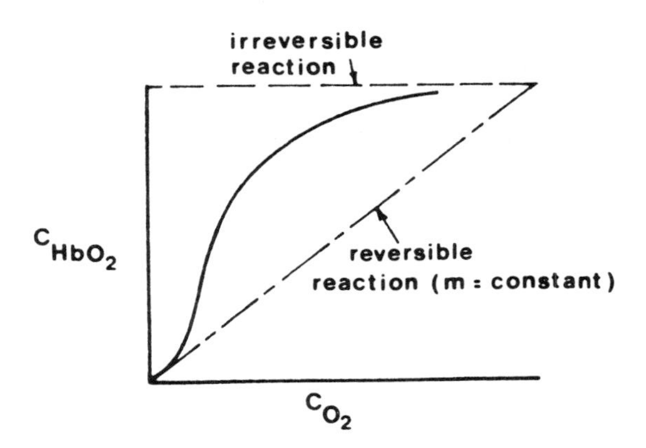

FIG. 11.7. Limiting approximations to the oxyhemoglobin dissociation curve.

where $m = dC_{HbO_2}/dC_{O_2}$, the slope of the equilibrium relationship between C_{HbO_2} and C_{O_2}. For m = const, we can easily solve this equation, since substitution of

$$X = 1 - \frac{C}{C_s}, \qquad \eta = \frac{z}{(4Dt)^{1/2}}(1 + m)^{1/2}$$

reduces it to the same form, with the same boundary conditions, as we had in the irreversible case above, except that η appears where ζ appeared previously. In this case, however, η' will always be infinity, due to the linear nature of the equilibrium (i.e., the second boundary condition is X = 1 at $\eta \to \infty$). Since erf ∞ = 1, the solution to this case is simply X = erf η. Because of the nature of this second boundary condition, the rate of frontal movement cannot be evaluated. However, we can determine the O_2 flux at z = 0 as follows

$$\text{Flux at surface} = -D \left.\frac{\partial C_{O_2}}{\partial z}\right|_{z=0} = C_s\left[\frac{D(1 + m)}{4t}\right]^{1/2} \left.\frac{dX}{d\eta}\right|_{\eta=0}$$

$$= C_s\left[\frac{D(1 + m)}{\pi t}\right]^{1/2}$$

It is interesting to note that the ratio of the flux computed in this case to that found in the irreversible case is $[2C_s(1 + m)/\pi(Hb)]^{1/2}$. However, since $m = (Hb)/C_s$, this is equivalent to $[2(1 + 1/m)/\pi]^{1/2}$, which, for large m, has the value $(2/\pi)^{1/2}$ or 0.798. Because the two theories bracket the actual behavior, and because they predict O_2 fluxes that are in agreement to within about 20%, it is apparent that either theory alone can represent the gas uptake rate reasonably accurately (for large m).

D. *Accounting for Hemoglobin Diffusion*

These treatments just presented all assume that $D_{Hb} = 0$ in the zone ahead of the advancing front. However, since $(Hb) = 0$ just behind the front and has a significant value ahead of the front, it is obvious that a considerable driving force for diffusion exists. Thus, in fact (Hb) diffuses toward the front where it meets O_2 diffusing from the opposite direction. In addition, there will be a curved concentration profile of Hb in the unreacted zone—albeit a very steep profile (owing to the large value of D_{Hb}). Analytical solutions do exist for the case of an instantaneous irreversible reaction between two species A and B, both of which can diffuse. The starting equations are

$$\frac{\partial C_A}{\partial t} = D_A \frac{\partial^2 C_A}{\partial z^2}$$

$$\frac{\partial C_B}{\partial t} = D_B \frac{\partial^2 C_B}{\partial z^2}$$

For

$$C_A = C_{Ai} \quad \text{at } z = 0,\ t > 0$$

$$C_B = q \quad \text{at } t = 0,\ z > 0$$

$$C_A = C_B = 0 \quad \text{at } z = z',\ t > 0$$

the following solutions pertain:

$$C_A = A_1 + B_1 \operatorname{erf} \zeta_A$$

$$C_B = A_2 + B_2 \operatorname{erf} \zeta_B$$

where $\zeta_A = z/(4D_A t)^{1/2}$, $\zeta_B = z/(4D_B t)^{1/2}$, and A_1, A_2, B_1, and B_2 are constants that can be evaluated by solving a set of simultaneous equations which arise from satisfying the boundary conditions. The analysis, too involved to be presented here, again predicts that the frontal position varies as $t^{1/2}$.

Figure 11.8 gives available graphical results for the case where $D_A/D_B = 2$. This is far from the type of situation one has with O_2 and Hb, but we present the profiles here to illustrate the type of behavior one finds. Note that the species with the lower diffusivity has the steeper profile (one would thus expect the profile for Hb to be quite steep).

All of these developments can be applied, of course, to situations in which the blood initially has a uniform nonzero O_2 and HbO_2 content. For these cases one merely replaces C_s by $C_s - C_0$ (where C_0 is the initial O_2 content) and lets (Hb) equal the correct initial value.

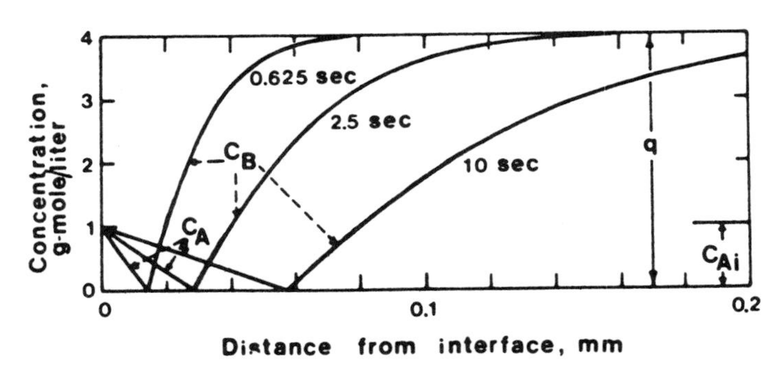

FIG. 11.8. Calculated concentration profiles during rapid second-order reaction in liquid film. Based on $D_A = 3.9 \times 10^{-5}$ ft^2/hr; $D_B = 1.95 \times 10^{-5}$ ft^2/hr. [From Sherwood and Pigford (1952).]

IX. ANALYSES OF GAS TRANSPORT IN MEMBRANE OXYGENATORS

Oxygen and carbon dioxide exchange in membrane devices can be characterized via the convective diffusion and reaction equation. For cylindrical coordinates this equation is

$$\frac{\partial C}{\partial t} + V\frac{\partial C}{\partial Z} - R = \frac{D_r}{r}\frac{\partial}{\partial r}\left(r\frac{\partial C}{\partial r}\right) + D_z\frac{\partial^2 C}{\partial Z^2}$$

where we have assumed that flow occurs only in the axial (Z) direction. D_r and D_z are effective radial and axial diffusivities, and R is a reaction production rate (mass/vol-time).

To characterize oxygen exchange in, say, a tubular device where blood is flowing inside the conduit and oxygen-rich gas surrounds the conduit, one writes the equation given above for both dissolved oxygen and combined oxygen (HbO_2) and adds them. If mole units are used, the sum of the reaction terms is identically zero and drops out. Assuming D_r and D_z for HbO_2 are negligibly small (this is true if the red blood cells do not migrate), and that reaction is fast compared to diffusion so that local equilibrium prevails, we end up with

$$\frac{\partial C}{\partial t}[1 + f(C)] + V\frac{\partial C}{\partial Z}[1 + f(C)] = \frac{D_r}{r}\frac{\partial}{\partial r}\left(r\frac{\partial C}{\partial r}\right) + D_z\frac{\partial^2 C}{\partial Z^2}$$

where C is the dissolved oxygen concentration, D_r and D_z refer to dissolved oxygen, and f(C) is the slope of the $HbO_2 - O_2$ equilibrium curve, i.e., dC_{HbO_2}/dC_{O_2}.

Since most practical systems reach steady state quickly one may ignore the time-dependent term. And, because axial diffusion effects are often small (especially as compared to axial convection), the axial diffusion term is frequently ignored. This leaves one with the following equation to solve:

$$V \frac{\partial C}{\partial Z}[1 + f(C)] = \frac{D_r}{r} \frac{\partial}{\partial r}(r \frac{\partial C}{\partial r})$$

The boundary conditions include

1. $C = C_i$ at $Z = 0$ for all r (inlet condition)
2. $\partial C/\partial r = 0$ at $r = 0$ for all Z (the concentration profile is radially symmetric in the tube)

and, at the tube wall ($r = R$), either

3a. $C = C_w$ for all Z
3b. $-D_r(\partial C/\partial r) = \text{const}$ for all Z, or
3c. $-D_r(\partial C/\partial r) = -D_m(\partial C_m/\partial r)$ for all Z.

Condition 3a, a constant concentration condition, would be valid for a uniform gas phase and negligible wall resistance (this would be true for oxygen if the blood-side resistance were high). Condition 3b, a constant flux condition, would hold where the membrane resistance predominates (e.g., for CO_2 transfer). The most general condition is 3c, which states conservation of flux between fluid and wall (membrane). This in essence reduces to 3a or 3b if the membrane resistance is very low or very high, respectively.

The velocity V is for most cases a function of radius. For laminar flow at sufficiently high shear rates, where blood is nearly Newtonian, a parabolic velocity profile is satisfactory, e.g.,

$$V(r) = V_{max}\left[1 - \left(\frac{r}{R}\right)^2\right]$$

A more accurate profile to use is that derived from the Casson equation for blood (see Chapter 3). For radial diffusion, use of the molecular diffusivity of O_2 in stagnant blood is erroneous since particle rotation in flowing blood can considerably augment diffusion. Perhaps the best way to determine D_r is by experiment under actual flow conditions.

Weissman (1967) has solved the steady-state convective diffusion equation for constant wall concentration and a parabolic velocity profile. Buckles (1966), Colton and Drake (1971), and Villarroel et al. (1971) all used the general wall condition 3c and a non-Newtonian velocity profile, but determined their D_r values differently.

Colton and Drake present results, shown in Figure 11.9, indicating how the oxygenation of blood in a 0.2-cm-internal-diameter tube varies with dimensionless length X for various choices of inlet blood and gas phase partial pressures (P_i and P_o). θ_T represents the dimensionless total (dissolved plus bound) oxygen concentrations, and C_T stands for the dissolved oxygen concentrations in cubic centimeters of O_2 (STP) per cubic centimeter of blood. Curves A provide results for zero Hb, for comparison purposes (i.e., no oxygen "source" or "sink"). Curves B and D depict oxygenation, while C and E show deoxygenation profiles. Clearly, oxygenation is a faster process, given the same P_i and P_o boundary conditions. This difference is related directly to the nonlinear nature of the HbO_2 saturation curve.

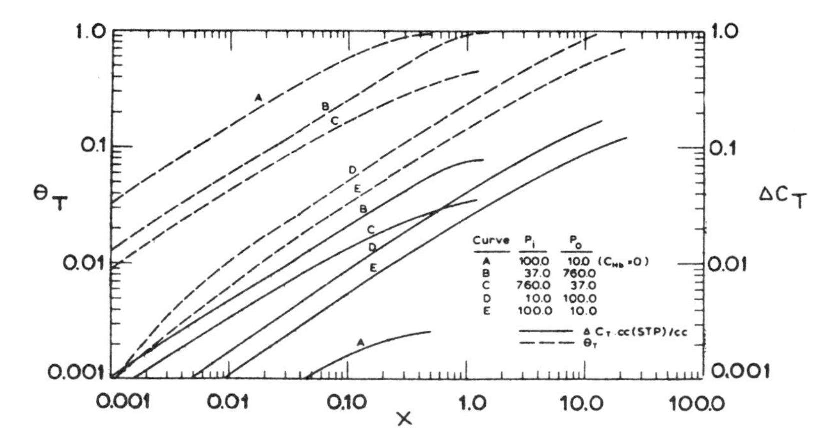

FIG. 11.9. Effect of boundary conditions on oxygen transport, θ_T, and ΔC_T as a function of X. [From Colton and Drake (1971).]

Colton and Drake also determined radial O_2 concentration profiles for oxygenation and deoxygenation, shown in Figures 11.10 and 11.11, at various axial (X) positions. The oxygenation curves indicate that there is a sharp transition from an outer fully saturated region to an inner unreacted region; i.e., the model one uses in the advancing front theory is borne out as valid. In deoxygenation, very gradual profiles develop, especially further along the tube, and the advancing front concept is obviously incorrect (one should note that deoxygenation is not of practical value). These differences again relate to the nonlinear shape of the HbO_2 saturation curve.

Villarroel et al. (1971) have pointed out that the function f(C) used above is dependent on CO_2 content. Thus, since CO_2 is given off by the blood during oxygenation, one must take into account the effect of changing P_{CO_2} on the HbO_2 saturation curve slope, f(C), as shown in Figure 10.9a. The real path followed by the blood will be on a transition line between a curve for P_{CO_2} = 46 mm Hg and

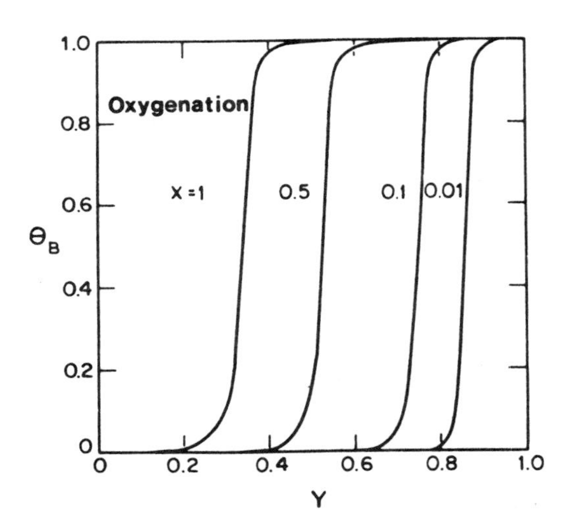

FIG. 11.10. Dimensionless radial saturation profiles at specified dimensionless lengths. Conditions: P_i = 10 mm Hg, P_o = 760 mm Hg. [From Colton and Drake (1971).]

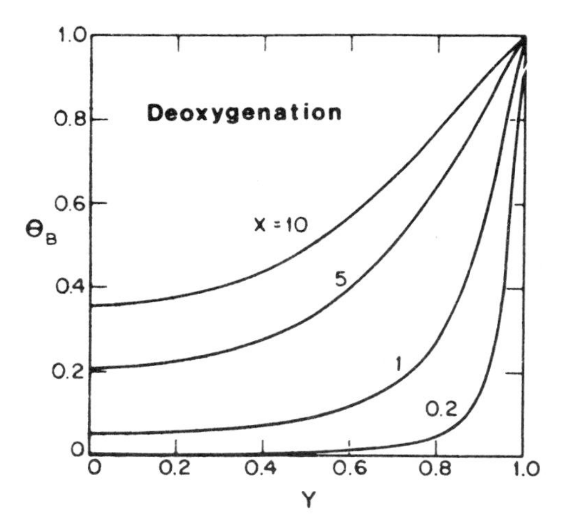

FIG. 11.11. Dimensionless radial saturation profiles at specified dimensionless lengths. Conditions: P_i = 760 mm Hg, P_o = 20 mm Hg. [From Colton and Drake (1971).]

a higher curve for P_{CO_2} = 40 mm Hg. The variation of P_{CO_2} which occurs, known as the Bohr shift, clearly acts so as to augment the uptake of O_2. A similar but much more significant effect of shifting P_{O_2} on the nature of the $HbCO_2$ saturation curves acts to aid CO_2 removal from blood. This effect (called the Haldane effect) is illustrated in Figure 11.12. In tissues, opposite processes occur which aid the extraction of O_2 from the blood and the uptake of CO_2 by the blood.

Therefore, to be accurate, one must solve the convective diffusion equations for CO_2 and O_2 transport simultaneously and keep track of these interactions. In doing this one should use the wall boundary condition 3c, since 3a is clearly invalid for CO_2 and 3b equally invalid for O_2. Villarroel has taken this approach, and obtained good agreement between data and theory. His analysis also incorporates a rotationally augmented diffusivity D_r, obtained by theoretical means. Additionally, Villarroel investigated the effects of pulsing the blood flow on gas transport, and found that enhance-

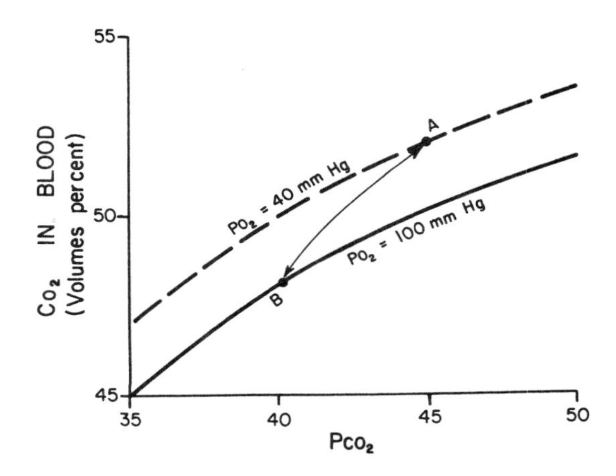

FIG. 11.12. Effect of P_{O_2} on the CO_2 content of human blood (the Haldane effect). [From Guyton (1971), p. 492.]

ment of transport occurred as a result of the action of unsteady convection on transient concentration profiles. Asymmetric flow pulses having sharp rises and longer drop-offs, as one has in the normal circulation, were found to be most effective. Figure 11.13 shows one result for a sinusoidal flow where the amplitude was 75% of the average flow rate and the frequency 1 Hz, compared to the steady-flow result.

Other means of augmenting gas transfer have been evaluated. Larsen and Dorson (1971), among others, have considered the effects of coiling tubes so as to promote the secondary flow patterns shown in Figure 11.14. Such patterns enhance radial mixing in the blood and give increased transfer. Figure 11.15 compares fractional hemoglobin saturation versus dimensionless tube length for coiled and straight tubes. Based on advancing front treatments it has been predicted that a coiled tube needs to be only 44% as long as a straight tube to give equivalent transfer of oxygen. Experimental data suggest the percentage is more like 55-81%, depending on flow

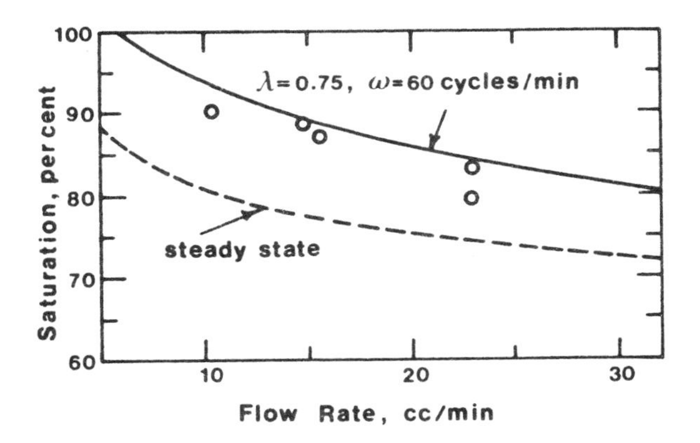

FIG. 11.13. Effect of pulsatile flow on oxygen transfer. [From Villarroel et al. (1971).]

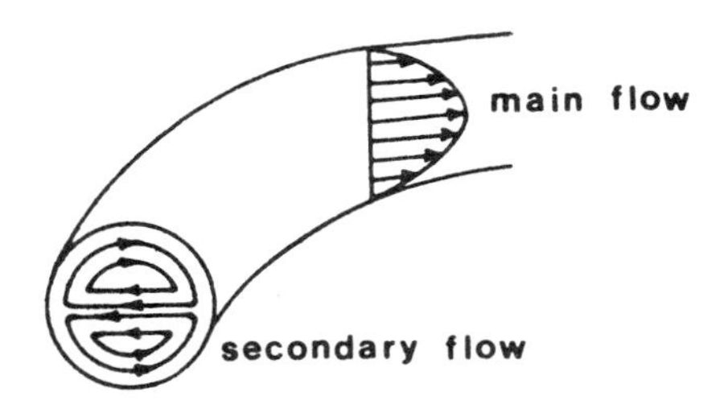

FIG. 11.14. Secondary flow patterns in coiled tubes.

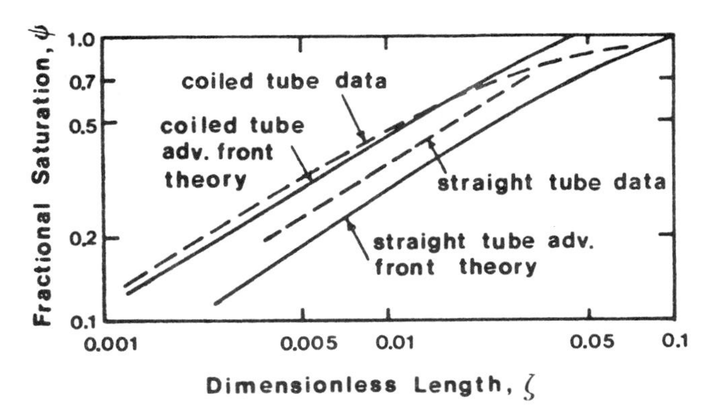

FIG. 11.15. Effect of coiling on oxygen uptake in tube oxygenators. [From Larsen and Dorson (1971).]

rate. Interestingly enough, it has been found that for water, the enhancement effect does not depend on the ratio of tube diameter to helix diameter, whereas for blood it does.

X. ADVANCING FRONT ANALYSIS OF OXYGENATION IN TUBES

Lightfoot (1968) has analyzed O_2 transfer to blood in straight tubes, assuming a reacted zone-unreacted zone model (see Figure 11.16). Recall here Colton and Drake's results, which show this to be valid. For the oxygenated zone, which extends from p to R, we may write from Fick's law

$$-N_{O_2} = D \frac{dC}{dr}$$

Since conservation of mass requires that

$$(N_{O_2})(2\pi r) = \text{const}$$

one can show that the oxygen flux at r = R (call it N_R) is

$$-N_R = \frac{D}{R} \frac{C_w - C_o}{\ln(R/p)}$$

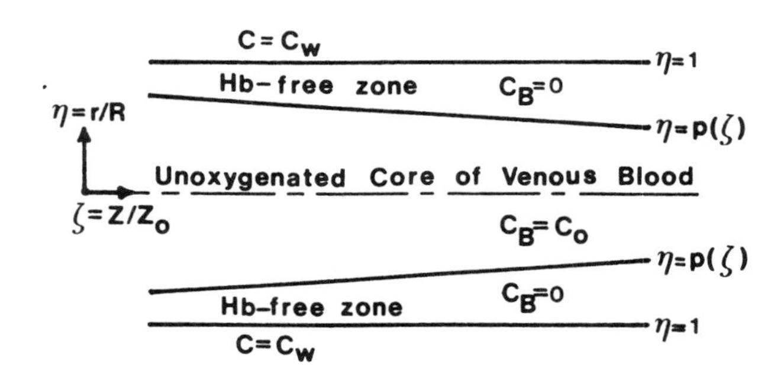

FIG. 11.16. Model for oxygen uptake in a tube. [From Lightfoot (1968).]

For the unreacted region

$$Q = 2\pi(\text{Hb})\int_0^p V(r)r\ dr$$

where Q is the flow rate of unreacted hemoglobin and V(r) is the velocity profile. For parabolic flow, $V(r) = V_{max}[1 - (r/R)^2]$, so

$$Q = 2\pi R^2 V_{max}(\text{Hb})\left[\frac{p^2}{2} - \frac{p^4}{4}\right]$$

Considering a differential slice dz of the tube, it is clear that the moles of O_2 entering in any time interval dt by radial diffusion will be $-N_R(2\pi R)$ dz. For each mole of O_2 entering a mole of Hb reacts, and the core volume therefore shrinks. The decrease in unreacted hemoglobin content during dt will be dQ; hence,

$$-N_R(2\pi R)\ dz = dQ$$

Substitution of dQ from the expression for Q and $-N_R$ from above gives

$$\zeta = \int_1^\eta (\eta - \eta^3)\ \ln \eta\ d\eta$$

where

$$\zeta = \frac{C_w - C_0}{(\text{Hb})}\ \frac{D}{R^2 V_{max}}\ Z \quad \text{and} \quad \eta = \frac{p}{R}$$

Integration yields

$$\zeta = \frac{3}{16} - \frac{1}{4}\left(\eta^2 - \frac{\eta^2}{4}\right) + \frac{1}{2}\ \ln \eta\left(\eta^2 - \frac{\eta^4}{2}\right)$$

The fractional saturation of the entering blood is obviously

$$\psi = \frac{Q_o - Q}{Q_o} = 1 - \frac{Q}{Q_o}$$

where Q_o is the rate at which unoxygenated hemoglobin enters the tube. From the equation for Q given earlier it follows that

$$\psi = 1 - 2\eta^2 + \eta^4$$

Figure 11.17 shows the thickness of the unreacted core and the fractional saturation of the blood, versus dimensionless distance ζ. Note that this model predicts that complete saturation is achieved at $\zeta = 3/32$. Lightfoot has compared this model (see Figure 11.18) with fractional saturation data obtained by Weissman and

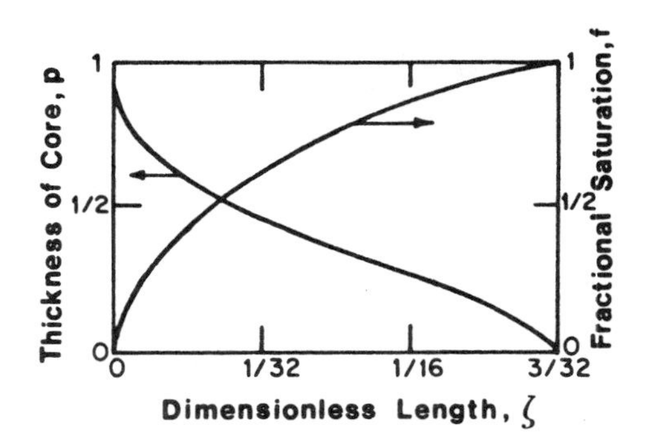

FIG. 11.17. Thickness of the venous core as a function of axial position. [From Lightfoot (1968).]

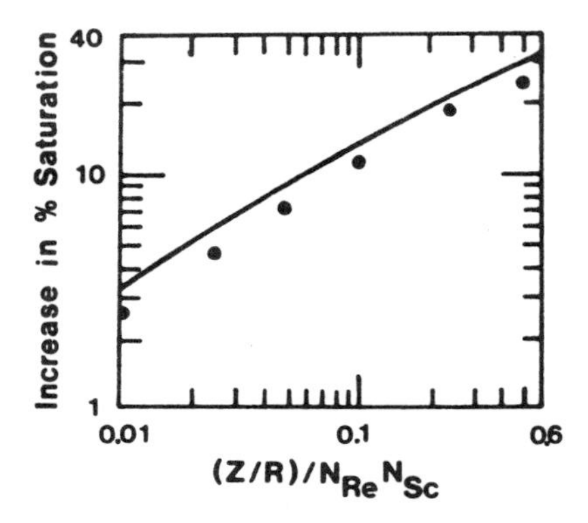

FIG. 11.18. Comparison of the unreacted-core model with the numerical results of Weissman and Mockros (1967), shown as the solid line. The points are predictions of the unreacted-core model. [From Lightfoot (1968).]

Mockros and shown the agreement to be fairly close, within about 20-30% (depending on the value of ζ).

PROBLEMS

1. *Blood-gas surface area in the rotating disc oxygenator.* For the Kay-Cross oxygenator described in the text (59 discs of 12.2 cm diameter, unit filled to a depth of one-third the disc diameter), calculate the amount of blood-gas interfacial area on the discs, in square meters, assuming thin, flat blood surfaces exist. Neglect the area of the top surface of the pool of blood.

At 120 rpm, what is the rate of generation of new surface in square meters per minute?

2. *Surface area in a bubble oxygenator.* A certain bubble oxygenator contains a blood-gas pool, in the bubble chimney, of 3-liters volume. The gas phase constitutes 10% by volume of this mixture. If the gas bubbles are roughly 1 mm in diameter, how much interfacial area for O_2 and CO_2 transfer will exist in this device?

3. *Performance of a membrane oxygenator.* A membrane oxygenator is to be used during open-heart surgery on a child. The membrane is 1/8-mil Teflon. Gas (pure O_2 saturated with water vapor at 37°C) is fed to the unit at the rate of 4 liters/min. The blood flow rate is 2 liters/min. The O_2 and CO_2 tensions in the entering blood are 40 and 46 mm Hg, respectively.

If it is desired that this device bring the blood O_2 and CO_2 tensions to normal arterial values (95 and 40 mm Hg, respectively), what area will be required? Assume that for CO_2 the membrane resistance is the only important resistance, and for O_2 that the membrane resistance is half of the total resistance. Calculate the area based on O_2 transport, and then based on CO_2 transport. Assume cocurrent flow of blood and gas.

If an oxygenator having the area required for the desired CO_2 transport rate is used, the actual O_2 transport rate will clearly be larger than specified. Will this cause any problems?

4. *Design of a film oxygenator using the advancing front theory.* Venous blood having an oxygen tension of 40 mm Hg is sent to a film type of oxygenator where it flows laminarly downward, while exposed to a gas phase of 1 atm total pressure and 98% O_2 - 2% CO_2 (dry basis) which has been saturated with water (37°C). Using the advancing front theory, calculate how deep the fully oxygenated zone will be into the blood at the bottom of the unit (it takes the blood 10 sec to reach the bottom). The diffusivity of O_2 in 45% hematocrit blood is about 1.2×10^{-5} cm^2/sec. Neglect counter-diffusion of hemoglobin and assume irreversible reaction.

REFERENCES

Buckles, R. G., *An Analysis of Gas Exchange in a Membrane Oxygenator*, Ph.D. Thesis, Massachusetts Institute of Technology, Cambridge, June 1966.

Colton, C. K., and Drake, R. F., Effect of boundary conditions on oxygen transport to blood flowing in a tube, *Chem. Eng. Prog. Symp. Ser.*, 67, No. 114, 88 (1971).

Forster, R. E., Rate of gas uptake by red cells, Chapter 32, *Handbook of Physiology*, Section 3, *Respiration*, Vol. 1, (W. O. Fenn and H. Rahn, eds.), Am. Physiol. Soc., Washington, D. C., 1964.

Galletti, P. M., and Brecher, G. A., *Heart-Lung Bypass*, Grune & Stratton, New York, 1962.

Galletti, P. M., Advances in heart-lung machines, in *Advances in Biomedical Engineering and Medical Physics*, Vol. 2 (S. N. Levine, ed.), Wiley-Interscience, New York, 1968.

Guyton, A. C., *Textbook of Medical Physiology*, 4th ed., Saunders, Philadelphia, Pennsylvania, 1971.

Larsen, K. G., and Dorson, W. J., Jr., Oxygen transfer to blood flowing in permeable tubes, *Proc. 24th Ann. Conf. Eng. in Med. and Biol.*, Las Vegas, 1971, p. 18.

Lightfoot, E. N., Low-order approximations for membrane blood oxygenators, *A.I.Ch.E. J.*, 14, 669 (1968).

Sherwood, T. K., and Pigford, R. L., *Absorption and Extraction*, McGraw-Hill, New York, 1952, pp. 332-337.

Villarroel, F., Lanham, C., Bischoff, K. B., Regan, T. M., and Calkins, J. M., Gas transfer to blood flowing in semipermeable tubes under steady and pulsatile flow conditions, *Chem. Eng. Prog. Symp. Ser.*, 67, No. 114, 96 (1971).

Weissman, M., *Analysis of Oxygen and Carbon Dioxide Diffusion into Flowing Blood*, Ph.D. Thesis, Northwestern University, Evanston, Illinois, 1967.

Weissman, M. H., and Mockros, L. F., Gas transfer to blood flowing in round tubes, *J. Eng. Mech. Div., Am. Soc. Civil Eng.*, 93, 225 (1967).

BIBLIOGRAPHY

Mockros, L. F., and Weissman, M. H., The artificial lung, in *Biomedical Engineering* (J. H. U. Brown, J. E. Jacobs, and L. Stark, eds.), Davis, Philadelphia, Pennsylvania, 1971.

Pierce, E. C., II, *Extracorporeal Circulation for Open-Heart Surgery*, Thomas, Springfield, Illinois, 1969.

APPENDIX

CONVERSION FACTORS AND CONSTANTS

$T(°C) = \frac{5}{9}[T(°F) - 32]$

$T(°R) = T(°F) + 460$

$T(°K) = T(°C) + 273.13$

1 in. = 2.54 cm; 1 m = 39.37 in.

1 ft^3 = 28,316 cc

1 lb = 453.6 g; 1 kg = 2.205 lb

1 g/cc = 62.44 lb/ft^3

1 atm = 760 mm Hg = 14.696 lb force/$in.^2$

1 $dyne/cm^2$ = 1 $g/cm\text{-}sec^2$ = 7.5×10^{-4} mm Hg

1 Btu = 252 cal

1 hp = 641.6 kcal/hr = 550 ft-lb force/sec

Gas constant, R = 1.987 cal/g-mol-°K

= 82.05 cm^3-atm/g-mol-°K

= 1544 ft-lb force/lb-mole-°R

Atomic weights:

C = 12.01	Cl = 35.45
H = 1.008	Na = 22.99
O = 16.00	K = 39.10
N = 14.01	Ca = 40.08
S = 32.06	He = 4.003
Fe = 55.85	I = 126.9
Mg = 24.31	P = 30.97

PHYSICAL PROPERTY DATA

Temperature		Water			Air
°C	°F	ρ (g/ml)	μ (cP)	Partial pressure (mm Hg)	ρ (g/liter)
0	32	0.9999	1.787	4.6	1.293
5	41	1.0000	1.519	6.5	1.270
10	50	0.9997	1.307	9.2	1.247
15	59	0.9991	1.139	12.8	1.226
20	68	0.9982	1.002	17.5	1.205
25	77	0.9971	0.890	23.8	1.185
30	86	0.9957	0.798	31.8	1.165
35	95	0.9941	0.719	42.2	1.146
37	98.6	0.9934	0.692	47.1	1.139
40	104	0.9922	0.653	55.3	1.128
45	113	0.9903	0.596	71.9	1.110
50	122	0.9881	0.547	92.5	1.093

Other Properties at 37°C

Thermal conductivities

k (liquid water) = 0.537 $kcal/hr\text{-}m^2\text{-}°C$

k (air) = 0.0232 $kcal/hr\text{-}m^2\text{-}°C$

Heat capacities

C_p (liquid water) = 0.9986 cal/g-°C

C_p (water vapor) = 0.484 cal/g-°C

C_p (air) = 0.238 cal/g-°C

Latent heat of vaporization of water = 576.6 cal/g

ANSWERS TO PROBLEMS*

CHAPTER 2

2. (a) 12.1 in. (b) 8.6 in.
3. 1.64 g/day
5. Cardiac output = 15 liters/min; stroke volume = 115 cm^3/beat

CHAPTER 3

1. 2.7 g iron
2. 0.078 dyn/cm^2
3. Shear rate = 132 sec^{-1}; torque = 877 dyn-cm
4. 2.43 cP
5. 2.19 cP; 3.3 laminae
7. H(core) = 58.9%; H(whole vessel) = 37.5%

*A manual containing detailed solutions to all problems in the text is available. Instructors may obtain copies directly from the author or publisher.

CHAPTER 4

4. 70 mm Hg
5. 101.6 mm Hg; 125.6 mm Hg (vigorous exercise)
6. 12.1%
7. 73,650 ft-lb force per day; 736.5 ft
8. 66,100 ft-lb force per day
9. 3.75 mm Hg
10. 384 mm Hg (feet) and -42.2 mm Hg (head), relative to 1 atm pressure

CHAPTER 5

2. 0.17°F; 0.85°F
3. Answers in kilocalories per hour are: (a) 377 (b) 673 (c) 132 (d) 1031 (e) 18 (f) metabolism = 1080; respiration loss = 102 (evaporation) plus 28 (sensible heat) (g) production plus gain = 1753; sum of losses = 1688
4. Skin = 14.4°C (57.8°F); 1020 kcal/hr convective loss rate; 18 min
5. 18.6 min
6. 3.3 quarts/day; 85 kcal/hr respiration heat loss
7. 6.9 cm (2.7 in.); 7.4 "clos"

CHAPTER 6

3. $k_1 = 0.05\ \text{min}^{-1}$ ($3.0\ \text{hr}^{-1}$); $k_2 = 0.0033\ \text{min}^{-1}$ ($0.2\ \text{hr}^{-1}$); $\alpha = -0.15$

CHAPTER 7

1. 7.115 atm (exact equation); 7.122 atm (Van't Hoff equation)
2. 0.722 (exact equation); 0.639 (dilute solution equation)
3. 41 g/m^2 per hour
4. 51.1 mV
5. 156.5 meq/liter (anions and cations each); totals are 313 meq/liter (interstitial fluid) and 314 meq/liter (blood); osmotic pressure difference = 19.3 mm Hg
6. 2.21

CHAPTER 8

1. 637 ml/min
2. 120 ml/min
3. 641 ml plasma per minute; 1165 ml blood per minute
4. 320 mg/min
5. 240 min

CHAPTER 9

1. K = 0.0182 cm/min; 59.9% removal (countercurrent flow); 57.7% removal (parallel flow); clearance = 119.8 cm^3/min (countercurrent flow) and 115.4 cm^3/min (parallel flow)
2. 502.5 min (8.38 hr)
3. 455.6 min (7.6 hr); save 47 min and about $3
4. 10.75 hr; save 143 min and lose about $54
5. 135 cm^3 of blood

CHAPTER 10

1. 2293 ml
2. 82.1%, 67.5%, 55.4%, 45.5%, and 37.4% after the first five expirations, respectively
3. 1.86×10^{-5} sec
4. 39% saturation
5. $P_{O_2} = 13.7$ mm Hg ($\psi = 13.6\%$); 65 breaths per minute
6. 4830 ml N_2 at BTP in the body fluids
7. About 60%
8. 96.0% saturation (97.3% for normal conditions)

CHAPTER 11

1. 0.824 m^2; 147.1 m^2/min
2. 1.8 m^2
3. Area = 1.0 m^2 (based on O_2 transport) and 2.83 m^2 (based on CO_2 transport)
4. 0.005 cm

INDEX

A

B

P